Pharmaceutical Biotechnology

Pharmaceutical Biotechnology

Edited by **Erica Helmer**

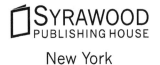

SYRAWOOD
PUBLISHING HOUSE

New York

Published by Syrawood Publishing House,
750 Third Avenue, 9th Floor,
New York, NY 10017, USA
www.syrawoodpublishinghouse.com

Pharmaceutical Biotechnology
Edited by Erica Helmer

International Standard Book Number: 978-1-68286-106-6 (Hardback)

Printed in the United States of America.

Contents

Preface

Every book is a source of knowledge and this one is no exception. The idea that led to the conceptualization of this book was the fact that the world is advancing rapidly; which makes it crucial to document the progress in every field. I am aware that a lot of data is already available, yet, there is a lot more to learn. Hence, I accepted the responsibility of editing this book and contributing my knowledge to the community.

Pharmaceutical biotechnology is an expanding field of science and technology which aims to design new therapeutic drugs, diagnose medical irregularities, etc. based on the tools and techniques of biotechnology. The objective of this book is to give a general view of the different areas of pharmaceutical biotechnology, and its applications. It strives to provide a fair idea about this discipline and to help develop a better understanding of the latest advances within tissue culture, bioengineering, drug design and development. While understanding the long-term perspectives of the topics like clinical trials and recombinant DNA technology, the book makes an effort in highlighting their significance as a modern tool for the growth of the discipline. The book is appropriate for students seeking detailed information in this area as well as for experts, and professionals engaged in this field.

While editing this book, I had multiple visions for it. Then I finally narrowed down to make every chapter a sole standing text explaining a particular topic, so that they can be used independently. However, the umbrella subject sinews them into a common theme. This makes the book a unique platform of knowledge.

I would like to give the major credit of this book to the experts from every corner of the world, who took the time to share their expertise with us. Also, I owe the completion of this book to the never-ending support of my family, who supported me throughout the project.

Editor

Comparative phytochemical screening and biological evaluation of n-hexane and water extracts of *Acacia tortilis*

D. Kubmarawa[1], M. E. Khan[2]* and A. Shuaibu[1]

[1]Department of Chemistry Federal University of Technology, P. M. B. 2076, Yola, Nigeria.
[2]Department of Chemistry Adamawa State University, P. M. B. 25, Mubi, Adamawa State, Nigeria.

N-Hexane and water extracts of the leaves, stem-bark and roots of the indigenous plant *Acacia tortilis* locally reputed for the treatment of cough, malaria, asthma and stomach pain in Girei Local Government Area (LGA), Adamawa State were phytochemically screened and biologically tested against *Escherichia coli*, *Shigella* sp., *Pseudomonas aeruginosa*, *Staphylococcus aureus*, *Streptococcus pyogene* and *Salmonella typhii*. Disc diffusion method was used for the analysis and both fractions were compared. The water extract was quite active on most of the microbes while some of the micro-organisms developed resistance against the N-hexane extract. The comparison of their activity indicated that there is a statistical difference, which is statistically significant. This confirms the fact that *Acacia tortilis* is used by the indigenes in forms of concoctions and decoction using water as the extracting solvent. It equally ascertains the bioactive components in the plant, thus, agreeing with the potential therapeutic significance of the plant as a natural source of drug development

Key words: N-Hexane, *Acacia tortilis*, Michika, phytochemically, therapeutic.

INTRODUCTION

The medicinal flora in the tropical eco-region has a preponderance of plants that provide raw material for addressing a range of medical disorders and pharmaceutical requirements. Nigeria is long recognized for her grass land savanna vegetation with a very rich botanical diversity (Jones et al., 2001; Hepper and Keay, 2000). Ethnic diversity in this temperate zone reflects an untapped wealth of indigenous uses of medicinal plants for the treatment of various health problems (Conuteix, 1961). Their secondary metabolites (Active ingredients) are a source of our sustenance (Ghani, 1990; Dobelis, 1993; Fatope, 2001; Kubmarawa et al., 2007) and are due to the presence of some valuable phytochemicals that combat most of the human maladies (Chidambara et al., 2003).

For a long period, plants have been a valuable source of natural products for maintaining human health and according to the World Health Organization (WHO); medicinal plants would be the best source to obtain a variety of drugs.

The success story of chemotherapy lies in the continuous search for new drugs to counter the challenges posed by resistant strains of microorganisms. The investigation of certain indigenous plants for their antimicrobial properties may yield useful results. A large number of plants are used to combat different diseases and are known to possess antimicrobial activity (Arora and Kaur, 1999).

Though the pharmaceutical industries have tried producing some new antibiotics in the last three decades, the resistance to them by microorganisms has instead increased (Cohen, 1992). In general, bacterial have the genetic ability to transmit and acquire resistance to drugs which are utilized as therapeutic agents. Such a fact is a cause for concern because of the number of patients in

*Corresponding author. E-mail: emamulu@yahoo.com.

hospitals who have suppressed immunity due to new bacterial strains, which are resistant (Bisset, 1994). There is now growing evidence that indicates a strong relationship between ethnic knowledge and sustainable use of biodiversity (Sullivan and Shealy, 1997). The time- tested ethnic knowledge when supplemented with the latest scientific insights can offer new models of economic development, that are both eco-friendly and socially acceptable (Croom, 1983). For-instance, the Nomadic Fulani's of Adamawa highlands, Nigeria, choose faith healing first, traditional herbal medicine next and modern medicine only when the first two have failed (Shariff, 2001; Sudhakar et al., 2007).

Thus, the use of traditional medicine and medicinal plants in most developing countries as a normative basis for the maintenance of good health has been widely observed (UNESCO, 1996). Furthermore, an increasing reliance on the use of medicinal plants in the industrialized societies has been traced to the extraction and development of several drugs and chemotherapeutics from these plants as well as form traditionally used rural herbal remedies (UNESCO, 1998). Isolation of medicinal agents less susceptible to regular antibiotics and recovery of increasing resistant isolates during antibacterial therapy is on the rise throughout the world (Gerding, 1991; Gold and Moellering, 1996; Archibald et al., 1997; O'Brien et al., 1999; Cookson, 2000; WHO, 2001; Cohen, 2002; FridkinS et al., 2002). One of the measures to minimize the increasing rate of resistance in the long- run is to have continuous in-depth investigation for new safe and effective antimicrobials as alternative agents to substitute the non effective ones. Natural resources, especially plants and microorganisms are potent candidates for such purposes.

Umbrella thorn, *Acacia totilis* also called umbrella thorn or Israeli Babool, is a medium to large canopied tree native primarily to the Savannah and Sahel of Africa but also occurring in the Middle East. Locally, it is reputed for its numerous medicinal and social uses as a cure for malaria, asthma, cough (concoction and decoction) and the pods used by natives for decoration, furniture, wagon wheels, fences, cages and pens.

The plant, *Acacia tortilis* (forsk) (mimosaceae), is called, umbrella thorn acacia (in English), Samar, sammar, smor, samra, sayyal (in Arabic), haak-en-steek (in Afrikaans), Kindil (in Kanuri), Gabaruwa (in Hausa), and Chilluki (in Fulani).

This research work is aimed at filling the knowledge gaps in this important sub-area of cultural biodiversity, directly relevant to the livelihood of the tribal communities, since the need for the integration of local knowledge for a sustainable management and conservation of natural resources receives attention on a daily bases (Posey, 1992). Also in mind is the constitution of compendium of all the medicinal plants, their cures and the parts used and where they are found, the statistical comparison

of the reactivity of the active ingredient(s) in the plant parts in various solvents. It was also prompted by the strong push in the chemical industries to move away from the use of large amounts of organic solvents and when possible, to perform chemical reactions in water so that there is less organic waste, a paradigm of green chemistry (Eric and Denis, 2006) and consequently to produce drugs from plants after clinical studies. This will reduce the distance of the patient to the drug and equally render the drugs affordable.

MATERIALS AND METHODS

Collection of plant materials

Fresh samples of the leaves, stem-bark and roots of the indigenous plant *Chilluki* were collected in Girei LGA, Adamawa State and were identified in the Biological Sciences Department Federal University of Technology Yola. The FHI number is 0796 and a specimen of the plant was deposited in the herbarium. The samples (1.00 kg) each were air dried in the laboratory before pounding to a fine powder using pestle and mortar to about 70 mesh sizes and then stored in dry containers.

Extraction

The powdered sample (150 g each) was accurately weighed and percolated with 2.0 L each of water and distilled ethanol for 72 h. After which there was decantation, filtration, and concentration using rotary evaporator (R110) at 35°C to obtain water and N-hexane soluble fractions, (F_W^1), and (F_H^1) labeled, F_W^L (11 g), F_W^S (09 g) F_W^R (7.6 g) and F_H^L (07 g), F_H^S (5.8 g), F_H^R (4.3 g) for water and N-Hexane fractions, respectively. The various fractions were divided into two portions each for phytochemical screening and the biological evaluation.

Qualitative chemical test

Standard methods described by Evans and Abulude (Sofowara 1993; Evans, 2000; Abulude et al., 2001, 2007) were used to test for the presence of phytochemical compound(s) (saponins, tannins, volatile oils, alkaloids, phenols and flavonoids) in the fractions.

Microorganisms

Organisms used for this study were, gram- negative (*Pseudomonas auroginosa* SHY3005, *Escherichia coli* SHY 3007, *Shigella dysentryae* SHY 3001, *Salmonella typhi* SHY 3002) and gram-positive (*Staphylococcus aureus* SHY 3004, *Streptococcus pyogene* SHY3001) bacteria. These organisms were clinical isolates obtained from Yola Specialist Hospital, Adamawa State, Nigeria.

Determination of antibacterial activity

The antibacterial activity of the extracts was determined using the agar well diffusion technique (Adeniyi and Ayepola, 2008). Sensitivity test agar plates were seeded with 0.1 ml of an overnight culture of each bacterial isolate (equivalent to 10^7 to 10^8 cfu ml⁻¹).

Table 1. Phytochemical constituents of the water extract of *A. tortilis.*

Phytochemical component	Plant extract		
	Leaf	Stem-bark	Root
Saponin	+	+	+
Tannin	+	-	+
Volatile oil	+	+	-
Alkaloid	+	+	+
Phenol	+	+	+
Flavonoid	+	+	-

+ = present; - = absent.

Table 2. Phytochemical constituents of the N -Hexane extract of *A. tortilis.*

Phytochemical component	Plant extract		
	Leaf	Stem-bark	Root
Saponin	-	+	+
Tannin	+	-	+
Volatile oil	+	+	-
Alkaloid	+	+	+
Phenol	+	+	+
Flavonoid	-	-	-

+ = present; - = absent.

The seeded plates were allowed to set and a standard cork borer of 8 mm diameter was used to cut uniform wells on the surface of the agar. The wells were then filled with 0.1 ml of each extract at a concentration of 0.025 mg / ml. The antibiotic Ampicillin at concentration of 0.01g /ml was used as positive control and distilled water as negative control. The plates were incubated at 37°C for 24 h after which the diameter of the zones of inhibition were measured (Fereshteh et al., 2005).

Statistical analysis

The one way ANOVA test (using coupled MS-Excel-Analyse-it® (Analyse-it®, 2010)) was used to analyze and compare the water and N-hexane results at a 95% confident level. Values of P≥0.05 were considered significant. Results were expressed as Mean ±SE of mean.

RESULTS

Phytochemical investigation

The phytochemical analysis of the water and N-hexane extracts from the leaves, stem bark and roots of the indigenous plant, *A. tortilis* are shown in Tables 1 and 2; the antimicrobial activities of the fractions against some gram-positive and gram-negative bacteria are shown in Tables 3 and 4.

DISCUSSION

The data obtained were subjected to statistical analysis using coupled MS-Excel-Analyse-it® (Analyse-it®, 2010). Independent Student's *t*-test at p≥0.05 was considered significant for the comparison of the antimicrobial activities of the water and N-hexane extracts.

Tables 1 and 2 indicate the presence of most of the pharmacologically useful classes of compounds (saponnins, tannins, volatile oil, alkaloids, phenols and flavonoids) tested for, except that in the N-hexane fraction; flavonoids were completely absent.

These secondary metabolites have been shown to have therapeutic activities in plants and function in a synergistic or antagonistic fashion for the treatment of diseases (Trease and Evans, 1996). Saponins, a special class of glycosides, have expectorant action which is very useful in the management of upper respiratory tract inflammation; saponins present in plants are cardiotonic in nature and are reported to have anti-diabetic and anti-fungal properties (Finar, 1989; Trease and Evans, 1989; Kamel, 1991). Tannins are reported to possess physiological astringent and haemostatic properties, which hasten wound healing and ameliorate inflamed mucus membrane and also inhibit the growth of microorganisms by precipitating microbial proteins and making nutritional

Table 3. Antimicrobial activity of the water extracts of *A. tortilis* on some (clinical isolates) gram-positive and gram-negative microorganisms.

Microorganism	Zone of growth inhibition (mm)				
	Leaf	Stem-bark	Root	Ampicilin	Distilled water
S. typhi	20	16	NA	26	-
E. coli	24	17	12	25	-
S. pyogene	20	15	6	25	-
S. dysentryae	21	15	6	24	-
P. auroginosa	15	17	13	21	-
S. aureus	NA	9	13	20	-

NA = Non active; Concentration of the extract used = 0.025 mg/ml. Concentration of the ampicillin = 0.01 mg/ml.

Table 4. Antimicrobial activity of the N-Hexane extracts of *A. tortilis* on some (clinical isolates) gram-positive and gram-negative microorganisms.

Microorganism	Zone of growth inhibition (mm)				
	Leaf	Stem-bark	Root	Ampicilin	Distilled water
S. typhi	4	6	10	26	-
E. coli	2	NA	11	25	-
S. pyogene	NA	17	14	25	-
S. dysentryae	NA	NA	1 6	24	-
P. auroginosa	NA	11	10	21	-
S. aureus	NA	NA	5	20	-

NA = Non active; Concentration of the extract used = 0.025 mg/ml. Concentration of the ampicillin = 0.01 mg/ml.

proteins unavailable for them; they form irreversible complexes with proline rich proteins, resulting in the inhibition of the cell protein synthesis. They have important roles such as stable and potent anti-oxidants (Trease and Evans, 1983; Tyler et al., 1988; Awosika, 1991; Ogunleye and Ibitoye, 2003).They act as binders and for treatment of diarrhea and dysentery (Dharmananda, 2003). Alkaloids are reported to have analgesic, anti-inflammatory and adatogenic activities which help to alleviate pains, develop resistance against diseases and endurance against stress (Gupta, 1994). Plant phenolic compounds especially flavonoids are currently of growing interest owning to their supposed properties in promoting health (anti-oxidants) (Rauha et al., 2000).

Thus, the present investigation clearly reveals the antibacterial nature of this plant and portrays it as a potential source of useful drug thereby suggesting that it could be exploited in the management of diseases caused by these bacteria in human and plant systems (Raghavendra et al., 2006).

Antimicrobial activities of the extract

The biological activities of the plant extracts and the measured diameters of zone of inhibition in (mm) against the microorganisms are shown in Tables 3 and 4. Zones of inhibition indicate the effect of the extracts on the microorganisms. The result showed that the water extract of the plant parts have more antimicrobial activity on the microbe than the N-hexane extract. The roots and the stem-bark are the most effective, though there is no activity on *S. typhi* and *S. aureus*.

Comparative classical statistical analysis of variance and comparing values of the Kruskal Walis (post hoc) test was carried. From the analysis, it was realized that in comparing the variables of the control (Ampicilline) with the variables water and N-hexane, the results were all statistically significant ($p \geq 0.0004$). This shows that water is the best proposed solvent of extraction - the much advocated "green chemistry paradigm" (Eric and Denis, 2006).

This is a confirmation of the usage of *A. tortolis* by the indigenes in forms of concoctions and decoction using the universal solvent, water as the medium of extraction. N-hexane on the other hand is a good solvent (but water better) for extraction but not as good as ordinary water.

The aforementioned is a clear indication that the plant can treat cough, malaria, asthma, stomach pain and other diseases. This is inconsonance with the activity of plant secondary metabolites of medicinal plants as they play a significant role in the anti-microbial, bacteriostatic and bactericidal activities (Lin et al., 2001). This thus, supports the use of the plant by herbalists and Girei LGAs indigenes for the treatment of their human ailments. Ampicillin (positive control) is higher in performance, with greater zones of inhibition than the extract(s) probably because impurities are interfering with extract's activity. When active compounds are isolated from the extracts, they may give higher activity than ampicillin.

Conclusion

Knowledge of the healing systems of plants is transferred orally from generation to generation without any written documentation and many of the traditional methods have a superstitious element. More so, lack of documentation of traditional healing methods has resulted in confusion amongst users. Thus, this piece of work strongly recommends the necessity of proper documentation of the actual healing methods, along with the main charac-teristic feature of the medicinal plants. It strongly sug-gests that the indigenous plant, Gabaruwa because of its phytochemical content and biological activity, could be a good source for alternative drugs specially when extracted with the universal solvent water.

REFERENCES

Abulude FO (2007). Phytochemical Screening and mineral contents of Leaves of Some Nigerian Woody plants. Res. J. Phytochem. 1:33 - 39

Abulude FO, Akajagbor, Dafiehware (2001). Distribution of trace minerals, phosphorus and phytate in some varieties of mushrooms found in Nigeria. Adv. Food Sci. 23:113–116

Adeniyi BA, Ayepola OO (2008). The phytochemical and Antimicrobial Activity of Leave Extracts of Eucalyptus camaldulensis and Eucalyptus torelliana (Myrtaceae). Res. J. Med. Plants 2(1):34 – 38.

Analyse-it® (2010). General and Clinical Laboratory Analyses Software (Version 1.73), Analyse-it Software Ltd., Leeds, England.

Archibald L, Phillips L, Mnnet D (1997). Antimicrobial resistance in isolates from inpatients and outpatients in the United States: increasing importance of the intensive care unit. Clin. Infect. Dis. 24:211 -215.

Arora D, Kaur J (1999). Antimicrobial activity of species. Int. J. Antimicrob. Agents 12:257 -266

Awosika, F, (1991). Local Medicinal plants and health of consumers. Clin. Pharm. Herbal Med. 9:28 -29.

Bisset NM (1994). Herbal Drugs and Phytopharmaceuticals. CRC Press, London. pp. 106 -108.

Chidambara K, Vanitha A, Mahadeva M, Ravishankar G (2003). Antioxidant and Antimicrobial activity of Cissus quandrangularis L. J. Med. Food 6:2.

Cohen ML (1992). Epidemiology of drug resistance: Implications of a post-microbial era. Science 257:1050-1055.

Cohen ML (2002). Changing patterns of infectious diseases. Nature 406:762-767.

Conuteix PJ (1961). The Major Significance of Minor Forest Products. In: Kappel RSC (Ed.), Local Value and Use of Forest in West Africa

Humid Forest Zones. FAO, Rome. pp. 81-86.

Cookson BD (2000). Methicillin-resistant Staphylococcus aureus in Community. New battlefronts or are the battles lost? Infect. Control Hosp. Epidemiol. 2:398-403.

Croom EM (1983). Documenting and evaluating herbal remedies. Ecol. Bot. 37:13 -27.

Dharmananda S (2003). Gallnuts and the uses of tannins in Chinese medicine. A paper Delivered at the Institute for Traditional Medicine, Portland, Oregon.

Dobelis IN (1993). Magic and medicine of plants. The Readers Digest Association Inc. Pleasant, New York. pp. 8-48.4(1):15-21.

Eric VV, Denis AD (2006). Modern Physical Organic Chemistry. University Science Books, Sausalito, California. p 151.

Evans WC (2000). Trease and Evans Pharmacology, 4th Edn. WB Saunders Company Ltd. pp. 224- 239.

Fatope MO (2001). "Natural Products Science: Looking Back and Looking Forward". A Professorial Inaugural Lecture, Bayero University Kano, Nigeria.

Fereshteh E, Morteza Y, Tafakori V (2005). Antimicrobial activity of Datura innoxia and Datura stramonium. Fitoterapia 76:118 -119.

Finar IL (1989). Chemistry; Stereochemistry and the Chemistry of Natural products, 5th Edn, Vol. 2. Longman Group, UK. pp. 517-605.

Fridkin S K, Hill HA, Volkava NV, Edwards JR, Lawton RM, Gaynes RP (2002). Temporal changes in prevalence of antimicrobial resistance in 23 U. S Hospitals. Emerg. Infect. Dis. 8:697-700.

Gerding DN, Larson TA, Hughes RA (1991). Aminoglycoside resistance and aminiglycosde usage: ten years of experience in one hospital. Antimicrob. Agents Chemther. 35:1284-1290.

Ghani A (1990). Introduction to Pharmacognosy. Ahmadu Bello University Press, Ltd. Zaria, Nigeria. pp. 45-47, 187-197.

Gold HS, Moellering RC (1996). Antimicrobial drug resistance. New Engl. J. Med. 335:1445-1453.

Gupta SS (1994). Prospects and prospective of natural products in medicine. Indian J. Pharmacol. 26:1-12.

Hepper FN, Keay R (2000). History of the flora of West Tropical Africa. Niger. Field 65:141-148.

Jones AM, Govan JR, Doherty CJ, Doherty CJ, Dodd ME, Isalska BJ, Stanbridge T N, Webb AK (2001). Spread of a multiresistant strain of Psseudomonas aeruginosa in an adult cystic fibrosis clinic. Lancet 358:557-558

Kamel JM (1991). An extract of the mesocarps of fruits of Balanite aegyptiaca exhibited a prominent anti-diabetic properties in Mice. Chem. Pharmacol. Bull. 39:1229 -1233.

Kubmarawa D, Ajoku A, Enwerem M, Okorie A (2007). Preliminary phytochemical and antimicrobial screening of 50 medicinal plants from Nigeria. Afr. J. Biotechnol. 6(14):1690-1696.

Lin YM, Flavin MT, Cassidy CS, Mar A, Chen FC (2001). Bioflavonoid as novel anti-tuberculosis agents. Bioorg. Med. Chem. Lett. 11(16):2101-2104.

O'Brien FG, Pearman JW, Gracy M (1999). Community strain of methicillin-resistant Staphylococcus aureus involved in a hospital outbreak. J. Clin. Microbiol. 37:2858-2862.

Ogunleye DS, Ibitoye SF (2003). Studies of antimicrobial activity and chemical constituents of Ximenia Americana. Trop. J. Pharm. Res. 2:239-241.

Posey D (1992). Traditional knowledge, Conservation and the Rain Forest Harvest In: Potkin M, Famolare L (Eds.), Sustainable Harvest and Marketing of Rain Forest Products. Island Press, Washington DC. pp. 46 -50.

Raghavendra MP, Satish S, Raveesha KA (2006). Phytochemical analysis and antibacterial activity of Oxalis corniculata; a known medicinal plant. Agriculture Microbiology Laboratory, Department of Studies in Botany, University of Mysore, Manasagangotri, Mysore, 570 006, India. (mySCIENCE 1(1), 2006, 72–78. http://myscience.uni-mysore.ac.in

Rauha JP, Remes S, Herinonen W, Hopia M, Kgjala T, Pitinlaja K, Vaorela H, Vaorela P (2000). Antimicrobial effects of finished plant extract containing flavanoids and other phenolic compounds. Int. J. Food Microbiol. 56:3 -12

Shariff ZU (2001). Modern Herbal Therapy for Common Ailments.

Nature pharmacy Series, Spectrum Books Limited, Ibadan, Nigeria in Association with Safari Books (Export) Limited, United Kingdom. pp. 9 -84.

Sofowara A (1993). Medicinal plants and Traditional medicine in Africa. Spectrum Books Ltd. Ibadan, Nigeria. p 289.

Sudhakar RC, Reddy KN, Thulsi RK, Chiranjibi P (2007). Ethnobotanical Studies on Medicinal plants Used by the Chenchus of Nallamalais in Kunool District, Andhra Pradesh, India. Res. J. Med. Plants (4):128-133.

Sullivan K, Shealy CN (1997). Complete Natural Home Remedies. Element Books Limited, Shaftesbury, UK. pp. 3-4.

Trease GE, Evans MD (1989). A text book of Pharmacognosy, 13th Edn. Baillier, Tindal and Caussel, London. pp. 144 -148.

Trease GE, Evans WC (1983). Textbook of Pharmacognosy, 12th Edn. Balliere, Tindall, London.

Trease GE, Evans WC (1996). Pharmacognosy. Alden Press, Oxford. pp. 213 -232.

Tyler VE, Brady LR, Roberts JE (1988). Pharmacology. Lea and Ferbiger, Philadelphia. pp. 85 -90.

UNESCO (1996). Culture and Health Orientation texts- World Decade for Cultural Development (1988 -1997). Document CLT/DEC/PRO-1996, Paris, France. 129 p.

UNESCO (1998). FIT/504-RAF-48 Terminal Report: Promotion of Ethnobotany and Sustainable Use of Plant Resources in Africa. 60 p.

WHO (2001). WHO Global Strategy for Containment of Antimicrobial Resistance. Accessed at: www.who.int/emc-documents/antimicrobial_resistance/docs/Global Start.Pdt

Validation and stability indicating RP-HPLC method for the determination of tadalafil API in pharmaceutical formulations

B. Prasanna Reddy[1]*, K. Amarnadh Reddy[2] and M. S. Reddy[3]

[1]Department of Quality control, Nosch Labs Pvt Ltd, Hyderabad-500072, A.P, India.
[2]Department of AR and D, Aurigene Discovery Technologies Ltd, Bangalore, India.
[3]Department of Plant Pathology and Entomology, Auburn University, USA.

The present study describes the development and subsequent of a stability indicating RP-HPLC method for the analysis of tadalafil. The samples separated on an Inertsil C_{18}, (5 μ , 150 mm x 4.6 mm i.d) by isocratic run using acetonitrile and phosphate buffer as mobile phase), with a flow rate of 0.8 ml/min, and the determination wavelength was 260 nm for analysis of tadalafil. The described method was linear within range of 70 - 130 μg/ml (r^2 = 0.999). The precision, ruggedness and robustness values were also within the prescribed limits (< 1% for system precision and < 2% for other parameters). Tadalafil was exposed to acidic, basic, oxidative and thermal stress conditions and the stressed samples were analyzed by the proposed method. Chromatographic peak purity results indicated the absence of co-eluting peaks with the main peak of tadalafil, which demonstrated the specificity of assay method for estimation of tadalafil in presence of degradation products. The proposed method can be used for routine analysis of tadalafil in quality control laboratories.

Key words: RP-HPLC, tadalafil, validation, stability indicating assay, forced degradation.

INTRODUCTION

Tadalafil hydro-2-methyl-6-[3,4-(methylenedioxy)phenyl] pyrazino-[1',2':1,6]pyrido[3,4-b]indole-1,4-dione (Figure 1), is a phosphodiesterase type 5 inhibitor used in the management of erectile dysfunction. It is not officially included in any of the pharmacopoeias. It is listed in the Merck Index (Budavari et al., 2001) and Martindle and complete drug reference (Sean et al., 2002). There are several (Cheng et al., 2005) methods for determination of tadalafil such as HPLC-EIMS (Zhu et al., 2005) and capillary electrophoresis methods (Aboul-Enein, 2005) and by HPLC (Aboul, 1994). The present work was designed to develop a simple, precise and rapid analytical LC procedure, which would serve as stability indicating assay method for analysis of tadalafil active pharmaceutical ingredient.

EXPERIMENTAL

Chemical and reagents

Tadalafil standard and API were provided from Smilax laboratories limited. HPLC grade sodium dihydrogen phosphate (NaH_2PO_4), disodium hydrogen phosphate (Na_2HPO_4), acetonitrile, hydrogen peroxide and sodium hydroxide were procured from Merck Ltd. High pure water was prepared by using Millipore Milli Q plus purification system.

HPLC instrumentation and conditions

A high performance liquid chromatograph system, with LC solutions data handling system, with an auto sampler was used for the analysis. The data was recorded using LC 2010 solutions software. The samples separation was performed on a Shimadzu Inertsil C_{18}, (5 μ, 150 mm x 4.6 mm, Japan) with the mobile phase consisting of acetonitrile and phosphate buffer (pH 7.0) with a ratio of 60: 40 (v/v) at ambient temperature. The flow rate was kept at 0.8 ml/min and the determination wavelength was 262 nm.

*Corresponding author. E-mail: drbpkreddy@gmail.com.

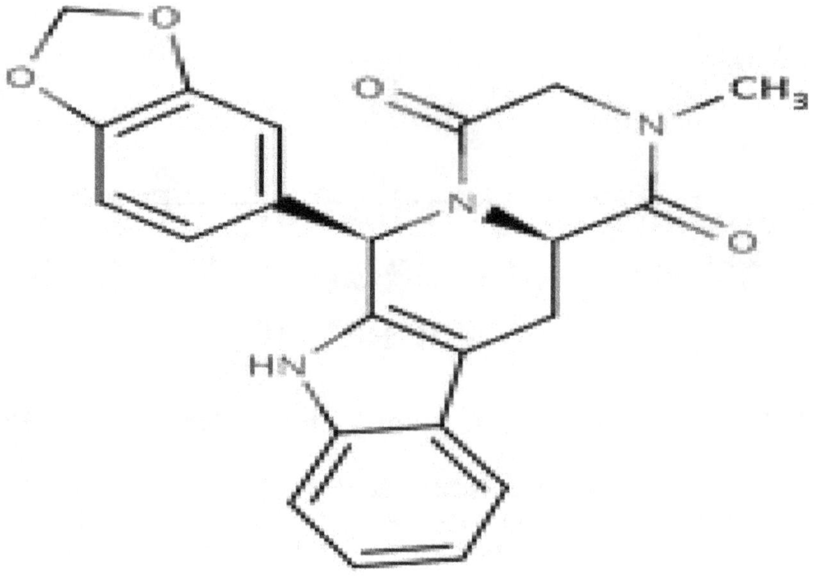

Figure 1. Structure of Tadalafil.

Standard and sample preparation

Mobile phase

Mix 700 ml of acetonitrile to the buffer, the mobile phase was sonicated for 15 min and then it was filtered through 0.45 µm membrane filter paper.

Standard solution

The standard was dissolved with mobile phase to 0.5 mg/ml. The test samples were dissolved with mobile phase. With the optimized chromatographic conditions, a steady baseline was recorded, the standard solution was injected and the chromatogram was recorded. This procedure was repeated for the sample solution.

Forced degradation studies

Tadalafil was allowed to hydrolyze in different strengths of base (0.005 N and 0.05 N NaOH), acid (0.05 N, 0.5 N and 1 N HCl) and hydrogen peroxide (30%, 10, 3 and 1%). Tadalafil was also studied for its thermal degradated at 80, 100, 120 °C for 1 h respectively. An accurately weighed 50 mg of tadalafil API was dissolved in 1 ml of respective base (NaOH), acid (HCl) or hydrogen peroxide and kept for specified period after which the volume was made up to 50 ml with water: acetonitrile (70:30, v/v). Five milliliters of the above solution were diluted with water: acetonitrile (70:30, v/v) to get a concentration of 100 ppm. Blank was also treated in same way.

Validation

Linearity was determined by injecting different concentration of sample solutions (50 - 150 µg/ml). For system precision, standard solution (100 µg) was injected to six replicates injections to check %RSD (relative standard deviation) and for method precision six time samples were prepared and each of those were injected in duplicate. Mean of all of these values gives to assay value.

To establish the within-day (intra-assay) and between-day (inter-assay) accuracy and precision of the method, tadalafil was assayed on one day and three separate days. Intra-assay and inter-assay were calculated.

Robustness of method was investigated by varying the chromatographic conditions such as change of flow rate (± 10%), organic content in mobile phase (± 2%), wavelength of detection (± 5%) and pH of buffer in mobile phase (± 0.2%). Robustness of the developed method was indicated by the overall %RSD between the data at each variable condition.

Limit of detection (LOD)

The detection limit is determined by the analysis of samples with the known concentrations of analyte and by establishing the minimum level at which the analyte can be reliably detected. The LOD was calculated as follows:

$$LOD = 3.3 \ (\sigma/S)$$

Limit of quantitation (LOQ)

The quantitation limit is determined by the analysis of sample of known concentration of analyte and by establishing the minimum level at which the analyte can be quantified with acceptable accuracy and precision.
The LOQ was calculated as follows:

$$LOQ = 10 \ (\sigma/S)$$

where S: Slope of the calibration curve, σ: Average standard deviation of the response

RESULTS

Chromatographic conditions

In order to separate tadalafil API, phosphate buffer-acetonitrile mixtures were used as the mobile phase. Satisfactory resolution was obtained using the mobile phase system of acetonitrile/phosphate buffer (70:30, v/v, pH 7.0) at a flow rate of 0.8 ml/min with UV detection at

Validation and stability indicating RP-HPLC method for the determination of tadalafil API in pharmaceutical formulations

9

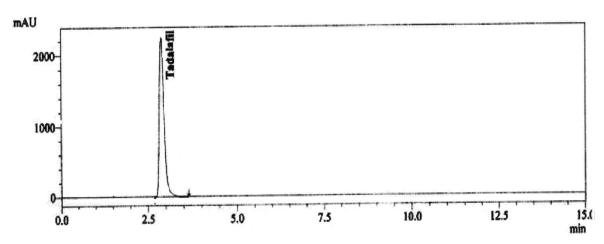

Figure 2. Chromatogram of Tadalafil API.

Table 1. Results of force degradation studies of Tadalafil.

Stress condition/duration/solution	Degradation %
Alkaline degradation (0.005 N NaOH, 1 hr)	10%
Alkaline degradation (0.05 N NaOH, 2 hr)	20%
Oxidative degradation (1 % H_2O_2)	0
Oxidative degradation (3 % H_2O_2)	0
Oxidative degradation (10 % H_2O_2)	0
Oxidative degradation (30 % H_2O_2, 80 °C for 10 min)	35
Acidic degradation(0.05 N HCl)	0
Acidic degradation(0.5 N HCl)	0
Acidic degradation(1 N HCl)	15
Thermal degradation (Solid sample, 80 °C, 1 hr)	15
Thermal degradation (Solid sample, 100 °C, 1 hr)	20
Thermal degradation (Solid sample, 120 °C, 1 hr)	26

260 nm. Under these conditions tadalafil with the retention time of tadalafil was 2.88 min. Figure 2 showed a typical chromatogram obtained under these conditions shown.

Forced degradation studies

During the study it was observed that upon treatment of tadalafil with different strengths of base (0.005 N and 0.05 N NaOH), acid (0.05 N, 0.5 N and 1 N HCl) and hydrogen peroxide (30, 10, 3 and 1%) the degradation was observed only with the higher strengths (0.05 N NaOH), acid (1 N HCl) and hydrogen peroxide (30%), where as with the lower strengths of alkali (0.005 N NaOH), acid (0.05 N and 0.05 N HCl) and hydrogen peroxide (1, 3 and 10%) no degradation was observed (Table 1).Further it is important to note that from the chromatograms (Figure 3a to c), it is evident that although the degraded peaks are observed. The tadalafil

stable under the applied stress conditions like heat, acid and alkaline and oxidative degradation states.

Linearity

The calibration curve showed good linearity in the range of 50 - 150 μg/ml, for tadalafil API with correlation co-efficient (R^2) of 0.9998 (Figure 4). A typical calibration curve has the regression equation of y = 23646x +568057 for tadalafil.

Precision

The results of system precision (% RSD = 0.26), method precision (% RSD = 0.10) are found within the prescribed limit of ICH guidelines (% RSD < 1%, and % RSD < 2 % respectively in case of system precision and method precision).

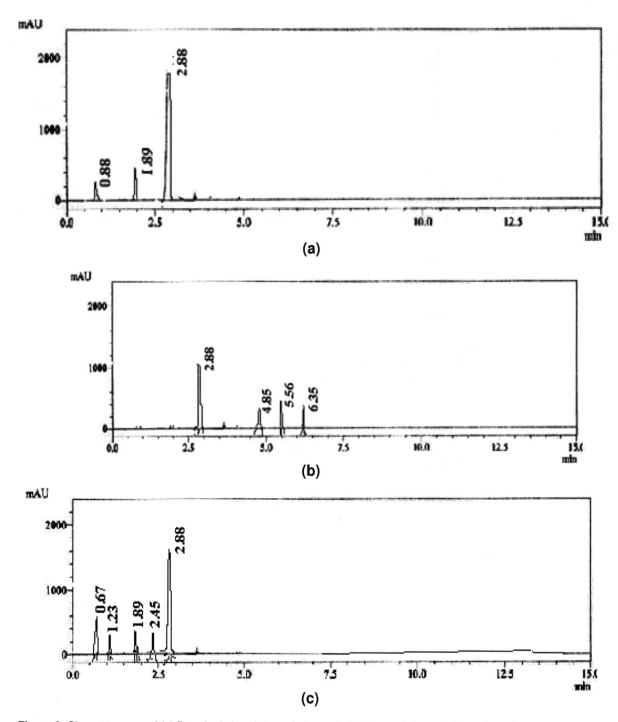

Figure 3. Chromatograms of (a) Base hydrolyzed-degraded sample (b) Thermal degraded sample and (c) Acid hydrolyzed degraded sample.

Intra-assay and Inter-assay

The intra and inter-day variation of the method was carried out and the high values of mean assay and low values of standard deviation and %RSD (%RSD < 2%) within a day and day to day variations for tadalafil revealed that the proposed method is precise in (Table 2 and 3).

Method robustness

Influence of small changes in chromatographic conditions such as change in flow rate (± 10%), organic content in mobile phase (± 2%), wavelength of detection (± 5%) and pH of buffer in mobile phase (± 0.2%) studied to determine the robustness of the method are also in favor (Table 4, %RSD < 2%) of the developed RP-HPLC

Validation and stability indicating RP-HPLC method for the determination of tadalafil API in pharmaceutical formulations

11

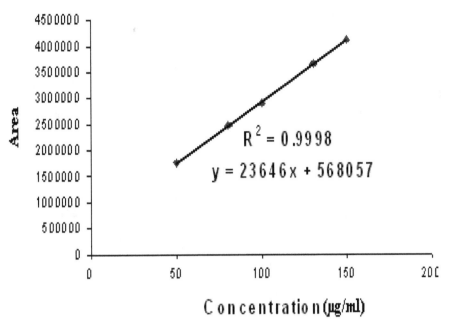

Figure 4. Linearity curve for Tadalafil.

Table 2. Intra-assay precision data of proposed RP-HPLC method (Method Ruggedness).

	Mean (% w/w)	SD	% RSD
Assay-1	99.75	0.450	0.45
Assay-2	99.30	0.230	0.24
Intra assay	99.53	0.410	0.40

Table 3. Inter-assay precision data of proposed RP-HPLC method.

	Mean (% w/w)	SD	% RSD
Assay-1	99.35	0.090	0.08
Assay-2	99.20	0.240	0.26
Intra assay	99.43	0.310	0.20

Table 4. The influence of changes in chromatographic parameters on RP-HPLC analysis of Tadalafil API (Method robustness).

Change in parameter	% RSD
Flow (0.7 ml/min)	0.65
Flow (0.9 ml/min)	0.92
Wavelength (255 nm)	0.74.
Wavelength (265 nm)	0.56
pH (6.8)	0.04
pH (7.2)	0.48
Organic phase composition (-2%)	0.58
Organic phase composition (+2%)	0.80

method for the analysis of tadalafil API.

LOD and LOQ

The minimum concentration level at which the analyte can be reliably detected (LOD) and quantified (LOQ) were found to be 0.05 and 0.5 µg/ml, respectively.

Specificity and stability in analytical solution

The results of specificity indicated that the peak was pure in presence of degraded sample. It is important to mention here that the tadalafil API was stable in solution from up to 24 h at 25°C.

The results of linearity, precision, inter and intra-assays, method robustness, LOD, LOQ and specificity and stability in analytical solution established the validation of the developed RP-HPLC assay for the analysis of tadalafil.

DISCUSSION

The present study is the first time report on stability indicating assay of tadalafil in presence of degradation products by HPLC. In this method isocratic elution method is selected for the analysis of tadalafil API because it gave better base line separation and peak width, which is suitable for the routine analysis of tadalafil. The developed method was validated as per ICH guidelines (ICH, 1996) and its updated international convention (ICH, 2002).

Stability testing forms an important part of the process of drug product development. The purpose of stability testing is to provide evidence on how the quality of a drug substance varies with time under the influence of a variety of environmental factors such as temperature, humidity and light, and enables recommendation of storage conditions, retest periods, and shelf life to be established (Avarez-Lueje et al., 2003; Abdul-Fattah et al., 2002; Lambropouls et al., 1999; Bebawy, 2003). The assay of tadalafil API (Active Pharmaceutical Ingredient) in stability test sample needs to be determined using stability indicating method, as recommended by the International Conference on Harmonization (ICH) guidelines (ICH, 1993) and (USP, 2003).

REFERENCES

Aboul-Enein HY, Ali I (2005). Talanta 65(1): 276-280.
Aboul-Enein HY (1994). Chromatographia 60(3-4): 187-191.
Abdul-Fattah AM, Bhargava HN (2002). A new high performance liquid Chromatography (HPLC) method for the analysis of halofantrine (HF) in Pharmaceuticals. J. Pharm. Biomed. Anal. 29: 901-908.
Avarez-Lueje A, Pujol S, Squella JA, Nunez Vergara LJ (2003). A Selective HPLC method for determination of lercanidipine in tablets. J. Pharm. Biomed. Anal. 31: 1-9.
Bebawy L (2003). I. Spectrophotometric and HPLC determination of linezolid in the Presence of its alkaline-induced degradation products and in pharmaceutical Tablets. Anal. Lett. 36: 1147-1161.
Budavari S, Eds (2001): In, The Merck Index, 13th Edn, Merck & Co., Inc., White House Station., NJ: p. 218.
Cheng CL, Chou CH (2005). J. Chromatogr. B Analyt. Technol. Biomed. Life Sci. 822(1-2): 278-284.
ICH (1996). Validation of Analytical Procedures: Methodology, in: Proceeding of the International Conference on Harmonization, Geneva. March.
ICH (2002).Guideline on Analytical method Validation, in: Proceeding of International Convention on quality for the pharmaceutical industry, Toronto, Canada, September.
ICH (1993). Stability testing of new drug substances and procedure in: Proceeding of the International conference on Harmonization, Geneva, October.
Lambropouls J, Spanos GA, Lozaridis (1999). V.N. Method development and Validation for the HPLC assay (potency and related substances) for 20 mg paroxetine tablets. J. Pharm. Biomed. Anal. 19: 793-802.
Sean C, Sweetman Eds. (2002). In., Martindale, The Complete Drug Reference, 34th Edn., The Pharmaceutical Press: London p. 875.
The United States Pharmacopoeia" 26th ed. (2003). US Pharmacopoeia convention, Rockville, MD. p. 1151.
Zhu X, Xiao S, Chen B, Zhang F, Yao S, Wan Z, Yang D, Han H (2005). J. Chromatogr A., eb25;1066(1-2): 89-95.

3

Cinnamomum zeylanicum extract inhibits proinflammatory cytokine TNF∝: *in vitro* and *in vivo* studies

Kalpana Joshi[1*], Shyam Awte[2], Payal Bhatnagar[2], Sameer Walunj[3], Rajesh Gupta[3], Swati Joshi[4], Sushma Sabharwal[3], Sarang Bani[5] and A. S. Padalkar[1]

[1] Department of Biotechnology, Sinhgad College of Engg, Pune, India-411041.
[2] Poona College of Pharmacy, Pune 411029, India-411029
[3] Division of Biochemistry, Department of Chemistry, University of Pune, Pune, India 411007.
[4] National Chemical Laboratory (NCL), Pune, India- 411007.
[5] Indian Institute of Integrative Medicine, Canal Road, Jammu-180 001, India.

Cinnamomum zeylanicum, a commonly used spice and well-known medicinal plant has been reported to have anti-diabetic, anti-oxidant and anti-microbial properties. We have investigated its anti-inflammatory activity using ethanol extract obtained from bark. *In vitro* and *in vivo* experiments were performed targeting TNF-α using flow cytometry. Ethanol extract of *C. zeylanicum* showed suppression of intracellular release of TNF-α in murine neutrophils as well as leukocytes in pleural fluid. The extract was found to inhibit TNF-α gene expression in LPS-stimulated human PBMCs at 20 μg/ml concentration. A potent anti-inflammatory activity of cinnamon extract is suggestive of its anti-arthritic activity, which could be confirmed in various models of arthritis.

Key words: *Cinnamomum zeylanicum*, TNF-α, flow cytometry, anti-inflammatory, gene expression.

INTRODUCTION

Inflammation is a process involving multiple factors acting in a complex network. The ingress of leukocytes into the site of inflammation is crucial for the pathogenesis of inflammatory conditions. Neutrophils and macrophages are known to recruit and play pivotal roles in acute and chronic inflammation, respectively (Wajant et al., 2003). Recruited cells are activated to release many inflammatory responses, causing a change from the acute phase of inflammation. Therefore, inhibition of the cellular reactions is one of the targets that are generally used as an *in vitro* model for anti-inflammatory testing.

TNF-α is a pro-inflammatory cytokine, mainly produced by activated monocytes and macrophages. Excessive production of TNF- α is believed to underlie the progression of many serious inflammatory diseases, such as rheumatoid arthritis (RA), Crohn's disease and psoriasis.

Therefore, anti- TNF-α therapy would be a possible tool for treatment of acute and chronic inflammatory diseases (Tracey and Cerami, 1993; Graninger and Smolen, 2002). Botanical substances having TNF-α inhibitory properties could be one of the therapeutic approaches for inflammatory disorders.

Cinnamomum zeylanicum (Lauraceae), which originates from the island of Sri-Lanka (formerly called Ceylon) southeast of India, has been used for its anti-diabetic, anti-nociceptive, astringent and diuretic activities. It has been demonstrated that bark and leaves of *C. zeylanicum* contain antifungal substances (Mishra et al., 2009). Its aqueous extract possessed antioxidant properties and it could be a potential therapeutic approach for the pathologies associated with the damage due to free radicals (Hasani-Ranjbar et al., 2009). It was found to have inhibitory effects on osteoclastogenesis through the suppression of nuclear factor of activated T cells, cytoplasmic1 (NFATc1) mediated signal transduction (Tsuji-Naito, 2008). In combination with other botanical

---

*Corresponding author. E-mail: joshikalpana@gmail.com.

products, *C. zeylanicum* showed potential clinical utility in patients with allergic rhinitis (Corren et al., 2008). It exhibited insulin-mimetic action in 3T3-L1 adipocytes while inhibiting the secretion of adiponectin (Roffey et al., 2006) and decreased blood glucose levels in glucose tolerance test (GTT) (Verspohl et al., 2006). It is also reported to have a role in wound healing (Kamath et al., 2003). Additionally, it has insecticidal activity (Abdel, 2006). Present investi-gation was carried out to evaluate the anti-inflammatory potential of hydro alcoholic bark extract of *C. zeylanicum* (OA4-50) and its effect on Tumor necrosis factor-a (TNF-α) secretion and gene expression. In the preliminary experiments all the extracts; aqueous, 50% ethanolic, 80% ethanolic and hexanoic extracts were evaluated for TNF-α inhibitory properties. As 50% ethanolic extract showed inhibitory effect on TNF-α release from human peripheral blood mono-nuclear cells (PBMCs), it was further evaluated in acute and chronic models.

MATERIALS AND METHODS

Chemicals

Histopaque-1077 density gradient solution, sterile Phosphate Buffered Saline (PBS), Trypan blue (0.4%), RPMI-1640 medium, HEPES, Glutamine, Fetal Bovine Serum (FBS), Penicillin, Strepto-mycin, Dimethylsulphoxide (DMSO), Ethylene Diamine Tetra Acetic acid (EDTA), Rolipram, Lipopolysaccharide (LPS), γ-cargeenan typeIV, Toluene, Ethyl acetate, Ethanol and Cinnamaldehyde were procured from Sigma-Aldrich (St. Louis, MO, USA), TNF-α enzyme-linked immunosorbent assay kit was purchased from R and D systems (Minneapolis, MN, USA). cDNA synthesis kit from Invitrogen (California, USA). SYBR Green RT-PCR reaction kit from Applied Biosystems (California USA). Phycoerythrin labeled mouse TNF-α monoclonal antibody, FACS lysing solution, permeabilizing solution and Golgi plug were obtained from BD Biosciences (California, USA). All the biological studies were done at Indian Institute of Integrative Medicine, Jammu.

Plant material and extract preparation

C. zeylanicum bark was collected from Green pharmacy (Pune), authenticated and a voucher specimen was submitted at the Bota-nical Survey of India, Western Circle, Pune (No. SPCIV7). Plant material was dried under shadow and extraction was carried out by cold maceration. Dried coarse powder was macerated overnight with 50% ethanol in orbital incubator shaker (Orbitek, Scigenics) at 20°C at 60 rpm. The extract was then filtered and centrifuged at 800 g for 10 min. Solution was allowed to dry by lyophilisation. The percentage yield was calculated on the basis of the dried plant material weight for testing. The extract was dissolved in vehicle and diluted to the desired concentration.

HPTLC analysis

High performance thin layer chromatography (HPTLC) characteri-zation of the cinnamon bark extract was done. Presence of volatile oil in the extract was confirmed during preliminary phytochemical screening of the extract. The hydro-alcoholic extract was charac-terized by HPTLC (F_{254}-Merk-silica gel plates) using reported TLC method for volatile oil (Colditz, 1985). Chromatographic separation

was carried out using solvent system of toluene: ethyl acetate (9:1.5) and plates were viewed at 225 and365 nm (Camag Multi wavelength scanner III, version IV). The spots were developed with vanillin - sulphuric acid and scanner at visible range (wavelength of 300 - 800).

Stock solution was prepared by dissolving the extract in 50% ethanol (26.27 ng/μl). Standard was prepared by dissolving the extract in 50 μl, then dissolve in 10 ml of ethanol. Injection volume was 5 μl (500 ng/spot).

Biological activity testing

Animals

Swiss albino mice and Wistar rat were obtained from the Indian institute of Integrated medicine, Jammu. They were kept in stan-dard environmental conditions and maintained on a standard rodent diet with water given *ad libitum*.

Isolation of human peripheral blood mononuclear cells

After obtaining written informed consent, venous blood sample was obtained from healthy adult donors. Human PBMCs were isolated from heparinized blood samples using histopaque density gradient, washed and were suspended in complete RPMI-1640 medium sup-plemented with 10 mM HEPES, 2 mM *l*-glutamine, 10% fetal bovine serum (FBS), 100 U/ml of penicillin, 100 μg/ml of streptomycin.

TNF-α inhibition in human PBMCs

Cell treatment

The stock solution of extracts (aqueous, 50% ethanolic, 80% etha-nolic and hexanolic) and pure compound were prepared in DMSO and then diluted to the desired concentration in which the final maximum concentration of DMSO in the media was not more than 0.1% DMSO. Cells were seeded at a density of 10^6 cells/ml in 96-well microtiter plate. Cells were pretreated with different extracts at 20 μg/ml and then stimulated with LPS (1 μg/ml). Positive controls were treated only with LPS where as in negative control wells me-dium containing 0.1% DMSO was added. Cells were maintained at 37°C in a humidified incubator under an atmosphere supplemented with 5% CO_2.

Quantitation of cytokines

Supernatants were collected for cytokine analysis. Cytokine levels were quantitated using enzyme-linked immunosorbant assay (ELISA) kit from R and D systems, according to the manufacturer's instructions. Supernatant (100 μl) was added to antibody-coated polystyrene wells and incubated for 2 h. After washing, the plates were incubated with biotin-labeled anti-cytokine antibody for 2 h. The plates were washed and incubated for 20 min with a streptavidin/horseradish peroxidase conjugate.

The plates were washed and incubated with trimethylbenzidine (TMB) and peroxide, to detect the horse radish peroxide. The reaction was stopped by the addition of 2N sulphuric acid and the absorbance read at 540 and 450 nm on a titertek Multiskan MCC/340 microplate reader (Palladino et al., 2003).

Gene expression studies

RNA isolation

Human PBMCs were washed in 6-well plates twice with 1 ml of

sterile-ice cold PBS and lysed directly with 1 ml of monophasic lysis reagent. RNA concentration and integrity were determined using Biophotometer and formaldehyde gel (Wagner, 1988).

cDNA synthesis

The mixture (20 µl) contained 1 µg total RNA, 1 µl oligo(dt) primer, 2 µl dNTP mix, 0.1 M DTT, 1 µl RNase out, 1 µl thermoscript RT (invitrogen) in 5X cDNA synthesis buffer. The synthesis reactions were preceded at 50°C for 60 s and 85°C for 20 min.

PCR primers

The primers were designed using complete cDNA sequence of human TNF-α gene available at NCBI (accession number NM_00594). The sequence (5' to 3') of the forward primer and reverse primer for amplification of Human TNF-α gene are A G C CCATGTTGTAGCAAACC and TGAGGTACAGGCCCTCTGAT respectively.

Real time polymerase chain reaction

Reaction mixture (50 µl) contained 10 µl of RNA-derived cDNA, 1 µl each of forward primer and reverse primer with 2X of 25 µl SYBR Green PCR master mix (ABI kit). The reactions were performed in 96-well plates in Opticon 2 real time PCR instrument. The thermal cycle conditions were as follows: 30 s each at 94, 50, 72°C for denaturation, annealing and polymerization reaction for 40 cycles, respectively.

Fluorescence signals measured during amplification were considered positive if the fluorescence intensity was 20-fold greater than the standard deviation of the baseline fluorescence. The C_T method of relative quantification was used to determine the fold change in expression (Wagner, 1988).

Cell viability assay

Viability of cells were determined by MTT [3-(4, 5-Dimethylthiazol-2-yl)-2, 5-Diphenyltetrazolium Bromide] colorimetric assay. After removing the supernatant, treated and control cells were incubated with MTT (5 mg/ml) for 4 h at 37°C and solubilized in DMSO. The amount of formazan production was determined spectrophotometrically at 545 nm.

Flow cytometric study (Prabhakar, 2002; Yin et al., 2001)

Sample preparation

OA4-50 was prepared as homogenous suspension in 0.1% gum acacia. Rolipram was used as a reference compound for comparison and validation of test model applied.

In vitro experiment: TNF-α estimation in neutrophils

Neutrophils were separated from whole blood taken from retro-orbital plexus of normal Swiss albino mice; added 2.5 µl of protein transport inhibitors, centrifuged and histopaque was added, incubated for 10 min and then centrifuged, added fluorescence-activated cell sorting (FACS) lysing solution. After subsequent washing with PBS, acquisition was done on the flow cytometry.

LPS was added to the isolated murine neutrophils. Drug sample at different doses was added and incubated for 3 h at 37°C with 5%

CO_2 concentration. After incubation permeabilizing solution (10X) was added. Sample was thoroughly washed with PBS and spun at 900 rpm. Anti-TNF-α monoclonal antibody was added and analyzed by flow cytometer (BD LSR).

In vivo experiment: TNF-α estimation in pleural leukocytes

In vivo studies were carried out using Pleurisy model for assessment of effect of OA4-50 extract on inflammatory parameter TNF-α. Wistar rats having a weight range of 120 - 180 g were employed for the study. Drug was administered orally using metal drug feeding cannula at the concentration of 5, 10, 20 mg/kg, 1 h before injection of 0.5 ml carragenan into the pleural cavity of rat.

After 4 h of carragenan challenge pleural fluid (50 µl) was taken in heparinized tubes and Golgi stop was added. Then it was treated with FACS lysing solution for the elimination of red blood cells if any. After 3 washes with PBS, 500 µl of permeabilizing solution was added and incubation was carried out for 15 min. Then samples were incubated for 30 min after addition of anti-TNF-α monoclonal antibody and were analyzed on flow cytometer (BD-LSR) using Cellquest Pro software.

Data analysis

Data were analyzed using Excel and GraphPad Prism 5. Statistical analysis was done using One-way ANOVA complemented with Dunnet test. $P < 0.05$ was considered as indicative of significance. Percentage inhibition of TNF-α release in human PBMCs was calculated using the formula:

% Inhibition = 100 - [(TNF-α levels in test - TNF-α levels in negative control)/ (TNF-α levels in positive control - TNF-α levels in negative control)] x 100

Percentage inhibition of TNF-α expression in murine neutophils and pleural leukocytes was calculated using the formula:

% Inhibition=100 - (Test/Control) x 100

RESULTS

Preparation of extract

Cold maceration procedure was followed to obtain hydro-alcoholic extract. Percentage yield was 80%. Extracts were light brown in colour, sparingly soluble in water and highly hygroscopic in nature.

Phytochemical analysis

Figure 1 depicts the HPTLC analysis of the HPTLC profile shows the presence of 4 peaks at RF 0.1, 0.4, 0.6 and 0.9. Three minor peaks with peak height 61.1, 13.7 and 10.4 with peak area 658.8, 158.9 and 169.7 were observed. Major component (Cinnamaldehyde) was observed at RF 0.6 with peak height and area 108.2 and 5214 respectively, which was confirmed by comparing with the HPTLC profile of standard Cinnamaldehyde. From calibration curve it was observed that concentration of major component (cinnamaldehyde) in extract was 2.3%.

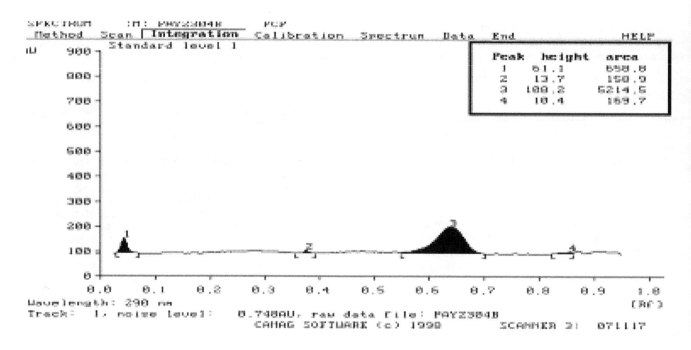

Peak	height	area
1	61.1	658.8
2	13.7	150.9
3	100.2	5214.5
4	10.4	169.7

Figure 1. HPTLC analyses of hydro-alcoholic cinnamon bark extract OA4-50.

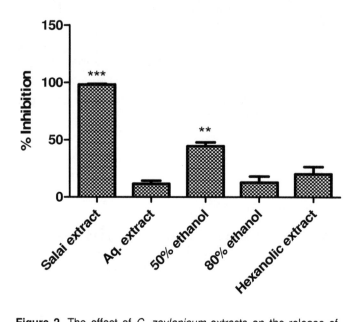

Figure 2. The effect of *C. zeylanicum* extracts on the release of TNF-α in hPBMCs.

Estimation of TNF α secretion form hPBMCs by ELISA

The extracts, including aqueous, 50% ethanolic, 80% ethanolic and hexanolic, were tested for inhibition of TNF-α secretion in human PBMCs (hPBMCs). Salai Guggul(Khan et al., 2006) was used as reference compound.

Fifty percentage ethanolic extract (OA4-50) was found to inhibit significantly the TNF- release form human PBMCs with a maximum inhibition of 44.38% at a concentration of 20 µg /ml (Figure 2). Salai extract, the reference compound gave a 98% inhibition in the same experimental setup.

Cell viability

Effects of OA4-50 on viability of human PBMCs and neutrophils were evaluated using MTT. The survival of cells was not significantly affected by treatment for 24, 48 or 72 h with hydro-alcoholic extracts at concentration ranging from 1 - 20 µg/ml. However, higher doses of extract (25 -100 µg/ml) decreased cell survival by over 80%. Thus, non-cytotoxic concentration of extract was used in subsequent studies.

RNA isolation from hPBMCs

RNA was isolated from human PBMCs (10^6 cells /ml), treated with LPS (1 µg/µl) and OA4-50 using the method described. Yield of RNA was 2 - 4 µg/ 10^6 hPBMCs. Integrity of RNA samples was checked on formaldehyde gel. Presence of 28s and 18s bands indicated intactness of RNA is intact. This RNA was used for cDNA synthesis.

Standardization of PCR

cDNA was amplified with TNF-α and β-actin specific primers. Reaction conditions were standardized using

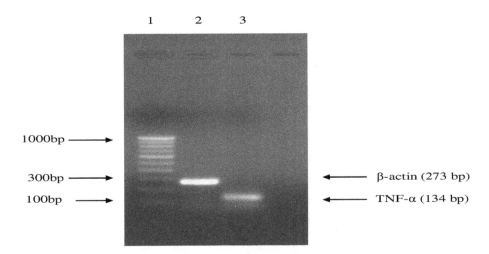

Figure 3. PCR standardization using β-actin and TNF-α primers on 2% agarose gel. Lane 1: Molecular weight marker (100 bp ladder); Lane 2: β-actin; Lane 3: TNF-α.

Table 1. Effect of cinnamon bark extract (OA4-50) on TNF-α expression in murine neutrophils.

Treatment group	Conc. (µg/ml)	Values of gated cell			Mean ± SE	% Inhibition
		n1	n2	N3		
OA4-50	1	2.26	2.01	2.04	2.10 ± 0.07	19.54
	2.5	1.84	2.14	2.42	2.13 ± 0.16	18.39
	5	1.88	2.44	1.89	2.07 ± 0.18	20.68
	10	1.68	1.93	1.67	1.76 ± 0.08	32.56
	20	1.3	1.38	1.48	1.38 ± 0.05	47.12
Control		2.59	2.58	2.68	2.61 ± 0.03	

various concentrations of primers, cDNA concentration and
taq polymerase. These conditions were used further for real time PCR. Figure 3 depicts the amplification of cDNA with TNF-α primer (Lane 2) and β-actin primer (Lane 3). Desired product of sizes 134 and 273 bp were obtained without any non-specific amplification. 100 bp ladders was used as molecular weight marker (Lane 1).

Real time PCR

Real time PCR was carried out on Opticon 2 RT PCR machine using SYBR Green. Melting curve analysis was carried out at 60 to 95℃ at 1℃ time intervals. SYBR Green is very non specific dye and can bind to any contaminant of the reaction and gives rise to non-specific products and multiple peaks appear on melting curve. Single peak indicated pure PCR product obtained after amplification on real time PCR and absence of non-specific products. Thermal cycling conditions optimized for PCR were met for real-time PCR. Lower the Ct value–more transcript abundance and vice versa. OA4-50 was

found to inhibit TNF-α gene expression by three fold as compared to LPS+ control.

Flow cytometric study

Intracellular TNF-α level in murine Neutrophils were estimated by Flow cytometer employing anti-TNF-α monoclonal antibody; data is summarized in Table 1. The test substance (OA4) was used at different concentrations ranging from 1 to 20 µg/ml. OA4 showed significant inhibition of intracellular expression with the maximum inhibition of 47.12% at 20 µg /ml concentration (Figure 4). Effect of cinnamon extract (50%) on TNF-α production in carrageenan induced inflammation Model (Table 2).

Carrageenan-induced pleurisy in wistar rat was used to evaluate the effect of test compound on TNF-α expression in pleural leukocytes (Figure 5). Animals were treated with different doses of 50% ethanolic extract (5, 10 and 20 mg /kg) administered by intaperitoneal route. Carrageenan treated animals were taken as vehicle control. The test compound showed suppression of TNF-α expression at 10 and 20 mg/kg (20.94 and 44.60%).

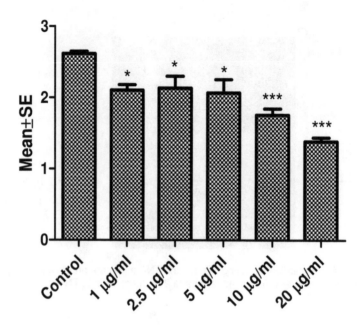

Figure 4. Effect of cinnamon bark extract (OA4-50) on TNF-α expression in murine neutrophils.

Table 2. Effect of cinnamon bark extract (OA4-50) on TNF-α expression in leukocytes from rat model of pleurisy.

Treatment group	Dose (mpk)	Values of gated cell			Mean ± SE	% Inhibition
		n1	n2	n3		
	5	21.85	21.7	22.27	21.94 ± 0.17	9.71
OA4-50	10	19.55,	16.98	21.1	19.21 ± 1.20	20.94
	20	13.53	13.32	13.53	13.46 ± 0.07	44.6
Vehicle control		24.23	24.09	24.58	24.3 ± 0.14	

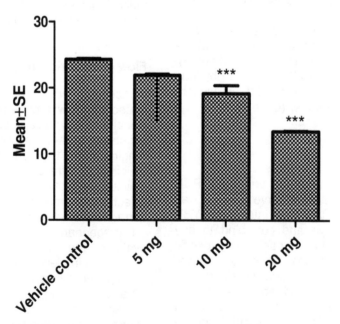

Figure 5. Effect of cinnamon bark extract (OA4-50) on TNF-α expression in leukocytes from rat model of pleurisy.

These results indicated that cinnamon bark is a potent anti-inflammatory drug.

DISCUSSION AND CONCLUSION

C. zeylanicum bark extract was found to have anti-inflammatory activity. *Cinnamomum* species including *Cinnamomum osmophloeum* (Fang et al., 2005; Rao et al., 2007; Tung et al., 2008), *Cinnamomum camphora* (Lee et al., 2006), *Cinnamomum insularimontanum* (Lin et al., 2008) and *Cinnamomum cassia* (Li et al., 2007) have also been demonstrated to have anti-inflammatory properties. The extract was tested with the standard models for both acute and chronic inflammation. For the acute inflammatory model, the *in vitro* test was performed using LPS-stimulated mice neutrophil model by Flow cytometer. It was found that the extract inhibited TNF-α and probably accounted for its anti-inflammatory effect. The inhibitory effect of the extract on TNF-α was supported by rat pleurisy model.

The present study shows that the 50% ethanol extract of cinnamon, at the highest dose (20 mg/kg) has an inhibitory effect on edema formation in carrageenan-induced rat pleurisy model. The edema induced by the injection of carrageenan into the pleural cavity of rat. Additionally, it was found to inhibit the release of TNF- α in human PBMCs. The result suggests that the inhibitory effect of the extract on edema formation is probably due to the inhibition of release of TNF-α. Therefore, the release of TNF-α after stimulation of neutrophils with LPS is a valid model system to test novel compounds for potential anti-inflammatory effects (Nazir et al., 2007). Inhibitory effect of the extract on TNF-α release from neutrophils was demonstrated in a dose-dependent manner. TNF-α plays a critical role in both acute and chronic inflammation. TNF-α facilitates inflammatory cell infiltration by promoting the adhesion of neutrophils and lymphocytes to endothelial cells. Additionally, TNF-α stimulates neutrophils to transcribe and release cytokines and chemokines biosynthesis (Khanna et al., 2007). Inhibition of TNF-α release can reduce the severity of inflammation. TNF-α is shown to accelerate both angiogenesis and matrix degradation by induction of vascular matrix metalloproteinase. Therefore, the inhibition of tissue granuloma by the extract at least in part, may be through interference with TNF-α release (Pandey et al., 2005).

It is interesting to know if the extract acted at expression level for TNF-alpha inhibition. Cinnamon (50%) inhibited the expression of TNF-α. It may inhibit either the initiation of transcription or the stability of the mRNAs encoding these molecules. It has been also shown that activation of transcription factor NF-κβ by TNF-α is required for the transcriptional activation of endothelial cell adhesion molecules. Thus, NF-κβ is believed to play an important role in the regulation of inflammatory response. NF-κβ activation was associated with the phosphorylation and degradation of Iκβ- α and the nuclear translocation of p[65] (Eigler et al., 1997). NF-κβ, a key transcription factor is implicated in the regulation of a variety of genes participating in immune and inflammatory responses. Effect of the herbal extract on transcription factor NF-κβ could be studied to understand mechanism of TNF- α expression inhibition.

C. zeylanicum has been reported to increase the hydroxyproline content in tissues, which is reduced in degenerative diseases like Osteoarthritis (OA) and thus promotes damaged cartilage repair and healing (Chakrabarti et al., 2006).

Potent anti-inflammatory activities of cinnamon extract at *in vitro* and *in vivo* experiments along with cartilage protecting activity is suggestive of its anti-inflammatory, anti-arthritic activity, which could be confirmed in various models of arthritis.

ACKNOWLEDGEMENTS

We are indebted to Dr. G. N. Qazi for providing IIIM facilities for various studies and thank NMITLI team Manish, Dnyaneshwar, Preeti and Yogita.

REFERENCES

Abdel Halim AS (2006). Efficacy of Cinnamomum zeylanicum on third stage larvae and adult fecundity of Musca domestica and Anopheles pharoensis. J. Egypt Soc. Parasitol. 38: 475-482.

Chakrabarti S, Zee JM, Patel KD (2006). Regulation of matrix metalloproteinase-9 (MMP-9) in TNF-stimulated neutrophils: novel pathways for tertiary granule release. J. Leukoc. Biol. 79: 1-9.

Colditz IG (1985). Kinetics of tachyphalaxis to mediators of acute inflammation. Immunology 55: 149-156.

Corren J, Lemay M, Lin Y, Rozga L, Randolph RK (2008). Clinical and biochemical effects of a combination botanical product (ClearGuard) for allergy: a pilot randomized double-blind placebo-controlled trial. Nutr. J. 7: 20.

Eigler A, Sinha B, Hartmann G, Endres S (1997). Taming TNF: strategies to restrain this proinflammatory cytokine. Immunol. Today 18: 487.

Fang SH, Rao YK, Tzeng YM (2005). Inhibitory effects of flavonol glycosides from Cinnamomum osmophloeum on inflammatory mediators in LPS/IFN-gamma-activated murine macrophages. Bioorg. Med. Chem. 13(238): 1-8.

Graninger W, Smolen J (2002). Treatment of rheumatoid arthritis by TNF-blocking agents. Int. Arch. Allergy Immunol. 127: 10-14

Hasani-Ranjbar S, Larijani B, Abdollahi M (2009). A systematic review of the potential herbal sources of future drugs effective in oxidant-related diseases. Inflamm. Allergy Drug Targets. 8: 2-10.

Kamath JV, Rana AC, Chowdhury AR (2003). Pro-healing effect of Cinnamomum zeylanicum bark. Phytother. Res. 17: 970-972.

Khan B, Ahmad AF, Bani S Kaul A, Suri KA, Satti NK, Athar M, Qazi GN (2006). Augmentation and proliferation of T lymphocytes and Th-1 cytokines by Withania somnifera in stressed mice. J. Int. Immunopharmacol. 6: 1394-1403.

Khanna D, Sethi G, Ahn KA, Pandey MK, Kunnumakkara AB, Sung B, Aggarwal A, Aggarwal BB (2007). Natural products as a gold mine for arthritis treatment. Curr. Opin. Pharmacol. 7: 344-351.

Lee HJ, Hyun EA, Yoon WJ, Kim BH, Rhee MH, Kang HK, Cho JY, Yoo ES (2006). *In vitro* anti-inflammatory and anti-oxidative effects of Cinnamomum camphora extracts. J. Ethnopharmacol. 103: 208-216.

Li TJ, Qiu Y, Mao JQ, Yang PY, Rui YC, Chen WS (2007), Protective effects of Guizhi-Fuling-Capsules on rat brain ischemia/reperfusion

Injury. J. Pharmacol. Sci. 105: 34-40.

Lin CT, Chen CJ, Lin TY, Tung JC, Wang SY (2008). Anti-inflammation activity of fruit essential oil from Cinnamomum insularimontanum Hayata. Bioresour. Technol. 9: 8783-8787.

Mishra AK, Mishra A, Kehri HK, Sharma B, Pandey AK (2009). Inhibitory activity of Indian spice plant Cinnamomum zeylanicum extracts against Alternaria solani and Curvularia lunata, the pathogenic dematiaceous moulds. Ann. Clin. Microbiol. Antimicrob. 7: 8-9.

Nazir N, Koul S, Qurishi MA, Sachin C, Taneja SC, Sheikh FA, Bani S, Qazi GN (2007). Immunomodulatory effect of bergenin and norbergenin against adjuvant-induced arthritis—A flow cytometric study. J. Ethnopharmacol. 112: 401-405.

Palladino MA, Bahjat FR, Theodorakis EA, Moldawer LL (2003). Anti-TNF-α therapies: the next generation. Nat. Rev. Drug Discov. I2: 736-746.

Pandey R, Maurya R, Singh GB, Sathiamoorthy, Naik S (2005). Immunosuppressive properties of flavonoids isolated from Boerhaavia diffusa Linn. Int. Immunopharmacol. 5: 541-553.

Prabhakar (2002). Simultaneous quantification of proinflammatory cytokines in human plasma using the LabMap assay. J. Immunol. Methods 260: 207-218.

Rao YK, Fang SH, Tzeng YM (2007). Evalution of the anti-inflammatory and anti-proliferation tumoral cells activities of Antrodia camphorata, Cordyceps sinensis, and Cinnamomum osmophloeum bark extracts. J. Ethnopharmacol. 114: 78-85.

Roffey B, Atwal A, Kubow S (2006). Cinnamon water extracts increase glucose uptake but inhibit adiponectin secretion in 3T3-L1 adipose cells. Mol. Nutr. Food Res. 50: 739-745.

Tracey K, Cerami A (1993). Tumor necrosis factor, other cytokines and disease. Annu. Rev. Cell Biol. 3: 317-343.

Tsuji-Naito K (2008). Aldehydic components of cinnamon bark extract suppresses RANKL-induced osteoclastogenesis through NFATc1 downregulation. Bioorg. Med. Chem. 16: 9176-9183.

Tung YT, Chua MT, Wang SY, Chang ST (2008). Anti-inflammation activities of essential oil and its constituents from indigenous cinnamon (Cinnamomum osmophloeum) twigs. Bioresour. Technol. 99: 3908-3913.

Verspohl EJ, Bauer K, Neddermann E (2006). Antidiabetic effect of Cinnamomum cassia and Cinnamomum zeylanicum in vivo and in vitro. Phytother. Res. 19: 203-206.

Wagner H (1988), in A plant drug analysis, Springer- Verlag, Berlin-Heidelberg. 226 pp.

Wajant H, Pfizenmaier K, Scheurich P (2003). Tumor necrosis factor signaling. Cell Death Differ. 10: 45-65.

Yin JL, Shackel NA, Zekry A, McGuinness PH, Richards C, Van Der Putten K, McCaughan GW, Eris JM, Bishop GA (2001). Real-time reverse transcriptase–polymerase chain reaction (RT–PCR) for measurement of cytokine and growth factor mRNA expression with fluorogenic probes or SYBR Green. Immunol. Cell Biol. 79: 213–221.

4

Synthesis, antimicrobial potential and toxicological activities of Ni(II) complex of mefloquine hydrochloride

Joshua A. Obaleye[2], Johnson F. Adediji[1]*, Ebenezer T. Olayinka[1] and Matthew A. Adebayo[1]

[1]Department of Chemical Sciences, Ajayi Crowther University Oyo, P. M. B 1066, Oyo, Oyo State, Nigeria.
[2]Department of Chemistry, University of Ilorin, Ilorin, Kwara State, Nigeria.

Transition metal complex of Ni(II) with mefloquine hydrochloride (antimalaria drug) was synthesized using a template method. Chemical analysis including conductivity measurements and spectroscopic studies were used to propose the geometry and mode of binding of the ligand to metal ion. From analytical data, the stoichiometry of the complex has been found to be 1:1. Infrared spectral data also suggest that the ligand (mefloquine hydrochloride) behaves as a tridentate ligand with N:N:O donor sequence towards the metal ion. The complex generally showed octahedral coordinate geometry. Molar conductance of 10^{-2} mol dm^{-3} methanol solution of the complex indicated non-electrolytic nature of metal complex. It also revealed that the ligand anions were covalently bonded to the complex. *In vivo* evaluation of antimalarial studies of the metal complex shows greater activities when compared to the free ligand. Mefloquine and its metal complex increased significantly ($p < 0.05$) serum alanine aminotransferase (ALT), aspartate aminotransferase (AST) and alkaline phosphatase (ALP) and significantly reduced these enzymes in the liver and kidney when compared to the control. This revealed that both mefloquine and its metal complex might show toxicity particularly on the liver and kidney with the metal complex group being mild.

Key words: Transition metal, antimicrobial, antimalarial drug, complexation, toxicological studies.

INTRODUCTION

Complexation chemistry is quite simply the chemistry of coordination compounds containing a central atom or ion to which are attached molecules or ions whose number usually exceeds the number corresponding to the oxidation number or valence of the central atom or ion. They are of great theoretical importance and they are also of great practical utility as well (Nadira et al., 1987).

Over the past three decades, intensive efforts have been made to design novel compounds to confront new strains of resistance micro-organisms. The ongoing intense search for novel and innovative drug delivery systems is predominantly a consequence of the well established fact that the convectional dosage forms are not sufficiently effective in conveying the drug compound to its site of action and this have necessitated the needs to search for more potent drugs.

The recognition of the potential employment of metal complexes and chelates in therapeutic application provides useful outlet for basic research in transition metal chemistry (Obaleye et al., 1997; Ogunniran et al., 2008). Mefloquine Hydrochloride (Ligand employed in this study) is (±)-erythro-α-(2-piperidyl)-2,8-bis(triflu-oromethyl)-4-quinoline methanol and it is known for antimalarial activity. The choice of quinoline moiety was as a result of the success with the case of chloroquine. Mefloquine was the only candidate drug that came off successfully during Vietnam war. Its total synthesis was first reported by Ohnmacht et al. (1971). More than 10,000 synthesized compounds, most of which were based on the quinoline moiety, were screened for antimalarial activity during the Vietnam War at the Walter Reed Army Institute (WRAI) in U.S.A (WHO, 1987). Mefloquine is a white or slightly yellow, crystalline powder, very soluble in water, freely soluble in methanol and alcohol. It melts at about 260°C with decomposition. It shows polymorphism. Since the ligand (mefloquine) consists of potential binding sites such as oxygen and two nitrogen atoms, this work set out

---

*Corresponding author. E-mail: dijijohnson@yahoo.com.

to study out the coordination tendencies, characterization after complexing with metal and the biological activities of mefloquine hydrochloride.

MATERIALS AND METHODS

Materials

Metal salt, Nickel(II) chloride hexahydrate used for the complexation was obtained from British Drug Houses chemical limited, Poole, England and was used as supplied. The ligand (mefloquine hydrochloride) was obtained from SWISS Pharmaceuticals Company Lagos, Nigeria. ALP, ALT and AST assay kits were obtained from Randox Laboratories Limited, Antrim, United Kingdom. Isolates of *Escherichia coli, Klebsiella pneumonia* and *Staphylococcus aureus* were obtained from the Department of Microbiology, University of Ilorin, Nigeria. Albino rats (Wistar strain) were obtained from the Department of Biochemistry, University of Ilorin, Ilorin, Nigeria. This study was carried out in the Department of Chemical Sciences Laboratory, Ajayi Crowther University, Oyo, Nigeria.

Synthesis of the metal complex

The complex was prepared based on previous reported procedures with slight modifications (Nadira et al., 1987; Ogunniran et al., 2008). 0.01 mol of ethanolic solutions of Nickel (II) chloride ($NiCl_2.6H_2O$) were prepared in a round bottomed flask. 0.01 mol (4.148 g) of mefloquine hydrochloride was dissolved in 20 cm³ ethanol and added to the solution of the metal salt in 10 cm³ ethanol in a round-bottomed flask fitted with a condenser and refluxed with constant stirring for 2 h. The chelate were separated out after leaving it for four days. The metal chelates thus separated were filtered and washed with methanol and then with distilled water to remove unreacted ligand and metal. Finally, the solid complex was dried in a dessicator. 10% methanolic ammonia (buffer) solution was used to maintain the pH of the reacting solution of metal salt and ligand under reflux.

Determination of physical properties of the complex

Infra-red spectra of the ligand and complex were recorded in KBr disc in the range 4000 - 600 cm⁻¹ on PUC Scientific model 500 FTIR Spectrometer. Electronic spectra were done on Aquamate Spectrophotometer Model V4.60. The metal estimation was done using an Alpha4 Atomic Absorption Spectrophotometer with PM 8251 simple-pen recorder. Conductivity measurements were carried out using WTW Conductometer Bridge. Thin layer Chromatography was carried out using TLC plate coated with silica gel.

Antimicrobial screening of the ligand and metal complex

The stimulatory or inhibitory activity of the ligand and the metal complex synthesized were determined according to the procedure previously reported by Obaleye and Famurewa (1989) as modified by Mohamed and Abdel-Wahab (2005). The bacteria species used for this test include clinical sample of *E. coli, S. aureus* and *K. pneumonia*. The antibacterial activities of the compounds were estimated on the basis of the size of the inhibition zone formed around the wells on sensitivity media. Antifungal activity of each compound was determined using culture of three fungi species; they are *Aspergillus niger, Aspergillus flavus* and *Rhizopus* species. They were cultured on potato dextrose agar. The plates were incubated aerobically at 28 ± 2°C for 96 h.

Treatment of animals

Male albino rats (Wistar strain), weighing between 160 - 180 g were obtained from the Department of Biochemistry, University of Ilorin, Ilorin and housed in the animal house of the Department of Chemical Sciences, Ajayi Crowther University, Oyo, Nigeria for acclimatization. They were kept in wire meshed cages and fed with commercial rat chow (Bendel Feeds Nigeria Ltd) and water *ad libitum*.

Eighteen rats were divided into three groups of 6 rats per group. The first group was used as control and received distilled water. The second group of rats was treated with free ligand (mefloquine), while the third group was treated with metal complex [Ni(Mef)Cl₂]. The distilled water, ligand and solution of metal complex were administered orally to the rats of various groups two times daily, morning and evening for seven days at the dose of 6.66 mg/Kg body weight. The animals were sacrificed 24 h after the last treatment.

Preparation of serum and tissue homogenate

The method described by Yakubu et al. (2005) was used to prepare the serum. The rats were sacrificed by stunning. Blood samples were collected by cardiac punctures into clean, dry centrifuge tubes after which they were left for 10 min at room temperature. The tubes were then centrifuged for 10 min at 3000 x g in an MSC (Essex, UK) bench centrifuge. The clear supernatant (serum) was aspirated using a Pasteur pipette into clean, dry sample bottles and then frozen overnight before use. The liver and kidney excised from rat, blotted of blood stains were rinsed in 1.15% KCl and homogenized in 4 volumes of ice-cold 0.01 mol dm⁻³ potassium phosphate buffer (pH 7.4). The homogenates were centrifuged at 12,500 x g for 15 min at 4°C and the supernatants, termed the post-mitochondrial fractions (PMF) were aliquoted and used for enzyme assays.

Determination of serum and tissue AST, ALT and ALP activities

Serum and tissues AST, ALT and ALP activities were determined using Randox diagnostic kits. Determination of AST and ALT activities were based on the principle described by Reitman and Franke (1957). ALP activity determination was based on the method of Wright et al. (1972). The yellow coloured p-nitro phenol formed was monitored at 405 nm. Protein determination of serum and all fractions was estimated by the method of Lowry et al. (1951) as modified by Yakubu et al. (2005) using bovine serum albumin as standard.

Statistical analysis

The data were analyzed using one way ANOVA followed by Duncan multivariable post-hoc test for comparison between control and treated rats in all groups. P values less than 0.05 were considered statistically significant.

RESULTS AND DISCUSSION

The metal chloride salt reacts with the ligand, L (L = Mefloquine) to form a compound ([M(II)LCl₂]). By using the proposed equation:

$$MX_2 \cdot nH_2O + L \rightarrow ML \cdot X_2 + nH_2O$$

Table 1. Some physical properties of mefloquine and its metal complex.[8,5]

Compounds	Melting point (°C)	Colour	% yield	Conductivity (Ω^{-1} cm^{-1} dm^{-3})
Mefloquine(Mef)	259 - 260	White	-	3.221×10^{-5}
Ni(Mef)Cl$_2$.6H$_2$O	242 - 244	Green	66.0	1.297×10^{-4}

Where:

M = Ni^{2+} metal salt;
L = mefloquine and
X$^-$ = Chloride ion.

The complex synthesized was found to be a non-hygroscopic solid with a light green colour (Table 1). The complex is very soluble in ethanol, methanol and distilled water. It has a sharp melting point and no decomposition was observed. The average percentage yield was 66.0%. The retention factor (R$_f$) values were calculated from the developed single spot for the complex indicating the purity of the compound (Mohamed and Abdel-Wahab, 2005). The R$_f$ of the metal complex was found to be higher than the ligand. Comparing the conductivity of the ligand with that of the metal complex at a room temperature suggests that it is non-electrolytic in nature. The analytical data of the anti-malarial metal complex showed 1:1 stoichiometry. The UV-spectra of the ligand and its metal complex have been interpreted in terms of charge transfer transitions from the metal to the anti-bonding orbital of the ligand and of the $\pi \rightarrow \pi\square\square$ transitions of the ligand (William et al., 1980). The ultraviolet spectrum of the free mefloquine HCl shows two absorption bands at 272.0 and 207.0 nm (Table 2). These transitions involve energies of 36765 and 48309 cm^{-1}. The bands have been assigned to the n $\rightarrow \pi\square$ and $v \rightarrow \sigma*$, transition respectively. These bands undergo hypsochromic shifts in the metal complex due to complexation. The infrared data (Table 3) showed the results of the most informative and indicative region. The assignments have been interpreted based on literature values obtained for similar structural com-pounds (Obaleye et al., 1999). The shifts observed in the absorption bands between mefloquine and its metal complex show that there is coordination. Metal-Ligand bands (Table 4) were observed in the ranges of 610 - 950 cm^{-1} in the metal complex. The Ni(II) complex shows a μ_{eff} value of 3.0 BM, which corresponds to high spin (octahedral) stereochemistry (Kamaruddin and Roy, 2001).

Figures 1 and 2 show the results of antibacterial and antifungal activities of free mefloquine and the metal complexes. The studies of the ligand and its metal complex gave the antimicrobial activity of the compounds. The Metal complex was found to be more active at higher (1.0 g/dm^3) concentration than its corresponding ligand. The synthesized complex was active against the three bacteria used, while they were found to be active against only two of the fungi used, A.niger, and A. flavus. Reports

Table 2. Ultraviolet/Visible spectral assignment of mefloquine and its metal complex.

Compound	Wavelength (nm)	Wave number (cm^{-1})
Mefloquine(Mef)	272.00	36765
	207.00	48309
Ni(Mef)Cl$_2$	317.0	31546
	284.0	35211
	222.0	45045
	207.0	48309

Table 3. IR spectral assignment of mefloquine and its metal complex.

Mefloquine (cm^{-1})	Ni(Mef)Cl$_2$ (cm^{-1})	Tentative assignment
3447.4 w, b	3346.8 b	N(OH), v(N–H) stretch
2925.1 s, b	2939.5 w, b	N(C–H) stretch of CH$_3$
1586.2 s	1580.0 s	N(C=N)
1380.9 s	1340.2 s	N(C–N) stretch

have shown that NiCl$_2$.6H$_2$O has no inhibitory activity on bacteria and fungi species (Obaleye et al., 1999).

Figures 3 - 5 show the results of ALT, AST and ALP activities of the serum, kidney and liver of rat. There was a significant increase (p < 0.05) in serum ALT, AST and ALP activities of mefloquine and its metal complex treated rats compared with the control, with the mefloquine group higher than the metal complex. The data also indicate that there was a significant reduction (p < 0.05) in the liver and kidney ALT, AST and ALP activities of mefloquine and its metal complex treated rats compared with the control, with the mefloquine group lower than the metal complex. The observed significant increase in the serum ALT, AST and ALP activities with a concomitant significant reduction in the same enzymes activities in the liver and kidney of rats administered with mefloquine and the metal complex may be as a result of extra-cellular fluid. ALP is a membrane-bound enzyme often used to assess the integrity of the plasma membrane stress imposed on the tissue by the drug, which may lead to loss of the enzyme molecule through leakage into and endoplasmic reticulum (Akanji et al., 1993). AST and ALT are enzymes associated with liver parenchymal cells. They are raised in acute liver damage. They are also

Table 4. Magnetic moment of the ligands and metal complexes.

Compound	Empirical formula	Formular weight	μ_{eff} (BM)	% Metal content found (calculated)
Mefloquine	$C_{17}H_{16}F_6N_2O$	414.80	-	-
Ni(Mef)Cl$_2$	Ni($C_{17}H_{16}F_6N_2O$)Cl$_2$.6H$_2$O	652.80	3.00	8.89 (9.04)

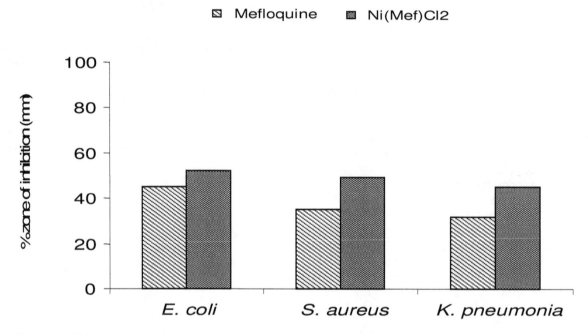

Figure 1. Inhibitory activity of the ligands and metal complexes against *Escherichia coli; Staphylococcus aureus,* and *Klebsiella pneumonia.*

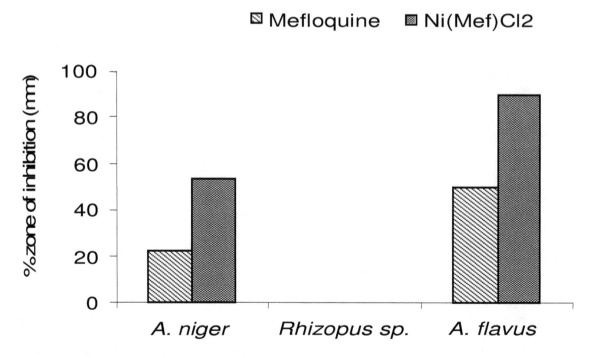

Figure 2. Inhibitory activity of the ligands and metal complexes against *Aspergillus niger, Rhizopus species* and *Aspergillus flavus.*

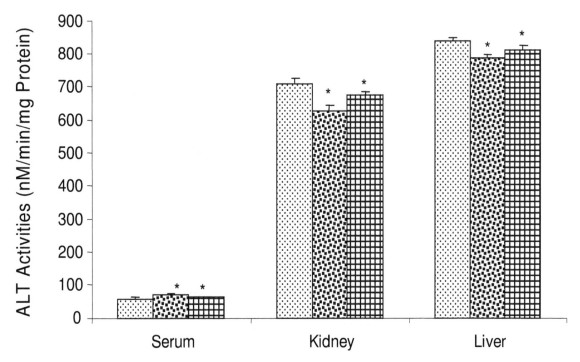

Figure 3. Effect of administration of ligands and metal complexes on the activities of alanine amino transferase (ALT) of rat serum, kidney and liver. * Significantly different from the control ($p < 0.05$).

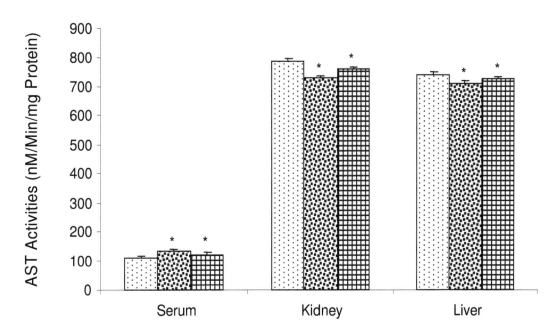

Figure 4. Effect of administration of ligands and metal complexes on the activities of aspartate amino transferase (AST) of rat serum, kidney and liver. * Significantly different from the control ($p < 0.05$)

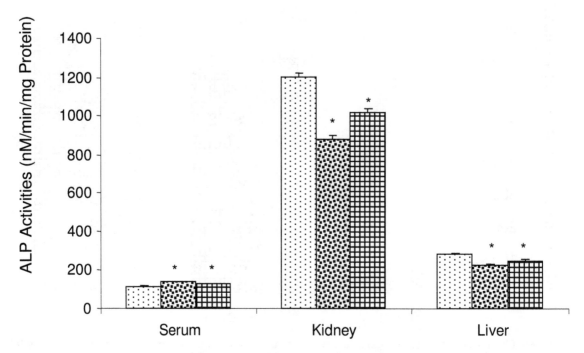

Figure 5. Effect of administration of ligands and metal complexes on the activities of alkaline phosphatase (ALP) of rat serum, kidney and liver. * Significantly different from the control (p < 0.05).

present in red blood cells, heart cells, muscle tissue, pancreas and kidneys. When body tissue or an organ such as the heart or liver is diseased or damaged, additional AST and ALT are released into the bloodstream. Both ALT and AST levels are reliable indicators of liver damage. In short, increase in serum ALT and AST has been reported in conditions involving necrosis of hepatocytes (Macfarlane et al., 2000), myocardial cells, erythrocyte and skeletal muscle cells (Halworth and Capps, 1993). Alteration in serum/tissue levels of AST, ALT and ALP as recorded in this studies are indications of derangement in cellular activities and hence toxicity, however, the toxicity is mild in the metal complex group compared to the mefloquine group.

Conclusion

The results of the chemical and physical analysis from this study show that the ligand (mefloquine) employed in this work coordinated with Ni(II). The metal complex possesses better physical properties than the parent compound. The toxicological studies revealed that both mefloquine and its metal complex might show toxicity particularly on the liver and kidney with the metal complex group being mild.

ACKNOWLEDGEMENTS

The authors appreciate the financial support of Science and Technology Education Post Basic (STEPB), University of Ilorin, Ilorin and Ajayi Crowther University, Oyo, Nigeria.

REFERENCES

Akanji MA, Olagoke OA, Oloyede OB (1993). Effects of chronic consumption of metabisulphate on the integrity of the rat kidney cellular system. Toxicol. 81: 173-179.
Halworth M, Capps N (1993). Therapeutic Drugs Monitoring and Clinical Biochemistry, ACB Ventures Publications, London.
Kamaruddin SK, Roy A (2001). Synthesis and characterization of Cr(III) Mn(II), Fe(III), Co(II), Ni(II) and Cu(II) complexes of 4-pyridy thioacetic acid and 2-pyrimidyl thioacetic acid. Indian J. Chem 40a(2): 211-212.
Lowry OH, Rosebrough NJ, Farr AL, Randall RJ (1951). Protein measurement with folin phenol reagent. J. Biol. Chem. 193:265-275.
Macfarlane I, Bomford A, Sherwood RA (2000). Liver Diseases and Laboratory Medicine. ACB Ventures Publications, London.
Mohamed GG, Abdel-Wahab ZH (2005). Mixed ligand complexes of bis (phenylimine) Schiff base ligands incorporating pyridinium moiety synthesis, characterisation and antibacterial activity. Spectrochimica Acta. Part A: Molecular and Biomolecular Spectroscopy. 9(61):2231-2238.
Nadira W, Singh HB (1987). Synthesis of metal complexes of antimalaria drugs and in-vitro evaluation of their activity. Inorg. Chim Acta. 135: 134-137.

Obaleye JA, Balogun EA, Adeyemi OG (1999). Synthesis and *in vitro* effect of some metal-drug complexes on malaria parasite. Biokemistri 9(1): 23-27.

Obaleye JA, Nde-aga JB, Balogun EA (1997). Some antimalaria drug metal complexes: Synthesis, characterization and their *in vivo* evaluation against malaria parasite. Afr. J. Sci. 1: 10-12.

Obaleye JA, Famurewa O (1989). Inhibitory effects of some inorganic boron triflouride complexes on some micro-organisms, Bios. Res. Comm. 1: 87-93.

Ogunniran KO, Ajanaku KO, James OO, Ajani OO, Nwinyi CO, Allansela (2008). Fe(iii) and Co(ii) complexes of mixed antibiotics: synthesis, characterization, antimicrobial potential and their effect on alkaline phosphatase activities of selected rat tissues. Int. J. Phy. Sci. 3(8): 177-182.

Ohnmacht CJ, Patel AR, Lutz RE (1971). Antimalarials, 7-bis. (Trifluoro methyl)-Cr-(2-piperidyl)-4-quinoline methanols. J. Med. Chem. 14: 926-928.

Reitman S, Frankel S (1957). A colorimetric method for the detection of serum glutamic oxaloacetic and glutamic pyruvic transaminases. Am. J. Chem. Path. 28:56-63.

WHO (1987). Drug Information 1(3). 127

Williams HD, Flemming I (1980). Spectroscopic Methods in Organic Chemistry, 4th ed. McGraw-Hill Book Ltd, London.

Wright PJ, Plummer DT, Leathwood PT (1972). Enzyme in rat urine Alkaline phosphatase. Enzymologia 42: 317-327.

Yakubu MT, Akanji MA, Oladiji AT (2005). Aphrodisiac potentials of aqueous extract of *Fadogia agrestis* (Schweinf. Ex Heirn) stem in male albino rats. Asia J. Androl. 7:399-404.

Determination of bioload of commercially available brands of fruit juice in Uyo, Nigeria

Clement Jackson[1]*, Emmanuel Ibezim[2], Agboke Akeem[1], Mfon Udofia[3] and Hilary Odo[2]

[1]Faculty of Pharmacy, University of Uyo, Akwa Ibom State, Nigeria.
[2]Faculty of Pharmaceutical Sciences, University of Nigeria, Nsukka, Enugu State, Nigeria.
[3]God's Glory Computers Institute, Uyo, Akwa Ibom Nigeria.

Six brands of fruit juice preparations made up of three different batches per brand were used for the study. The purpose of the experiment was to identify and characterize the microbial load (bioload) in these products using standard procedures. At the end of the study, none of the samples was found to contain any viable microorganism. These findings showed that the samples used in the study were of high quality standard, and therefore fit for human consumption. Foods with a pH lower than 4 are considered as high in acid and are generally regarded as not being susceptible to spoilage by a variety of microorganisms. At this low pH, acid – tolerant yeasts and mycelial fungi mostly cause spoilage, while bacterial spores will not germinate and grow under these acidic conditions. The acid or acidified foods with a pH below 4.6 are not subjected to heat – treatments at temperatures sufficient to destroy bacterial spores.

Key words: Bioload, fruit juice, viable, microorganism.

INTRODUCTION

Traditionally, fruit juices are considered susceptible to spoilage only by yeast, mycelial fungi and lactic acid bacteria (Chang and Kang, 2004). Foods with a pH lower than 4 are considered as high in acid and are generally regarded as not being susceptible to spoilage by a variety of microorganisms (Jay, 1998). The low pH is considered sufficient to prevent the growth of almost all bacteria spore – formers. Spores of *Clostridium botulinum* can not germinate or produce the lethal *botulinum* toxin in an environment with a pH below 4.6 (Chang and Kang, 2004).

The microorganisms present in fruit juice often originate from the natural flora of the raw materials used for the preparation and those introduced during the course of the processing (Splittstoesser et al., 1994). The number and types of organisms are determined by the properties of the food product and activity of the organisms in the product. In some cases, the micro-organisms have no discernable deleterious effects and the food is consumed without harm (Yeh et al., 2004). In other cases, however, the presence of microorganisms have manifested in form

of spoilage, food-borne illness and fermentation (Yeh et al., 2004). During the heat – treatment of foods, pathogens and most non – spore – forming micro – organisms are killed, but a heat process sufficient to destroy all the microbial spores will have a detrimental effect on the organoleptic quality of the product (Walls and Chuyata, 2000). The purpose of this study is to evaluate the purity of some brands of fruit juice in Uyo Nigeria. The presence of Registration Number from Regulatory Agencies may not necessarily give assurance of quality, as these can be faked.

MATERIALS AND METHODS

Brands of fruit juice used

The fruit Juices employed in this study were locally manufactured by companies in Nigeria and were purchased at Uyo market. A total of 6 brands were used in the study and each brand contains three samples of different batches (a, b and c). The various fruit juice preparations are shown on Table 1.

Microbial count

The experiment was carried out in three different phases. Each batch of the different brands of the fruit juice constituted a phase

*Corresponding author. E-mail: clementjackson1@yahoo.com.

Table 1. Various fruit juice preparations used.

Product code	Name of product	Manufacturer's address	Container type	Volume	NAFDAC reg. No	Batch No.
1a.	Apple extract drink (Chivita®)	9A, Block E Ind Estate, Badagry Express way, Amuwo Odofin Lagos Nigeria.	X	50 cl	01-4278	521032388
b.	"	"	"	"	"	732433210
c.	"	"	"	"	"	313489021
2a.	Yoghurt fruit drink	Chi Ltd, Chivita Avenue Ajao Estate Akpakun Oshodi Lagos	Y	250 ml	Nil	18;45;26
b.	"	"	"	"	"	"
c.	"	"	"	"	"	"
3a.	Orange fruit drink (Jucee ®)	3 Ladipo Oluwole Street, Ikeja, Lagos, Nig.	Y	1 L	Nil	09.06
b.	"	"	"	"	"	09.04
c.	"	"	"	"	"	09.01
4a.	Blackcurrant Fruitdrink (Ribena®)	Igbesa Rd, Agbara, Ogun State.	Y	200 ml	01-3699	01:39:02
b.	"	"	"	"	"	01:41:21
c.	"	"	"	"	"	02:04:31
5a.	Citrus drink (Tampico®)	Eleyele Ind. Layout, Ibadan, Nigeria.	Y	200 ml	01:3699	01:39:02
b.	"	"	"	"	"	01:32:11
c.	"	"	"	"	"	01:34:05
6a.	Greatson immense flavoured orange drink (Dansa®)	KM 10 Onitsha Expressing, Abeokuta	X	1 L	01-75163	001
b.	"	"	"	"	"	002
c.	"	"	"	"	"	003

X = plastic container, Y = paper pack, a, b and c = different batches.

made up of both positive and negative controls. For the positive control, a mixture of culture containing *Escherichia coli* and *Candida albicans* was inoculated on an over-dried agar plate and incubated in the same environment conditions as test. The negative control is made up of only the over-dried agar on which nothing was inoculated and was also placed at the same environmental conditions as the test.

For phase A, the experiment was carried out without further diluting of the fruit juice. This was to determine the presence or otherwise of viable microorganisms in the fruit juices at the concentration at which they were consumed. In phase B, the diluent used was sterile water while normal saline was used as the diluent in phase C. The use of both sterile water and normal saline are known to encourage growth of microorganisms in fruit juice under storage. The underside of an over-dried agar plate was divided into eight segments using a marker. 5 ml of the fruit juice was withdrawn from each sample in phase A and transferred to sterile test tubes. A sterile rubber teat was attached to a sterile pipette and used to suck up and down twice from the samples in the test tubes. The sample was finally collected and at a constant rate of one drop per second, one drop each was placed at the centre of each marked segment of the plates.

Bacterial numbers were estimated using the Pour Plate Technique. Using sterile distilled water, serial dilutions of (10-1-10-6) were prepared from each of the fruit juice samples and incubated at respective temperatures for 48 h. Total viable counts were determined on Plate Count Agar, *E. coli* on Macconkey medium, and *C.*

albicans on Sabouraud medium. Identification of microorganisms was done using the API 20E system (Analytical Profile Index, Biomerieux, Durham, NC, USA). The pH determinations were done using a pH meter (Orion Model 420A).

The plates were covered and kept until the drops permeated into the medium. The plate were labeled for the particular sample and incubated in an inverted position for 24 h at 37°C alongside of the positive and negative controls. For phase B, the diluent used was sterile water. A sterile pipette was used to aseptically transfer 1 ml of each sample in this group into sterile test tubes containing 9 ml of sterile water making a 10-fold serial dilution. The same procedure as in phase A was applied in the inoculation of the plates in phase B with samples and same environmental conditions were applied. For phase C, the diluent used was normal saline. A 10-fold serial dilution of the samples in this group was made using the normal saline. The same procedures as in A and B above were strictly followed also allying the positive and negative controls.

RESULTS

After a period of 24 h, no growth was seen on any of the test groups. There was also no growth on the negative control groups while there were some visible growths on positive groups which has plates containing the micro-organisms (*C. albicans* = 2.3×10^3, *E. coli* = 3.4×10^3 for

Apple drink, *C. albicans* = 2.1 × 103, *E. coli* = 3.5 × 103 for orange drink, *C. albicans* = 1.75 × 103, *E. coli* = 3.0 × 103 for black currant drink and *C. albicans* = 2.8 × 103, *E. coli* = 5.4 × 103 for yoghurt). The plates were left in the incubator for further 48 h. After the 72 h period, there were still no growths on any of the test groups as well as the negative controls.

Since there were no visible growths on any of the test samples, it therefore showed that, they do not contain any viable micro-organisms. They could contain dead microorganisms, however, but this did not show in form of growth. For the group in phase A which was undiluted and showed no visible growths, it implied that, either the preservative used did not allow the growth of the micro-organisms at that concentration or the manufacturers observed strict aseptic techniques to eliminate microbes at the time of production. The difference in packaging did not affect the quality of the six brands of fruit juice analyzed.

DISCUSSION

In spite of the potential benefits offered by fruit juices, concerns over their safety and quality have been raised. In the present investigation, there was visible growth only on the positive control. The results from positive control group showed that black currant has the least microbial count while yoghurt has the highest. Milk is an essential component; this might be responsible for the microbial count on positive control.

Overall, the preservatives used in the preparations could have put the microorganisms in their dormant stage which resulted in the lack of growth in the above two experiments. The effect of introduction of water and normal saline which has been shown to support the growth of micro-organisms was also checked. After 72 h of incubation, there were still no growths on the test samples. The result of this work has gone a long way in assuring the public of the safety of the six brands of the fruit juices produced and marketed in Nigeria.

In conclusion, it can be categorically stated that, within the limits of experimental error, the above brands of fruit beverages marketed in Uyo, Nigeria are pure and free from microbial contamination and, therefore, fit for human and animal consumptions.

REFERENCES

Chang S, Kang D (2004). *Alicyclobacillus* spp. in the fruit juice Industry: History, Characteristics and Current Isolation/Detection Procedures. Crit. Rev. Microbiol., 30: 55-74.

Jay JM (1998). Intrinsic and Extrinsic Parameters of Foods that affect Microbial Growth. In: Modern Food Microbiology, 5th ed. Chapman and Hah., New York, pp. 354-355.

Splittstoesser DF, Churey JJ, Lee CY (1994). Growth characteristics of aciduric spore-forming bacilli isolated from fruit juices. J. Food Prot., 57: 1080-1083.

Walls I, Chuyate R (2000). Isolation of *Alicyclobacillus acidoterrstris* from fruits juices. J. AOAC Int., 83: 1115-1120.

Yeh JY, Ellis H, Chen J (2004). Influence of calcium lactate on the fate of spoilage and pathogenic microorganisms in orange juice. J. Food Prot., 67: 1429-1433.

6

Evaluation of okro gum as a binder in the formulation of thiamine hydrochloride granules and tablets

G. C. Onunkwo

Department of Pharmaceutical Technology and Industrial Pharmacy, Faculty of Pharmaceutical Sciences, University of Nigeria, Nsukka, Nigeria. E-mail: ogo4justice@yahoo.com.

The aim of this study is to examine the suitability of okro gum as a binder for pharmaceutical tablet formulations. A comparative evaluation of *Abelmoschus esculentus* (okro) gum as a binder in the formulation of thiamine hydrochloride granules and tablets was performed. Gelatin, acacia and polyvinylpyrrolidone (PVP), were employed as standard binders for comparison. The properties of granules and tablets evaluated were; flow rate, angle of repose, density, weight uniformity, hardness, friability, disintegration time and dissolution rate. The granules had good flow properties. However, binder concentration influenced flow characteristics. Okro gum gave the highest hardness/friability ratios. It also prolonged disintegration time and dissolution time and dissolution rate. Hence, okro gum may not be useful as a binder in conventional tablet formulation. Nevertheless it could be a good candidate for evaluation as a binder or hydrophilic polymer in sustained release tablet formulation.

Key words: *Abelmoschus esculentus* gum, binder, granules, tablets.

INTRODUCTION

Research on many flowering plants growing in Nigeria as sources of pharmaceutical recipients have yielded interesting results. Recently, a polysaccharide gum from *Abelmoschus esculentus* popularly known as okro was shown to have favourable suspending and emulsifying properties (Brown, 1991). The plant belongs to the plant family Malvaceae. Okro fruits are edible. The generic name Abelmoschus is suggestive of the musky odour of the seed. The fruits are larger than those of the two other related species; *A. cannabis* and *A. sabdarifta*. It is both a tropical and temperate crop but grows more extensively in the tropics. It is an annual crop native to Africa, probably Ethiopia, but is now cultivated widely in other parts of the world like India and United States of America (Martin and Robert, 1965). The fruits are normally sliced into small bits or ground. Water is usually added to facilitate the production of mucilage. Okro gum produces high viscosity mucilage even at low concentrations. Nasipuri et al. (1996) have determined the molecular weight of okro gum mucilage by gel filtration chromatography and light scattering methods and obtained a value of about 150,000. The charge on the gum mucilage was also determined by paper electrophoretic method. The particles were found to be negatively charged. The results obtained from the surface and interfacial tension studies show that okro mucilage has little surface activity (Nasipuri et al., 1996).

The present investigation was aimed at comparing the effectiveness of this edible gum as a binder in tablet formulations. Thiamine hydrochloride was used as a soluble drug that can be easily assayed.

MATERIALS AND METHODS

Materials

The following materials were used as supplied by their manufacturers: maize starch, stearic acid, lactose (May and Bakers, England); acacia, gelatin, microcrystalline cellulose, polyvinylpyrrolidone (Merck, W. Germany); ethanol (95%), thiamine hydrochloride and acetone (BDH, England).

Methods

Processing of okro-gum: A one kg quantity of unripe and tender fruits of okro gum was used. The fruits were washed, sliced and ground by means of a blender. The crushed mass was soaked in distilled water to hydrate with occasional stirring six hours. A white muslin cloth was used to express the viscous solution to produce the gum extract. Acetone was used to precipitate the extract at a ratio of 3 parts of acetone to 1 part of extract. Filtration of the precipitated gum was performed using a vacuum pump, attached to a Buckner funnel with filter paper (Whatman, 12.5 mm). Finally, the gum was dried in a desiccator containing anhydrous calcium chloride. Size reduction and screening of the dried gum was carried out using an end runner mill (Manesty, England), and a 250 µm stainless steel sieve. Airtight powder bottles were used to store the undersized fraction (less than 250 µm).

Production of thiamine hydrochloride granules

The granules were produced using the moist granulation method. Four binders, gelatin, acacia, polyvinylpyrrolidone (PVP) and okro gum were used at five concentrations (1 - 5% w/w). Microcrystalline cellulose (5% w/w) was employed as the disintegrant. Lactose, microcrystalline cellulose and the drug were mixed intimately in a mortar for 10 min and binder solution added to obtain a damp mass. The moist mass was forced through a 1.7 mm sieve and the granules dried at 40°C in a hot air oven (Gallenkamp) for one hour. The dried granules were further forced through a 1.0 mm stainless steel sieve stored in clean air-tight powder bottles and evaluated for flow properties.

Compression of granules

The fines of the granules were first mixed with 3% w/w stearic acid and then the coarse fraction for 5 min. The tablets were compressed in a tabletting machine (Model F_3, Manesty) fitted with 9.5 mm concave faced punches at a tablet target weight of 300 mg.

Evaluation of granule properties

Flow rate determination: The funnel method of Carstensen and Chan, (1977) was employed. A funnel of specified dimensions having orifice and base diameters of 0.8 cm and 9.0 cm respectively was used and securely clamped to a retort stand. A 50 g sample was introduced into the funnel and the powder allowed to fall freely under gravity. The flow rate was calculated from the following expression.

$$\text{Flow Rate} = \frac{\text{Amount of powder}}{\text{Time of flow}} \quad (1)$$

Each experiment was conducted five times. The mean value and coefficient of variation was determined.

Angle of repose

A funnel of 0.8 and 8 cm in orifice and surface diameters respectively, was used, adopting the method of fixed funnel and free standing cone (Parrot, 1966). A 50 g sample was allowed to flow through the funnel to form a cone. A cathetometer (Eberbatch, England) was used to determine the height of the heap (h). The base of the cone was traced out using a pencil and its radius (r) determined. The angle of repose was determined from the following relationship:

$$\text{Tan } e = \frac{h}{r} \quad (2)$$

Each experiment was conducted five times. The mean value and coefficient of variation were determined.

Bulk and tapped densities

The bulk volume (V_B) was determined by recording the volume occupied by a 50 g sample introduced in a 100 ml measuring cylinder. The bulk density (P_B) was calculated from the equation:

$$P_B = \frac{w}{V_B} \text{ g/ml} \quad (3)$$

The tapped volume was determined by tapping the cylinder from a fixed height on a soft base, until there was no further reduction in volume (V_t). The tapped density (P_t) was calculated from the equation:

$$P_t = \frac{W}{V_t} \quad (4)$$

Tablet evaluation

Uniformity of weight determination

Twenty tablets were randomly selected from each batch and then weighed individually and collectively using an electronic weighing balance (Mettlers). The mean weight and standard deviation were determined.

Hardness test

The hardness of 10 tablets selected randomly from each of the batches after equilibrating at room temperature for 24 h was determined in an automatic hardness tester (Erweka, Model TBH - 28). The mean hardness was calculated.

Friability

The weight of 20 tablets selected from each batch at random was determined collectively as initial weight, W_A. The tablets were placed in a friabilator (Erweka Apparatabeau); set to rotate at 25 rpm for 4 min. At the end of the run, the tablets were de-dusted and weighed (W_B). Friability was calculated from the equation.

$$F = \frac{(W_A - W_B) \times 100}{W_A} \quad (5)$$

The test was repeated five times and the mean value determined.

Disintegration time determination

Erweka disintegration test apparatus (Model DT4) was used based on the British Pharmacopoeia, 2003 method. The disintegration medium was 0.1 N HCl, maintained at $37 \pm 0.5°C$. Five tablets from each batch were used for the test. The disintegration time was taken as the mean time needed for the tablets to break into particles small enough to pass through the screen into the disintegration medium.

Table 1. Physical properties of thiamine hydrochloride granulations.

Binder conc. (% w/w)	Bulk density	Tapped density	Angle of repose	Flow rate
Acacia				
1	0.4015	0.4625	37.75	3.32
2	0.3951	0.4580	37.60	3.36
3	0.3902	0.4515	37.42	3.40
4	0.3866	0.4478	37.45	3.43
5	0.3802	0.4395	36.65	3.41
Gelatin				
1	0.3825	0.4550	37.45	3.34
2	0.3770	0.4460	37.16	3.37
3	0.3722	0.4385	36.79	3.44
4	0.3689	0.4310	36.21	3.46
5	0.3656	0.4270	35.90	3.44
PVP				
1	0.4225	0.4821	38.75	3.26
2	0.4186	0.4775	38.40	3.30
3	0.4107	0.4710	37.90	3.38
4	0.4075	0.4660	37.55	3.55
5	0.4020	0.4605	37.06	3.52
Okro gum				
1	0.3750	0.4325	36.50	3.40
2	0.3702	0.4250	36.15	3.45
3	0.3675	0.4202	35.76	3.50
4	0.3608	0.4155	35.32	3.55
5	0.3555	0.4095	34.82	3.52

Dissolution rate determination

Erweka dissolution apparatus was used, employing the British Pharmacopoeia 2003 method. One tablet was placed in the apparatus and rotated at 100 rpm. The dissolution medium was 1000 ml 0.1 N HCL, maintained at $37 \pm 0.5\,°C$. Five milliliter portions of the dissolution medium were withdrawn using a pipette fitted with a non-adsorbent cotton wool at predetermined time intervals. Each 5 ml sample withdrawn was replaced by an equivalent fresh dissolution medium, maintained at $37 \pm 0.5\,°C$. The solution was analyzed after colour development using a Sp6-450 UV/VIS spectrophotometer at 430 nm.

RESULTS AND DISCUSSION

Granule properties

The flowability of thiamine hydrochloride granules was expressed as flow rate, angle of repose and density as shown in Table 1.

Flow rate

Flow rate increased with increase in binder concentration and then decreased after an optimum value. Granules formulated with okro gum had the highest flow rate at 1 - 2%w/w binder concentrations. The large average granule size formed at high binder concentration of the binder

may have affected the flow rate. Large granule size has been shown to obstruct flow through funnel orifice especially when the granule size approaches the size of the orifice diameter. The relationship between flow rate and orifice diameter has been reported by Danish and Parrot, 1977.

Angle of repose

Angle of repose decreased as binder content of the granules increased. This may be attributed to the reduced cohesive forces of the larger granules formed at higher binder concentration (Shotton and Ganderton, 1961). Granulations produced with okro gum demonstrated the highest reduction in angle of repose and the angle of repose values for all the granulations were below 42°. This suggests good flow properties (Shah and Mlodezeniex, 1977). Angle of repose is a measure of powder resistance to flow under gravity due to frictional forces resulting from the surface properties of the granules.

Tablet properties

Weight Uniformity: There was no significant variation in

Table 2. Content and weight uniformity of thiamine hydrochloride tablets formulated with different binders.

Binder conc. (% w/w) Acacia	Content uniformity drug content (mg)	Weight uniformity (mg)
1	25.50	306.0 (1.69)*
2	24.75	305.9 (1.55)
3	24.50	307.9 (2.80)
4	25.00	302.7 (1.98)
5	25.00	300.10 (1.70)
Gelatin		
1	25.25	304.80 (1.25)
2	24.75	295.70 91.57)
3	25.00	300.60 (12.70)
4	24.25	303.60 (1.87)
5	25.00	308.20 (1.32)
PVP		
1	26.00	301.25 (1.62)
2	25.00	303.05 (2.11)
3	24.50	298.05 (2.04)
4	24.75	300.45 (1.82)
5	24.75	306.75 92.15)
Okro gum		
1	25.25	301.75 (2.43)
2	25.00	300.35 (1.63)
3	25.25	303.33 (2.01)
4	24.25	303.10 (2.01)
5	24.75	301.60 91.67)

*Values in bracket represent standard deviations.

the mean weights of thiamine hydrochloride tablets since all showed low coefficient of variations of below 2% (Table 2). A good tablet weight uniformity is an indication of a good uniformity of tablet contents.

Hardness and friability

The effect of binder concentration on tablet hardness and friability are shown in Table 3. An increase in binder concentration increased the hardness of the tablets. On the other hand, friability decreased as binder concentration increased. An increase in binder concentration will enhance the formation of stronger interparticulate bonds between the granules during compression in a tabletting machine (Esezobo and Pilpel, 1976). This means that the tablets would offer greater resistance to shock and abrasion since there is a stronger adhesive bonding of the granules at high binder concentrations. In general, the tablets showed good friability profiles, since most had friability values of less than 1.0% (Harwood and Pilpel, 1968). Moreover, the tablets made from okro gum had high hardness/friability ratios, since the tablets recorded

the highest hardness and least friability values.

Disintegration time

The effect of binder concentration on tablet disintegration time is shown in Table 4. The tablets formulated with okro gum failed the British Pharmacopoeia 2003 disintegration time test. However, tablets containing polyvinylprrolidone (PVP), acacia, and gelatin as binders disintegrated in less than 15 min. The binders follow this order of increasing tablet disintegration time: PVP < acacia < gelatin < Okro gum.

Dissolution profile

The dissolution data of the tablets are presented in Table 5. Tablets made with PVP gave the highest drug release while okro gum had the lowest. As the binder concentration increased, there was a general decrease in the release rate of thiamine hydrochloride from the tablets Okro gum displayed a very remarkable delay in the

Table 3. Hardness and friability values of thiamine hydrochloride tablets formulated with different binders.

Binder Conc. (% w/w) Acacia	Hardness (N)	Friability (%)	Hardness / Friability Ratio
1	2.73 (2.27)*	0.95	2.87
2	2.54 91.69)	0.91	3.89
3	4.83 (1.26)	0.87	5.55
4	6.15 (0.85)	0.81	7.59
5	7.17 (0.45)	0.76	9.43
Gelatin			
1	3.33 (1.59)	0.92	3.62
2	3.90 (1.23)	0.89	4.38
3	5.04 (1.39)	0.85	5.93
4	6.65 (1.07)	0.80	8.31
5	7.55 (0.78)	0.74	10.20
PVP			
1	2.51 (1.59	1.02	2.46
2	3.12 (0.99)	0.98	3.18
3	3.95 (1.04)	0.90	4.39
4	4.81 (0.91)	0.85	5.66
5	5.51 (0.47)	0.82	6.72
Okro gum			
1	4.20 (0.93)	0.86	4.88
2	6.28 (1.00)	0.81	7.75
3	8.46 (0.79)	0.78	10.85
4	10.23 (1.86)	0.73	14.01
5	11.55 (0.95)	0.65	17.77

Table 4. Disintegration time of the thiamine hydrochloride tablets formulated with different binders.

Binder conc. (% w/w) Acacia	Disintegration time (min)
1	5.96 (0.36)*
2	7.12 (0.26)
3	10.36 (0.54)
4	12.46 (0.34)
5	14.24 (0.25)
Gelatin	
1	6.44 (0.29)
2	7.76 (0.30)
3	11.10 (0.26)
4	13.14 (0.59)
5	15.24 (0.63
PVP	
1	4.70 (0.29)
2	6.40 (0.60)
3	8.16 (0.38)
4	10.10 (0.31)
5	11.94 (0.33)

Table 4. Contd.

Okro gum	
1	21.60 (1.14)
2	31.20 (1.30)
3	51.20 (1.64)
4	76.60 (1.82)
5	111.80 (2.05)

* Values in brackets represent standard deviations.

Table 5. Dissolution rate data (per cent of drug released) of thiamine hydrochloride tablets formulated with different binders.

Binder Conc. (% w/w)	Dissolution Time (min)					
Acacia	5	10	15	20	25	30
1	47.06	58.82	75.49	85.29	98.04	101.96
2	40.40	50.51	65.66	11.78	84.85	94.95
3	38.78	44.90	57.14	69.39	78.57	88.76
4	32.00	38.00	50.00	60.00	70.00	78.00
5	28.00	34.00	44.60	56.00	66.00	72.00
Gelatin						
1	39.60	47.52	55.45	69.31	93.07	100.99
2	36.37	44.45	70.71	65.65	78.79	92.93
3	32.00	40.00	46.00	50.00	62.00	74.00
4	24.74	37.11	41.24	47.42	57.73	72.16
5	18.00	28.00	36.00	42.0	48.00	60.00
PVP						
1	42.31	57.69	76.92	98.08	101.92	105.77
2	40.00	54.00	70.00	92.00	100.00	100.00
3	36.73	51.02	65.31	83.67	95.92	97.96
4	30.30	46.46	56.57	74.75	84.85	90.91
5	26.26	40.40	52.53	68.69	76.77	84.85
Okro gum						
1	27.72	33.60	41.58	45.54	51.49	55.45
2	24.00	30.00	38.00	42.00	46.00	56.00
3	19.80	25.74	33.66	39.60	43.46	45.54
4	16.49	22.68	28.87	39.18	41.24	43.40
5	10.10	16.16	24.24	32.32	34.34	36.37

release rate at higher binder concentrations since none of the tablet batches formulated with okro gum released up to 75% of drug in 30 min (Esezobo and Pilpel, 1976).

Conclusion

A. esculentus gum could not be suitably employed in conventional tablet formulation as a binder since it prolongs tablet disintegration time and also remarkably delays drug dissolution rate. Perhaps it may be a good candidate for evaluation as a binder or hydrophilic polymer in sustained release tablet formulation.

REFERENCES

Brown SK (1991). PhD Thesis, University of Lagos. Application of okro gum in the formulation of pharmaceutical dosage forms. pp.1-30.

Martin FN, Robert N (1965). Chemistry of plant gums and mucilages. Reinhold Publishing Co-operation. New York Chapman and Hall, London. pp. 350 – 355.

Nasipuri RN, Igwilo CF, Brown SA, Kunle OO (1996). Mucilage from Abelmoschus esculentus (okro) fruits; a potential pharmaceutical raw material. Part 1. Physicochemical properties, J. Pharm. Res. Dev. 1: 22-28.

Carstensen JJ, Chan PC (1977). Flow rates and repose angles of wet processed granulations. J. Pharm. Sci. 60: 1235 – 1239.

Parrot EC (1966). Measurement of repose angle by a fixed funnel and free standing cone method. Amer. J. Pharm. Edu. 30: 205 – 209.

British Pharmacopoeia (2003). Her Majesty's Stationery Office, London.

Danish FO, Parrot EL (1977). Flow rates of solid particulate pharmaceuticals. J. Pharm. Sci. 60: 549-554.

Shotton WA, Ganderton D (1961). Coating of simple crystalline materials with stearic acid. J. Pharm. Pharmacol. 12: (1961) 87T-92T.

Shah AC, Mlodezeniex AB (1977). Mechanism of surface lubrication. Excipient mixing and processing characteristics of powders and properties of compressed tablets. J. Pharm. Sci. 66: 1377 – 1382.

Esezobo S, Pilpel N (1976). Some formulation factors affecting tensile strength, disintegration and dissolution of uncoated oxytetracycline tablets. J. Pharm. Pharmacol. 28: 6 – 15.

Harwood CF, Pilpel N (1968). Granulation of griseofulvin. J. Pharm. Sci. 57: 478-481.

Formulation and evaluation of paracetamol tablets manufactured using the dried fruit of *Phoenix dactylifera* Linn as an excipient

N. C. Ngwuluka*, B. A. Idiakhoa, E. I. Nep, I. Ogaji and I. S. Okafor

Department of Pharmaceutics and Pharmaceutical Technology, Faculty of Pharmaceutical Sciences, University of Jos, P. M. B. 2084, Jos, Nigeria.

Dried and milled date palm fruit was evaluated for its binding properties in comparison with acacia and tragacanth. Characterization of the granules in addition to quality control tests that included uniformity of weight, hardness, friability, disintegration and dissolution were undertaken. The granules manufactured using the binders had good flow properties and compressibility. As the concentration of the binders increased, the binding ability improved producing tablets with good uniformity of weight and hardness. The tablets manufactured using dried date palm was found to be less friable than tablets manufactured using acacia and tragacanth. Although, the tablets did not disintegrate, the drug release from the tablets passed the USP and BP specification for dissolution of paracetamol. Therefore, dried date palm fruit may be explored as a pharmaceutical excipient.

Key words: Date palm, quality control tests, disintegration, dissolution, weight variation, paracetamol.

INTRODUCTION

Natural polysaccharides are widely used in the pharmaceutical and food industry as excipients and additives due to their low toxicity, biodegradable, availability and low cost. Excipients are essential ingredients of a dosage form which are added to increase volume, aid flow, enable compactness and make a drug convenient to administer. They can also be used to modify the release of drug, thereby, influencing the absorption and subsequent bioavailability of the incorporated drug. Furthermore, they act as vehicles which transport the incorporated drug to the site of absorption and are expected to guarantee the stability of the incorporated drug, the precision and accuracy of the dosage, and also improve on the organoleptic properties of the drugs where necessary in order to enhance patient adherence (Pifferi et al., 1999). They should optimize the performances of dosage forms during manufacturing as well as when patients ingest them (Pifferi and Restani,

2003).

Date fruit is an edible fruit composed of amino acids and proteins, carbohydrates, fatty acids, salts and minerals, and dietary fibre (Al-shahib and Marshall, 2003). Carbohydrates make up to 44 - 88% of the fruit which include mainly reducing sugars such as fructose, sucrose, mannose, glucose and maltose in addition to small amounts of polysaccharides such as pectin (0.5 - 3.9%), starch and cellulose (Al-shahib and Marshall, 2003). The protein content is approximately 2.3 - 5.6% with 23 amino acids which include alanine, aspartic acid, serine, glutamic acid, threonine, proline and glycine. There are 15 types of fatty acids such as arachidic, palmitic, stearic, myristic, capric, lauric and behenic acids, which make up about 0.2 - 0.5% of the fruit. However, eight of the fatty acids are found in the fleshy part of the fruit. The mineral content includes iron, cobalt, calcium, potassium, fluorine, copper, magnesium, phosphorus, sodium and zinc. Some varieties of date palm can produce as much as 400 - 600kg fresh fruits per annum for a span of 60 years and these fruits are available 8 months of the year (Al-shahib and Marshall, 2003). The moisture content decreases as they ripen

---

*Corresponding author. E-mail: ngwuluka@unijos.edu.ng.

Table 1. Compositions of paracetamol tablets at different concentrations of the binder.

Ingredients	Batch I (%) 2% binder	Batch II (%) 5% binder	Batch III (%) 10% binder	Batch IV (%) 20% binder
Paracetamol	71.4	71.4	71.4	71.4
Lactose	19.6	16.6	11.6	1.6
Binder	2.0	5.0	10.0	20.0
Corn starch	5.0	5.0	5.0	5.0
Talc	1.0	1.0	1.0	1.0
Magnesium stearate	1.0	1.0	1.0	1.0

from 83.6% to as low as 12.7% in dried state. Date palm fruit has been studied for its antioxidative and antimutagenic activities (Vayalil, 2002). However, little is known of its use as a pharmaceutical excipient.

This study was undertaken to explore the ability of dried date palm fruit to act as a binder in tablet manufacturing. To evaluate the binding properties of date palm, characterization of granules and tablets and *in vitro* drug release studies were undertaken.

MATERIALS AND METHODS

Materials

Paracetamol BP (Zhengzhou United Asia Trading Co.,Ltd, Zhengzhou, Henan, China), corn starch (G Koepcek E and Co GMBH, Sachsenfeld, Hamburg, Germany), lactose (Milkaut, Rivadavia, Franck - Pcia. de Santa Fe), talc (Hopkins and Williams, Chadwell Health Essex, England), Magnesium stearate (Gurr Chemicals, Bell Sons and Co, Southport, England), acacia (BDH Chemical Ltd, Poole, England) and tragacanth (Steculia Gum Halewood Chemicals Ltd, Stanwell Moor, Staines, Middlesex, England). Hydrochloric acid was of analytical grade.

Preparation of dried powdered date palm

Date palm fruits were bought from a local market in Jos, Nigeria. The fruits are usually sold partially dried. The seeds were extracted from the fruit and discarded while the fleshy fruits were further dried over 24 h and milled to powder for use as a binder.

Manufacture of tablets employing wet granulation method

Wet granulation method of tablet manufacturing was employed with milled date palm as a binding agent and water as the granulating liquid. Batches of paracetamol tablets were formulated using 2, 5, 10 and 20%$^{w}/_{w}$ of date palm powder. Paracetamol, lactose, date palm mucilage and corn starch were blended to form a damp coherent mass which was screened through a sieve No 10 and dried at 60°C for one hour. Corn starch was divided into two and incorporated during wet blending and after drying of granules to act as an intragranular and extragranular disintegrant. For comparative purposes, acacia and tragacanth gums were also used as binders at the same concentrations as date palm. The compositions of the batches are shown in Table 1.

Evaluation of granules

Particle size distribution of the granules

Particle size distribution of the granules was determined by mesh analysis employing a stack of sieves after granules had been weighed (34 g) and the granules were shaken for 10 min. The quantities of granules on each sieve were obtained gravimetrically.

Evaluation of bulk and tapped densities of the granules

The volume of a known quantity of the granules from each batch was obtained before and after tapping. The volume before tapping was used to determine the bulk density while the volume after tapping was employed to determine the tap density mathematically. Furthermore, Hausner's quotient and Carr's compressibility index used to determine the flow and compressibility properties of granules were obtained from the equations:

$$\text{Hausner's quotient} = \frac{\text{Tapped density}}{\text{Bulk}} \qquad 1$$

$$\text{Carr's compressibility} = \frac{\text{Tapped density} - \text{Bulk density}}{\text{Tapped density}} \times 100 \qquad 2$$

Assessment of rate of flow and angle of repose

A simple method whereby weighed quantity of granules from each batch was allowed to flow through an orifice (funnel) at a fixed height was used to determine flow rate. The time taken for the weighed granules to flow out completely from the orifice was recorded. This was performed in triplicate. Flow rate was obtained by the equation below:

$$\text{Flow rate} = \frac{\text{Weight of granules}}{\text{Time (sec)}} \qquad 3$$

Furthermore, the angle of repose was determined by calculating tan θ from the height and radius of the cone formed by the granules as they flowed out of the orifice and subsequently obtaining the inverse of tan θ.

Compression of granules

The granules were blended with the disintegrant (corn starch), glidant (talc) and lubricant (magnesium stearate). The blend was compressed using a single punch tableting machine (Manesty Type F3, Liver Poole, England) with a punch diameter of 0.75 cm set at 933 Pa (N/m^2) compression pressure. The die volume was to correspond to the weight of the tablet to ensure that 500 mg paracetamol is obtained.

Evaluation of the batches of tablets

Compendial and non-compendial tests were undertaken to assess the quality and performance of the batches with different binders in comparison with one another. These tests include uniformity of weight and diameter, hardness, friability, disintegration time and dissolution.

Uniformity of weight and diameter of tablets

Twenty tablets were randomly selected from each batch and assessed gravimetrically on an individual tablet basis. The mean weight as well as standard deviation were calculated. The diameters of the tablets were determined by employing a micrometer screw gauge (Sterling Manufacturing Company, India).

Mechanical strength of tablets

Although, the crushing strength test is non-compendial, it is undertaken to determine the ability of the tablets to withstand pressure during handling, packaging and transportation. A monsanto tablet hardness tester (Copley Scientific Ltd, Nottingham, United Kingdom) was employed to determine the mechanical strength of the tablets. The average force required to crush the tablets from each batch was obtained.

Friability testing of tablets

To evaluate the degree of friability of the tablets from each batch, ten tablets were randomly selected, dusted and weighed. The tablets were placed in a Roche friabilator (Erweka Gmbh, Germany) and subjected to its tumbling actions at 25 revolutions per minute for four minutes. Afterwards, the tablets were once again dusted and reweighed to determine the percentage loss of weight.

Disintegration studies on the tablets

Six tablets from each batch were utilized for disintegration studies in distilled water at 37°C using an Educational Sciences Disintegration Apparatus (Es Eagle Scientific Limited, Nottingham, United Kingdom). The disintegration time was taken to be the time no granule of any tablet was left on the mesh of the apparatus.

In vitro drug release studies

In vitro drug release studies were undertaken using USP apparatus I (basket method). The dissolution medium was 1000 mL of 0.1 N HCl at 37°C for 30 min to depict the gastric medium where the tablets will disintegrate. In all experiments, 5 mL of sample was withdrawn at 5 min interval and replaced with fresh medium to maintain sink condition. Samples were filtered and assayed spectrophotometrically at 230 nm.

Data analysis

Simple statistical analysis was utilized for content uniformity of weight, uniformity of diameter and uniformity of thickness while dissolution efficiency (DE) was used for the in vitro dissolution studies.

RESULTS AND DISCUSSION

The powder obtained from milling dried fruit of phoenix Dactylifera was brown in colour. On hydration, rapid swelling was observed which generated viscous mucilage that was utilized as a binder for wet granulation method. Granulation is employed in pharmaceutical manufacturing due to the poor flow and compaction of powders (Krycer et al., 1983). Wet granulation is a pharmaceutical process of tabletting which provides better uniformity of content especially for low drug concentrations, controls product bulk density as well as compaction of even high drug contents (Faure et el., 2001). Furthermore, it improves flow and handling, appearance, mixture's resistance to segregation and reduces variation in tablet dissolution (Kristensen and Schaefer, 1987; Westerhuis and Coenegracht, 1997; McConville et al., 2004). The type of binder used in granulating influences the properties of the granules as well as the quality of the tablets produced (Becker et al., 1997). Wet granulation is basically the addition of a binder solution or a solvent to a powder mixture; sieving to generate granules and subsequent granule drying.

Evaluation of granules

Particle size distribution of granules is evaluated due to the impact of granule size on flowability, uniformity of weight and content, compression, dissolution and subsequently, drug release (Yalkowsky and Bolton, 1990; Fichtner et el., 2005; Rohrs et al., 2006; Virtanen et al., 2010). Particle size and particle size distribution affects the compatibility and rearrangement of particles (Virtanen et al., 2010). Though, there are exceptions, the flow properties of granules are improved when the particles are large and the particle size distribution is narrow. However, larger particles lead to less strong tablets due to the fact that they have lesser surface areas for bond formation as compared to smaller particles (Sun and Himmelspach, 2006). Hence, an optimal particle size and size distribution will be required to obtain good flow properties, compaction and hardness.

The particle sizes of the paracetamol granules increased as the concentration of the binders increased as shown in Figure 1. This applied for both date palm and tragacanth; however for acacia, particle size increased as concentration increased to 10% and then a decrease in particle size was observed at 20% concentration of acacia. It may be an indication that the binding mechanism of acacia changes above 10% (Becker et al., 1997). There were much less fine particles which implied that the granules may have good flow properties. However, less fine particles may indicate that there would be more unfilled voids during the process of compression

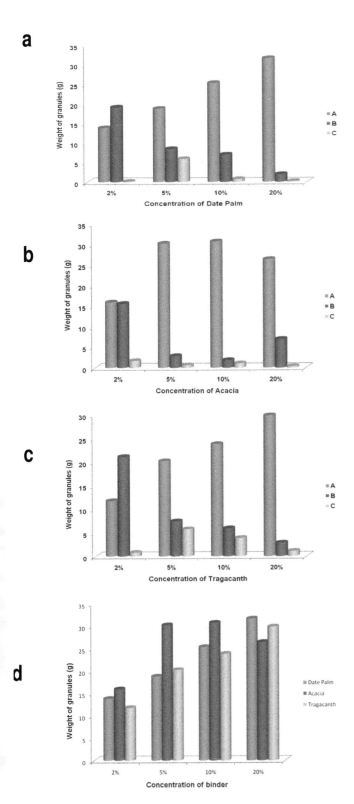

Figure 1. (a) Particle size distribution of granules employing date palm as a binder at different concentrations. NB: A, B, C depicts the weights of the granules on each sieve: A is for sieve with mesh number 60; B – mesh number 80 and C is 100. (b) Particle size distribution of granules employing acacia as a binder at different concentrations. (c) Particle size distribution of granules employing tragacanth as a binder at different concentrations. (d) comparative particel size distribution of the date palm, acacia and tragacanth at mesh number 60.

which may lead to less hard and friable tablets. Granules prepared with date palm as a binder compared more measurably with those prepared with acacia and more specifically with tragacanth.

Other parameters for assessing the properties of granules which include flow rate, angle of repose, bulk and tapped densities, Hausner quotient and Carr's compressibility are shown in Table 2. Compressibility of granules is determined so as to assess the ability of the granules to compact and decrease in volume when pressure is applied. This is needed to ensure that the suitability of the granules for tabletting in order to produce strong tablets which can withstand pressure. Compressibility index is also an indicative of the flow properties of granules while Hausner quotient relates to the cohesiveness of the granules (Mohammadi and Harnby, 1997). When the percentage compressibility is below 15% the granules have excellent flow properties while cohesive granules have percentage compressibility above 25% indicating poor flow properties (Endale et al., 2008; Bacher et al., 2008). Granules with Hausner ratio below 1.25 have good flow properties (Panda et al., 2008) and granules with angle of repose below 40° Cbut preferably below 30° Cexhibit good flow (Reddy et al., 2003) while granules with 50° would flow with difficulty (Reus-Medina et al., 2004).

Therefore, granules prepared by using different binders - date palm, acacia and tragacanth - exhibited good flow properties and satisfactory compressibility. Carr's compressibility and Hausner ratio were below 15% and 1.25, respectively, for the different concentrations of the binders while angle of repose was below 40°C for the different binder concentrations except 2% tragacanth. The flow properties of granules are determined due to its effect on the uniformity of weight of tablets. Hence, it is envisaged date palm as a binder would exhibit less variation in the uniformity of weight of tablets.

Evaluation of tablets

A summary of the properties of the tablets formulated for the batches employing the different binders are shown in Table 3 (Ferrari et al., 1996). Uniformity of weight, thickness and diameter are indication of the amount of active pharmaceutical ingredient (API) in the tablets, however, it is not a guarantee that the API is uniform in all tablets especially in formulations with low dose concentrations.

Furthermore, should weights, thickness or diameter of tablets in a batch vary, there will be variations in disintegration and dissolution. The compendial specifi- cation for uniformity of weight states that for tablets weighing more than 324 mg, weights of not more than two tablets should deviate from the average weight by more than 5% (USP, 1995). The tablets from the different batches which had different binders and at different

Table 2. Characterization of the granules prepared by the different binders.

	Date palm powder				Acacia gum				Tragacanth gum			
	2%	5%	10%	20%	2%	5%	10%	20%	2%	5%	10%	20%
Angle of repose (°)	29.74	28.02	26.66	29.62	32.25	31.56	31.27	31.51	42.73	28.90	26.72	28.99
Flow rate (g/sec)	5.90	5.63	5.86	5.37	6.99	5.01	5.67	5.05	0.86	7.05	5.84	5.52
Bulk density (g/mL)	1.06	0.69	0.51	0.49	0.85	0.43	0.48	0.62	1.26	0.59	0.51	0.44
Tapped density (g/mL)	1.15	0.74	0.55	0.52	0.94	0.45	0.51	0.67	1.33	0.65	0.54	0.47
Hausner quotient	0.92	0.94	0.92	0.94	0.90	0.94	0.94	0.93	0.94	0.91	0.94	1.07
Carr's compressibility (%)	8.47	6.52	8.94	6.06	11.11	6.00	5.97	7.84	5.88	9.52	6.35	6.85

Table 3. Compendial and non-compendial tests for tablets prepared by the different binders.

	Date palm powder				Acacia gum				Tragacanth gum			
	2%	5%	10%	20%	2%	5%	10%	20%	2%	5%	10%	20%
Uniformity of weight (g)	0.703	0.693	0.694	0.700	0.699	0.697	0.693	0.699	0.690	0.692	0.673	0.697
Std. dev.	0.008	0.014	0.015	0.007	0.007	0.004	0.010	0.006	0.010	0.019	0.024	0.024
Uniformity of diameter (mm)	0.954	0.956	0.965	0.985	0.964	0.966	0.967	0.965	0.967	0.966	0.965	0.966
Std. dev.	0.002	0.002	0.002	0.003	0.005	0.004	0.003	0.002	0.007	0.006	0.007	0.006
Uniformity of thickness (mm)	0.28	0.28	0.29	0.29	0.29	0.23	0.21	0.26	0.27	0.20	0.21	0.22
Std. dev.	0.003	0.002	0.002	0.002	0.004	0.004	0.003	0.003	0.005	0.006	0.007	0.006
Hardness (kg)	6.00	8.50	8.50	> 14	> 3.50	4.00	8.50	8.50	1.00	4.50	6.25	> 14
Friability (%)	24.89	11.34	7.22	0.93	23.18	12.44	18.52	26.65	-	9.89	11.15	24.89
Disintegration (min)	> 30	> 30	> 30	> 30	23	27	> 30	> 30	5	7	11	14

concentrations met the compendial specification.

Crushing strength test shows the ability of tablets to withstand pressure or stress during handling, packaging and transportation. It is the property of a tablet that is measured to assess its resistance to permanent deformation. Furthermore, the mechanical strength of a tablet determines the disintegration time and the rate of dissolution. As the concentration of the binder increases, the mechanical strength increases. This was obtainable for date palm and tragacanth while there was no further increase in mechanical strength when 20% acacia was used. For the mechanical strength of a tablet to be satisfactory, the minimum requirement is 4 kg (Allen et al., 2004). As shown in Table 3, 2% acacia and tragacanth did not comply with the specification. All the concentrations of date palm met the specifications implying that date palm produced tablets with good mechanical strength.

Friability is another mechanical property of a tablet with compendial (USP, 1995) specification not more than 1%. While crushing strength test is a bulk deformation of the tablet, friability is a surface deformation which may be enhanced by the morphology of the tablet (Riippi et al., 1998). The rougher the surface of the tablet, the more friable it will be. It was observed that paracetamol tablets prepared with acacia and tragacanth were friable though hard as the concentration of the binder increases. 2%

tragacanth could not withstand the friability test due to its softness. On the contrary, the friability of the tablets prepared with date palm decreases as the concentration of the binder increases. However, only 20% date palm met the compendial specification for friability.

Disintegration is a crucial step in release of drugs from immediate release dosage forms. The rate of disintegration is directly proportional to the rate of dissolution. The rate of disintegration is influenced by the rate of influx of water into the tablets which is also dependent on the porosity of the tablets. When the porosity is high, disintegration is hardly influenced by tablet formulation; otherwise, disintegration will be affected by the excipients (Bi et al., 1999). Although, the batches of the different types and concentrations of binders contained the same quantity of disintegrant (corn starch), only tragacanth at its different concentrations met the BP specification for disintegration which states that uncoated tablets should disintegrate within 15 min. Tragacanth in comparison with date palm and acacia produced relatively soft tablets which were friable and disintegrated rapidly. While, 2 and 5% acacia disintegrated in less than 30 min, none of the concentrations of date palm disintegrated in less than 30 min. The main mechanisms of disintegration proposed are swelling of disintegrant resulting in development of swelling force, capillary action and annihilation of intermolecular forces

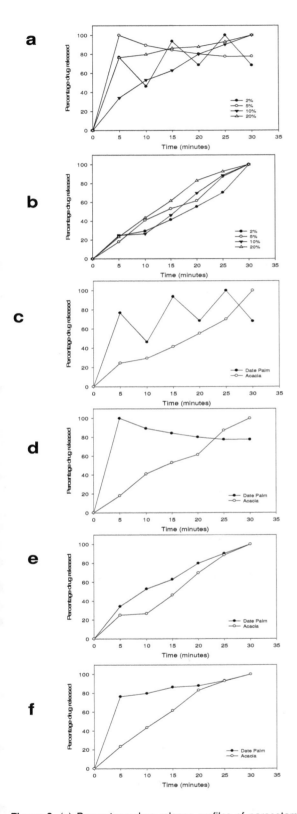

Figure 2. (a) Percentage drug release profiles of paracetamol tablets with date palm as the binding agent. (b) Percentage drug release profiles of paracetamol tablets with acacia as the binding agent. (c) Comparative drug release profiles of paracetamol tablets at 2% binder concentration. (d) Comparative drug release profiles of paracetamol tablets at 5% binder concentration. (e) Comparative drug release profiles of paracetamol tablets at 10% binder concentration. (f) Comparative drug release profiles of paracetamol tablets at 20% binder concentration.

resulting in development of a repulsive force between particles.

Some pharmaceutical excipients have inherent ability to disintegrate due to annihilation of bonds within which is enhanced by the penetration of a solvent (depending on its dielectic constant) that helps to weaken the bonds. The higher the dielectric constant of the solvent employed; the greater the weakening of bonds within the particles. Whichever the mechanism of disintegration in a given formulation, it should be adequate to overcome the impact of tablet hardness to disintegrating properties of a tablet. Basically, tragacanth did not produce very hard tablet and so the disintegrant, which employed swelling mechanism was able to induce disintegration. Perhaps increasing the quantity of disintegrant in the batches with date palm may enable disintegration of the tablets since it appeared that date palm may not be a self-disintegrating binder where annihilation of bonds is observed.

In vitro drug release studies

The rate of dissolution determines the rate and extent of absorption and subsequent therapeutic outcome of a drug. The factors that affect dissolution include type and concentration of binder, hardness, surface area, distance of diffusion, solubility of the drug, manufacturing process (wet granulation, dry granulation or direct compression) and diluents. The batches with date palm were compared with those of acacia for in vitro drug release studies. Although, tablets prepared with date palm as a binder did not disintegrate, the incorporated paracetamol was released from the tablets within 30 min. The drug release profiles of tablets with date palm was compared with those of acacia (Figure 2) and only tablets prepared with 10% date palm were comparable with tablets prepared with acacia producing a linear drug release profile. Tablets prepared with 2 and 20% date palm released over 70% of the drug in 5 min while 5% released 100% of the drug in 5 min as well. The rapid dissolution of paracetamol showed that date palm at 2, 5 and 20% did not control its rate of release. Furthermore, the drug release profile obtained from tablets with 2% date palm as a binder if utilized may produce erratic concentrations of paracetamol tablets in the plasma.

Solubility of paracetamol is 14 mg/mL and it is classified under the biopharmaceutical classification system, BCS class III – high solubility and low permeability, though, it may be said to have properties of BCS class I – high solubility and high permeability (Kalantzi et al., 2006). This indeed may explain the rapid release within 5 min from date palm batches though the tablets did not disintegrate which also attest to increased rate of hydration enabling rapid dissolution and diffusion out of the tablets. The USP and BP states that the quantity of drug released should not be less than 85% of the labelled amount of paracetamol in 30 min. Hence, all the batches of date palm and acacia complied with the specification. Furthermore, FDA guidance for industry, for the dissolution testing of immediate release solid oral dosage forms suggests that in some cases for class III drugs, 85% drug release in 0.1 N HCl in 15 min ensures that there would be no bioavailability problems. Based on this, tablets with 5 and 20% date palm may not have any bioavailability problems. However, to compare and determine the similarities or dissimilarities between the binders' dissolution profiles, dissolution efficiency was employed. Dissolution efficiency is known as area under the dissolution curve within a time range (t_1- t_2) expressed as a percentage of the dissolution curve at maximum dissolution y_{100}, over the same time frame (Anderson et al., 1998; Costa and Sousa Lobo, 2001) and is represented by the equation:

$$\text{Dissolution Efficiency (DE)} = \frac{\int_{t_1}^{t_2} y.\, dt}{y_{100}\,(t_2 - t_1)} \times 100 \qquad 4$$

Where, y is the percentage dissolved at time t.

The integral of the numerator which is the area under the curve was calculated using the trapezoidal method:

$$AUC = \sum_{i=1}^{i=n} \frac{(t_1 - t_{i-1})\,(y_{i-1} + y_i)}{2} \qquad 5$$

The dissolution efficiency is used to determine the dissolution performance of an individual formulation. The dissolution efficiencies of the different concentrations of date palm and acacia are shown in Table 4. The dissolution profiles of tablets formulated with date palm and acacia can only be said to be equivalent and be used interchangeably if the differences between them are within appropriate limits (± 10%, which is often used) (Anderson et al., 1998). The differences between the dissolution profiles from the binders for the same concentration exceeded by more than ± 10%; hence, the dissolution profiles are dissimilar. This is an indication of the paracetamol tablets formulated with date palm may be adjudged to be bio-inequivalent to those formulated with acacia.

Conclusion

Dried date palm fruit is a natural product which is non toxic, biodegradable and biocompatible that can be employed as a pharmaceutical binding agent for immediate release dosage forms. The granules manufactured with date palm had good flow properties and satisfactory compressibility which led to tablets with less variation in uniformity. The tablets had good uniformity of

Table 4. Dissolution efficiencies of the different concentrations of the binders.

Concentration of binder	Dissolution efficiency (%)
2% date palm	102.5
5% date palm	100.9
10% date palm	61.6
20% date palm	78.9
2% acacia	45.2
5% acacia	51.9
10% acacia	44.6
20% acacia	59.0

uniformity of weight, thickness and diameter, hard and less friable than acacia and tragacanth as its concentration increases; and a better binder than tragacanth.

REFERENCES

Allen LV, Popovich NG, Ansel HC (2004). Ansel's pharmaceutical dosage forms and drug delivery systems" in, 8th Edition edn, Lippincott Williams and Wilkins, Philadelphia. pp. 236.

Al-shahib W, Marshall RJ (2003). The Fruit of the Date Palm: its Possible use as the Best Food for the Future?. Intern. J. Food Sci Nutr., 54(4): 247.

Anderson NH, Bauer M, Boussac N, Khan-Malek R, Munden P, Sardaro M (1998). An evaluation of fit factors and dissolution efficiency for the comparison of in vitro dissolution profiles. J. Pharmac. Biomed. Analysis, 17 (4-5): 811-822.

Bacher C, Olsen PM, Bertelsen P, Sonnergaard JM (2008). Compressibility and compactibility of granules produced by wet and dry granulation. Intern. J. Pharm., 358(1-2):69-74.

Becker D, Rigassi T, Bauer-brandl A (1997). Effectiveness of Binders in Wet Granulation: A Comparison Using Model Formulations of Different Tabletability. Drug Dev. Ind. Pharm., 23(8):791-808.

Bi YX, Sunada H, Yonezawa Y, Danjo K (1999). Evaluation of Rapidly Disintegrating Tablets Prepared by a Direct Compression Method. Drug development and industrial pharmacy, 25(5):571-581.

Costa P, Sousa Lobo JM (2001). Modeling and comparison of dissolution profiles. Euro. J. Pharmac. Sci., 13(2): 123-133.

Endale A, Gebre-Mariam T, Schmidt P (2008). Granulation by Roller Compaction and Enteric Coated Tablet Formulation of the Extract of the Seeds of Glinus Lotoides Loaded on Aeroperl® 300 Pharma. AAPS Pharm. Sci. Tech., 9(1): 31-38.

Faure A, York P, Rowe RC (2001). Process control and scale-up of pharmaceutical wet granulation processes: a review. Euro. J. Pharmaceut. Biopharm., 52(3):269-277.

Ferrari F, Bertoni M, Bonferoni MC, Rossi S, Caramella C, Nyström C (1996). Investigation on bonding and disintegration properties of pharmaceutical materials. Inter. J. Pharma., 136(1-2): 71-79.

Fichtner F, Rasmuson Å, Alderborn G (2005). Particle size distribution and evolution in tablet structure during and after compaction. *Inter. J. o. pharmacy.*, 292(1-2): 211-225.

Kalantzi L, Reppas C, Dressman JB, Amidon GL, Junginger HE, Midha KK, Shah VP, Stavchansky SA, *Barends DM (2006). Biowaiver monographs for immediate release solid oral dosage forms Acetaminophen (paracetamol). J. Pharm. Sci., 95(1):4-14.

Kristensen HG, Schaefer T (1987). Granulation: A Review on Pharmaceutical Wet-Granulation. Drug Dev. Ind. Pharm., 13(4-5) 803-872.

Krycer I, Pope DG, Hersey JA (1983). An evaluation of tablet binding agents part I. Solution binders. Powder Technol., 34(1): 39-51.

McConville JT, Ross AC, Chambers AR, Smith G, Florence AJ, Stevens HNE (2004). The effect of wet granulation on the erosion behaviour of an HPMC–lactose tablet, used as a rate-controlling component in a pulsatile drug delivery capsule formulation. Euro. J. Pharmac. Biopharmac., 57(3): 541-549.

Mohammadi MS, Harnby N (1997). Bulk density modelling as a means of typifying the microstructure and flow characteristics of cohesive powders. Powder Technol., 92(1): 1-8.

Panda D, Choudhury NSK, Yedukondalu M, Si S, Gupta R (2008). Evaluation of gum of Moringa oleifera as a binder and release retardant in tablet formulation. Indian J. Pharmac. Sci., 70(5): 614-618.

Pifferi G, Restani P (2003). The safety of pharmaceutical excipients. Il Farmaco, 58(8): 541-550.

Pifferi G, Santoro P, Pedrani M (1999). Quality and functionality of excipients. Il Farmaco, 54(1-2): 1-14.

Reddy K, Mutalik S, Reddy S (2003). Once-daily sustained-release matrix tablets of nicorandil: Formulation and in vitro evaluation. AAPS Pharm. Sci. Tech,, 4(4): 480-488.

Reus-Medina M, Lanz M, Kumar V, Leuenberger H (2004). Comparative evaluation of the powder properties and compression behaviour of a new cellulose-based direct compression excipient and Avicel PH-102. J. Pharm. Pharmac., 56(8): 951-956.

Riippi M, Antikainen O, Niskanen T, Yliruusi J (1998). The effect of compression force on surface structure, crushing strength, friability and disintegration time of erythromycin acistrate tablets. Euro. J. Pharmac. Biopharmaceutics, 46(3): 339-345.

Rohrs BR, Amidon GE, Meury RH, Secreast PJ, King HM, Skoug CJ (2006). Particle size limits to meet USP content uniformity criteria for tablets and capsules. J. Pharmac. Sci., 95(5):1049-1059.

Sun, C, Himmelspach MW (2006). Reduced tabletability of roller compacted granules as a result of granule size enlargement. J. Pharmac. Sci., 95(1): 200-206.

US Pharmacopeia National Formulary USP 23/NF 18 (1995). UnitedStates Pharmacopeial Convention. Inc., Rockville, MD.

Vayalil PK (2002). Antioxidant and Antimutagenic Properties of Aqueous Extract of Date Fruit (Phoenix dactylifera L. Arecaceae). J. Agri. Food Chem., 50(3):610-617.

Virtanen S, Antikainen O, Räikkönen H, Yliruusi J (2010). Granule size distribution of tablets", J. Pharmac. Sci., 99(4): 2061-2069.

Westerhuis JA, Coenegracht PMJ (1997). Multivariate modelling of the pharmaceutical two-step process of wet granulation and tableting with multiblock partial least squares. J. Chemometrics, 11(5): 379-392.

Yalkowsky SH, Bolton S (1990). Particle Size and Content Uniformity. Pharmaceutical Research, 7(9):962-966.

8

Evaluation of *in vitro* antimicrobial effect of combinations of erythromycin and *Euphorbia hirta* leaf extract against *Staphylococcus aureus*

Michael Adikwu[2] Clement Jackson[1*] and Charles Esimone[2]

[1]Department of Pharmaceutics and Pharmaceutical Technology, University of Uyo, Akwa Ibom State, Nigeria.
[2]Department of Pharmaceutics, University of Nigeria, Nsukka, Enugu State, Nigeria.

The *in vitro* combined effects of erythromycin and methanol extract of leaves of *Euphorbia hirta* against clinical isolates of *Staphylococcus aureus* were investigated using the Checkerboard technique. The organism was susceptible to the extract with MIC of 25 mg/ml, while erythromycin had MIC of 0.005 mg/ml. The research aims to investigate the possible interaction that may exist when standardize herbal drugs are combined with synthetic antimicrobials. Previously, stock solutions of both the extract and erythromycin were prepared in appropriate volume of dimethylsulphoxide and water respectively to get a final concentration of 50 mg/ml each. Minimum inhibitory concentration was determined by method of serial dilution while interaction study was carried out according to the continuous variation checkerboard method. Upon combination, some ratios showed synergistic (9:1, 8:2, 7:3, 6:4, 3:7, 2,8, 1:9) while others indicated indifference (5:5, 4:6) activities against the isolates. These results indicate that some combinations of the extract with erythromycin could be synergistic in activity for some ratio combinations and indifferent for some others.

Key words: *In vitro*, erythromycin, *Euphorbia hirta*, *staphylococcus aureus*, MIC checkerboard.

INTRODUCTION

Several reasons have been advanced to justify the use of combination of two or more antibiotic treatment (Esimone et al., 2006; Ibezim et al., 2006).

For many years now; combination of two or more antibiotics has been recognized as an important method for, at least, delaying the emergence of bacterial resistance (Chambers, 2006). Besides, antibiotic combinations may also produce desirable synergistic effects in the treatment of bacterial infections (Zinner, 1981).

Two very distinct traditional methods of testing *in vitro* antibiotic interaction are the Checkerboard technique and the Time killing curve method (Eliopoulos et al., 1988). The checkerboard method will be used in this research. erythromycin is usually bacteriostatic, but can be bactericidal in high concentrations against very susceptible organisms. The antibiotic is most effective *in vitro* against aerobic gram-positive cocci and bacilli (Goodman and Gilman, 2001).

Euphorbia hirta belongs to the family Euphorbiaceae. It is a small annual herb common to tropical countries (Sofowora, 1982). *E. hirta* has various phytochemicals embedded in the plant parts.

The leaves are found to contain triterpenoids, sterols, alkaloids, glycosides and tannin (Anozie, 1991). In Nigeria, extracts of the plant are used as eardrops and in the treatment of boils, sore and promoting wound healing (Igoli et al., 2005).

In this study, the interaction between erythromycin and methanol extract of leaves of *E. hirta* has been investigated using Checkerboard method. The results of this research could provide rational basis for the use of standardized herbal drugs in combination therapy of prevailing diseases.

MATERIALS AND METHODS

Plant collection and identification

Fresh leaves of *E. hirta* were collected from Nsukka, Enugu State,

Nigeria. The plant was authenticated by Mr. A. O. Ozioko of Bioresources Development and Conservation Programme, Aku Road, Nsukka. Specimen vouchers were kept in the department of Pharmacognosy, University of Nigeria, Nsukka with number; E.h cco: 002

Sample preparation and extraction procedures

The fresh leaves were air dried for one week and ground into fine powder using a mechanical grinder. 25 g of the fine powder was macerated with 375 ml of methanol in a conical flask. This was covered and shaken every 30 min for 6 h, and then allowed to stand for 48 h.

The solution was subsequently shaken and filtered using Whatman filter paper. The filtrate was evaporated to dryness with the aid of a rotatory evaporator (Model type 349/2, Corning Ltd). The extract was then stored below ambient temperature.

Preparation of extract/drug stock solution

The stock solution of E. hirta leaf extract was prepared on each occasion by careful weighing and dissolving in suitable volume of Dimethylsulphoxide (DMSO) to get a concentration of 50 mg/ml. A tablet of erythromycin was dissolved in appropriate volume of water to get 50 mg/ml of stock solution.

Culture media

The media employed for the study was: Nutrient agar.

Test microorganisms

Clinical isolates of staphylococcus aureus were obtained from the Department of Pharmaceutical Microbiology, University of Nigeria, Nsukka.

Sterilization of materials

The Petri dishes and pipettes packed into metal canisters were appropriately sterilized in the hot air oven (Ov-335, Hareus) at 170°C for 1 h at each occasion. Solution of the extract and culture media were autoclaved at 121°C for 15 min.

Preparation of culture media

All culture media were formulated according to manufacturers' specification. Basically for nutrient agar, this involves appropriate weighing of nutrient agar, distributing into bijou bottles (in 20 ml) and then sterilization using autoclave at 121°C, 151 b/sq. inch for 15 min; then allowed to cool to 45°C before pouring into the agar plate. The pH of the agar medium was maintained at 7.4.

Maintenance and standardization of test organisms

The organism (S. aureus) was maintained by weekly sub culturing on nutrient agar slant. Before each experiment, the organism was activated by successive sub culturing and incubation. Standardization of the test microorganism was according to previously reported method (Chinwuba, 1991; NCCLS, 1990).

Sensitivity of test microorganism

The sensitivity of the test microorganism to the methanol extract and erythromycin was evaluated by determining the minimum inhibitory concentration (MIC) of both using the two fold broth dilution technique previously described (NCCLS, 1990; Esimone, 1999).

Evaluation of combined effects of E. hirta methanol extract and erythromycin

Stock solutions of E. hirta (50 mg/ml) and erythromycin (50 mg/ml) prepared in double -strength nutrient broth and autoclaved at 121°C for 15 min were employed. Varying proportions of the extract (Euph) and erythromycin (Eryth) were prepared according to the continuous variation checkerboard method previously described by NCCLS, 1990.

Each proportion of the herbal extract/ erythromycin combination was serially diluted (2 fold), inoculated with 0.1 ml of 10^6 cfu/ ml culture of test microorganism and then incubated for 24 h at 37°C. Interaction was assessed algebraically by determining the fractional inhibitory concentration (FIC) indices according to the equations below:

$$FIC_{index} = FIC_{Extract} + FIC_{Erythromycin} \dots\dots\dots\dots\dots\dots\dots\dots\dots\dots \quad (1)$$

$FIC_{Extract}$ (fractional inhibitory concentration of Extract)

$$= \frac{\text{MIC of Extract in combination with Erythromycin}}{\text{MIC of Extract alone}} \quad (2)$$

$FIC_{Erythromycin}$ (fractional inhibitory concentration of Erythromycin)

$$= \frac{\text{MIC of Erythromycin in combination with Extract}}{\text{MIC of Erythromycin alone}} \dots \quad (3)$$

RESULTS

Combined drug use is occasionally recommended to prevent resistance emerging during treatment and to achieve higher efficacy in the treatment of infections and diseases. The combination is hoped to achieve a desirable synergistic effect in this study.

Results of the systematic and scientific evaluation of the in vitro effects of E. hirta leaf extract and erythromycin have been presented in this paper (Table 1). FIC index values < 1 were considered as synergy and the degree of synergy increases as the value tends towards zero. FIC index values of 1 indicate additivity, values greater than 1, but less than 2 represent indifference while values greater than 2 show antagonism (Chinwuba, 1991; Esimone et al., 1999). Based on these, synergistic effect was obtained by combination of erythromycin and E. hirta against S. aureus in the ratios (9:1, 8:2, 7:3, 6:4, 3:7, 2:8, 1:9) while others (5:5, 4:6,) showed indifference.

DISCUSSION

The results reveal that E. hirta extract has promising antibacterial effects. A plausible mechanism of action could

Table 1. Combined activity of *E. hirta* leaf extract and erythromycin against *S. aureus*.

Ratio of drug combination Eryth : Euph	MIC Eryth (mg/ml)	MIC Euph (mg/ml)	FIC Eryth	FIC Euph	FIC Index	Inference
10 : 0	0.005	-	-	-	-	-
9 : 1	0.0045	1.25	0.9	0.05	0.95	Syn
8 : 2	0.004	2.5	0.8	0.1	0.9	Syn
7 : 3	0.0035	3.75	0.7	0.15	0.85	Syn
6 : 4	0.003	5.0	0.6	0.2	0.8	Syn
5 : 5	0.005	12.5	1.0	0.5	1.5	IND
4 : 6	0.004	15.0	0.8	0.6	1.4	IND
3 : 7	0.0015	8.75	0.3	0.35	0.65	Syn
2 : 8	0.001	10.0	0.2	0.4	0.6	Syn
1 : 9	0.005	11.25	0.1	0.45	0.55	Syn
0 : 10	-	25	-	-	-	-

MIC = Minimum inhibitory concentration; Eryth = erythromycin; Euph = *E. hirta*; FIC = fractional inhibitory concentration; Syn = synergism; IND = indifference.

could be suggested that the *E. hirta* leaf extract potentiated the activity of erythromycin, giving rise to synergism.

The results of these *in vitro* tests indicate that the combination of *E. hirta* leaf extract and erythromycin at a given ratio has a possible clinical significance in the treatment of bacterial infection caused by *S. aureus*. Unguided and indiscriminate combination may result to an effect or outcome which has no clinical significance.

Moreover, this herbal extract is widely available, cheap and quite safe. It also has mild side effects of nausea and vomiting.

In conclusion, it may be stated there is a favorable interaction between *E. hirta* leaf extract and erythromycin against *S. aureus* in some given combination ratios.

ACKNOWLEDGEMENT

We appreciate the members of technical staff of the division of Pharmaceutical microbiology, Department of Pharmaceutics, University of Nigeria, Nsukka. We also acknowledge members of staff of God's Glory Computers Institute, Uyo, Akwa Ibom State, Nigeria.

REFERENCES

Anozie VC (1991). God's healing power in Plants. Clin. Pharm. Herb Medium. 7: 23-25.
Chambers HF (2006). General principles of antimicrobial therapy. In Goodman and Gilman's pharmacologiced Basis of Therapeutics, Bruton LL (e+d), 11th Ed., mcGraw Hill: USA. 1102 – 1104

Chinwuba GN, Chiori Go, Ghobashy AA, OkorE VC (1991). Determination of Synergy of antibiotic combination by overlay inoculum susceptibility Research. 41:14 –150
Eliopoulos GM, Eliopons CT (1988). Antibiotic combinations: should they be tested? Clin. Microbiol. Rev. 1: 139–156.
Esimone CO, Adikwu MU, Uzuegbu DB, udeogaranya PO (1999). The effect of ethylenediaminetetraacetic acid on the antimicrobial properties of Benzoic acid and cetrimide J. pharm. Res. Dev. 4(1): 1-8.
Esimone CO, Iroha IR, CO Ude IG, Adikwu MU (2006). *In vitro* interaction of ampicillin with ciprofloxacin or spiramycin as determined by the Decimal assay for additivity technique. Niger. J. Health Biomed. Sci. 5(1): 12–16.
Goodman and Gilman's (2001). The Pharmacological basis of therapeutics. Tenth Edition Library of Congress Cataloging-in-Publication Limited. pp. 1250-1251.
Ibezim EC, Esimone CO, Okorie O, Obodo CE, Nnamani PO, Brown SA, Onyishi IV (2006). A study of the *in vitro* interaction of cotrimoxazole and ampicilin uding the checkerboard method. Afr. J. Biotechnol. 5(13): 1284–1288.
Igoli JO, Ogaji TA, Tor-Anyiin, Igoli NP (2005), Traditional medicine practice amongst the Igede People of Nigeria. Part 11, Afr J Tradit. Complement Altern. Med. 2(2): 134-152.
National Committee for Clinical Laboratory standards. Performance standards For Antimicrobial Disc susceptibility test 4th ed., approved Document M2 – A4 (NCCLS) villanova p. 1990.
Sofowora EA (1982). Medicinal Plants and Traditional Medicine in Africa, John Wiley and Sons, Chichester. p. 198.
Zinner SN, Klastersky J, Gaya BC, Riff JC (1981). *In vivo* and *in vitro* studies of three antibiotic combinations against gram negative bacteria and *Staphylococcus aureus*. Antimicrob. Agents chemother. 20: 463–469.

9

Evaluation of essential oils composition of methanolic *Allium sativum* extract on Trypanosoma *brucei* infected rats

Oluwatosin K. Yusuf[1]* and Clement O. Bewaji[2]

[1]Department of Biochemistry, Federal University of Technology, Trypanosomosis Research Unit, PMB 65, Minna, Nigeria.
[2]Department of Biochemistry, University of Ilorin, Ilorin, Nigeria.

The essential oils composition and anti – trypanosomal activity of fermented methanolic *Allium sativum* extract was investigated. The crude extract was partially purified using column chromatography to give fractions A, B and C, which were further characterized by gas chromatographic – mass spectral (GC/MS) analysis. The fractions identified thirteen, sixteen and seventeen compounds respectively. The main components were oxygenated hydrocarbon (palmitoleic and steric acid) and n – hydrocarbon (unsaturated).The crude extract show anti- trypanosomal activity on *Trypanosoma brucei* infected rats.

Key words: *Allium sativum*, essential oils, gas chromatographic – mass spectral analysis, retention index (KI, anti- trypanosomal).

INTRODUCTION

Allium sativum L., commonly known as garlic, belongs to family *Alliaceae*. Its close relatives include the onion, the shallot and the leek (McGee, 2004). Garlic has been used throughout recorded history for both culinary and medicinal purposes. It has a characteristics pungent, spicy flavour that mellows and sweetens considerably with cooking (McGee, 2004). It also has been taken as a tonic, a bactericide and a popular remedy for various ailments (Blackwood and Fulder, 1986). More recently, however, it has been recognized as a medicinal plant for the prevention of blood circulatory disorders (Fogarty, 1993; Steiner et al., 1996), cancer (Amagase and Milner, 1993; Nishino et al., 1989; Wargovich, 1986), memory loss (Moriguchi et al., 1994) and anti-trypanosomal (Yusuf and Ekanem, 2010).

It have been reported that garlic bulb contain two classes of antioxidant components namely flavonoids and polyphenol derivatives which are naturally occuring compound of gallic acid. Previous quantitative phytochemical analysis of fermented methanolic garlic extract shows that the plant contain secondary metabolite with high percentage of glycoside (21.088%), alkaloids (3.570%) and saponins (0.696%), moderate amount of phenol, tannins, flavonoid, steroids, terpenes and anthraquinone and trace amount of phlobatannin (Yusuf and Ekanem, 2010). Several chromatograms of the garlic have been published (Itakura et al., 2001) but so far no analysis of the volatile compounds in garlic that is responsible for its anti-trypanosomal activity has been reported.

Essential oils (EOs) are extremely complex mixtures containing compounds of several different functional-group classes. A specific aromatic profile should be determined by gas-chromatography-mass detection methods, to define their constituent for their safety and efficacy.

EXPERIMENTAL

Plant material

Fresh bulbs of *A. sativum* L., commonly known as garlic were

---

*Corresponding author. E-mail: toscue@yahoo.com.

Table 1. Compounds present in fraction a of fermented garlic extract.

KI	Compound	%
701	2,3 –Pentanedione	0.77
792	1- octane	1.15
1593	1- hexadecane	2.50
1900	Nonadecane	2.88
1984	Hexadecanoic acid	13.74
2009	Octadecanoic acid	15.92
2800	Octacosane	7.10
2600	Hexacosane	4.80
2456	Tetracosan-1-ol	5.57
	9-Octadecen-18-olide	15.93
	5-Octadecene	3.26
	Classification of compounds	
	Unknown compound	4.61
	n-hydrocarbon	21.70
	Oxygenated hydrocarbon	45.50
	Unknown compound	4.61
		71.81

The compounds were identified by the combination of both the mass spectra and retention indices on DB – 5 capillary coated column. Values (%) represent percentage composition, KI represent retention index.

purchased from Minna Central Market, Niger State, Nigeria in the months of March/April 2008 and authentication was carried out at Federal College of Forestry, Ibadan, Oyo state.

Preparation of plant

Garlic bulbs (A. sativum) were opened to reveal its fleshy sections called cloves. The cloves were peeled and blended. One hundred gram of A. sativium was soaked in 250 ml methanol for 24 h and filtered. The solvent was removed using rotary evaporator. The resulting yield (8.66 g) were subjected to column chromatography using silica gel (60 to 120 mesh) and eluted with n-hexane, n-hexane – ethylacetate, ethyl acetate, ethyl acetate – methanol and methanol. Thin layer chromatography was performed with precoated silica gel GF- 25- UV 254 plates and detection was done by spraying with sulphuric acid to give three fractions (A, B and C). The essential oils of the fractions were studied.

Parasite inoculum

Trypanosoma brucei was obtained from the Veterinary and Livestock Studies Department of the Nigerian Institute for Trypanosomiasis Research, VOM, Plateau State of Nigeria. The parasite was maintained by repeated passaging into other rats.

Parasitaemia determination

Parasitaemia count was carried out on infected rats at 24 h interval to monitor infection progress. The counting of the number of parasite was done under the light microscope at X40 magnification from thin blood smear freshly obtained from the tip of the tail of infected rats.

Administration of crude extract

Infected rats were administered intraperitoneally with 0.5 ml solution of fermented garlic methanolic extract in distilled water containing 300 mg/kg body weigh on the first day of sighting parasite in the blood (normally 3 days post infection) of infected rats (Yusuf and Ekanem, 2010). The control group for this experiment was infected untreated rats.

Gas chromatography-mass spectrometry analyses

Agilent 6890 N gas chromatography (GC) was interfaced with a VG analytical 70 – 250 s double-focusing mass spectrometer. Helium was used as the carrier gas. The MS operating conditions were: Ionization voltage 70 eV, ion source 250 °C. The GC was fitted with a 30 m x 0.32 mm fused capillary silica column coated with DB-5. The GC operating parameters were identical with those of the GC analysis.

The percentage compositions of the oil were computed in each case from GC peak areas and are shown in Table 1. Retention indices for all the compounds were determined according to the Kovats method relative to the n-alkanes series. The identification of the compounds was done by comparison of retention indices and by matching their fragmentation patterns in mass spectra with those of published mass spectra data (Jennings and Shibamoto, 1980; Adams, 1995; Joulain et al., 1998; Koenig et al., 2004). In a few cases, identification of components was carried out by means of commercial libraries (Wiley,NIST05 and Hochmuth) (Itakura et al.

Table 2. Compounds present in fraction b of fermented garlic extract.

KI	Compound	%
1065	1- Phenyl ethanone	3.44
1392	1-Tetradecene	1.84
1481	Tridecan-2-one	1.12
1524	2-methoxy-4-(2-propenyl) – phenol acetate	2.71
1676	Methyl-z(1R,2S)-3-oxo-2-(z)-pent-2-cyclopentyl-acetate	4.17
1841	2-Phemethyl benzoate	2.33
1994	1-Eicosene	5.91
2128	Octadecyl acetate	4.65
2195	1-Docosene	5.43
2370	9-Tetracosene	11.05
2400	Tetracosane	4.75
2800	Octacosane	3.68
2848	Hexacosanol	2.91
2852	Hexacosan-1-ol	8.63
	2S,3S-Methyi-2-amino-3-methyl pentanoate	1.07
	5-Octadecene	9.06
	Classification of compounds	
	n-hydrocarbon	41.70
	Oxygenated hydrocarbon	24.10
	Aromatic hydrocarbon	6.90
		72.70

The compounds were identified by the combination of both the mass spectra and retention indices on DB – 5 capillary coated column. Values (%) represent percentage composition.KI represent retention index.

al., 2001).

RESULTS AND DISCUSSION

The oil extracted was amber in colour. The analysis of the fractions A of extract showed the presence of sixteen compounds corresponding to 71.80% of the total fraction (Table 1). The compound comprises of n- hydrocarbon (21.70%), oxygenated hydrocarbon (45.50%) and unknown compound (4.60%). The prominent compound are oxygenated hydrocarbon (Octadecanoic acid (15.92%), Hexadecanoic acid (13.74%) and 9-Octadecen -8-olide (12.47%) (Table 1).

Also, the determination of compounds in fraction B identified sixteen compounds corresponding to 72.70% of the total fraction (Table 2). The compound comprises of n- hydrocarbon (41.70%), oxygenated hydrocarbon (24.10%) and aromatic hydrocarbon 6.90%). The prominent among the n- hydrocarbon are: 9- Tetracosene (11.05%) (Table 2).

While, the fractions C garlic extract showed the presence of seventeen compounds corresponding to 87.04% of the total fraction (Table 3). The compound

comprises of n- hydrocarbon (42.640%), oxygenated hydrocarbon (27.50%), aromatic hydrocarbon (10.30%) and nitrogen containing hydrocarbon (6.60%). The prominent among the n-hydrocarbon are: 1-Docosene (14.31%) and 1-Octadene (11.90%) (Table 3).

It is worth mentioning that compounds such as octadecanoic acid, hexadecanoic acid and 9-Octadecen-18-olide which were detected in the fermented extract are systematic name for monoenoic fatty acid (Palmitoloeic, oleic and linoleic acid) belonging to omega 6 and omega 7. The parasitaemia of infected treated with garlic bulbs extract oil showed a decrease in the proliferation of parasite and extension of surviving days of rats from 8 days of the control (infected untreated) to 17 days for infected garlic treated rats (Figure 1). The oil could be useful in the management of African trypanosomiasis.

ACKNOWLEDGEMENT

Authors are grateful to Dr Oladosu of chemistry department, University of Ibadan for his assistance in GC-MS analysis.

Table 3. Compounds present in fraction c of fermented garlic extract.

KI	Compound	%
2600	Hexacosane	6.02
2402	Integerrimine	2.67
2470	Senkirkine	3.88
2800	Octacosane	4.55
2500	Pentacosane	3.08
2456	Tetracosan-1-ol	3.61
2195	1-Docosene	14.31
2009	Hexadecyl acetate	6.55
1793	1-Octadene	11.90
1676	Methyl-z(1R,2S)-3-oxo-2-(z)-pent-2-cyclopentyl-acetate	6.55
1524	2-methoxy-4-(2-propenyl) – phenol acetate	3.74
1383	E-(3,7-Dimethyl-2,6-Octadienyl acetate	2.94
1116	Tetradecane	1.60
1094	Methyl-2-butenoate	1.74
642	Benzene	0.94
	Serkirkine acetate	4.81
	9-Octadecen-18-olide	7.62
	Classification of compounds	
	n-hydrocarbon	42.64
	Oxygenated hydrocarbon	27.50
	Aromatic hydrocarbon	10.30
	Nitrogen containing hydrocarbon	6.60
		87.04

The compounds were identified by the combination of both the mass spectra and retention indices on DB – 5 capillary coated column. Values (%) represent percentage composition, KI represent retention index.

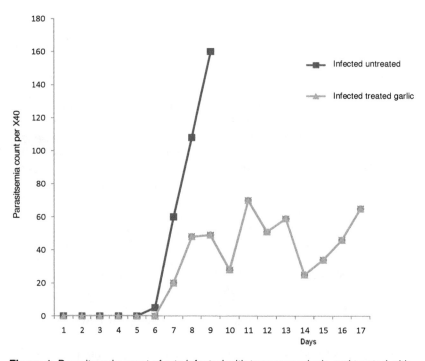

Figure 1. Parasitaemia count of rats infected with trypanosomiasis and treated with fermented menthanolic garlic extract.

REFERENCES

Adams RP (1995). Identification of essential oil components by gas chromatography-mass spectrometry. Allured Publishing Corporation, Carol Stream, Illinois, USA.

Amagase H, Milner JA (1993). Impact of various sources of garlic and their constituents on 7,12-dimethylbenz(a)anthracene binding to mammary cell DNA. Carcinog, 14: 1627-1631

Blackwood J, Fulder S (1986). Garlic; Nature's Original Remedy Javelin Books England.

Fogarty M (1993). Garlic's potential role in reducing heart disease. Br. J. Clin. Pract., 47: 64-65.

Itakura Y, Ichikawa M, Mori Y, Okino R, Udayama M, Morita T (2001). How to Distinguish Garlic from the Other Allium Vegetables. J. Nutri., 131: 963S-967S.

Jennings W, Shibamoto T (1980). Qualitative analysis of flavour volatiles by gascapillary chromatography. Academic Press, New York.

Joulain D, Koenig WA (1998). The atlas of spectral data of sesquiterpenehydrocarbons. E-B Verlag, Hamburg, Germany.

Koenig WA, Joulain D, Hochmuth D (2004). Terpenoids and Related Constituentsof Essential Oils. Library of Massfinder 3. Dr. Detler Hchmuth: Hamburg,Germany McGee H (2004). On food and cooking (revised edition) scribner. The Onion family; onions, garlic and leeks. pp. 310-313.

Moriguchi T, Takashina K, Chu PJ, Saito H, Nishiyama N (1994). Prolongation of life span and improved learning in the senescence accelerated mouse produced by aged garlic extracts. Biol. Pharm. Bull., 17: 1589-1594.

Nishino H, Iwashima A, Itakura Y, Matsuura H, Fuwa T (1989). Antitumor-promoting activity of garlic extracts. Oncol., 46: 277-280.

Steiner M, Kahn AH, Holbert D, Lin RIS (1996). A double-blind crossover study in moderately hypercholesterolemic men that compared the effect of aged garlic extract and placebo administration on blood lipids. Am. J. Clin. Nutr., 64: 866-870.

Wargovich MJ (1986). Dietary promoters and antipromoters. Antimutat. Anticancer. Mech., p. 409.

Yusuf KO, Ekanem JT (2010). Studies of phytochemical constituents and antitrypanosomal properties of fermented wheat germ and garlic bulbs extract on Trypanosoma brucei – infected rats. J. Med. Plants Res., 4(19): 2016-2020.

10

In vitro antiplasmodial and cyclin- dependent protein kinase (pfmrk) inhibitory activities of selected flavonoids in combination with chloroquine (CQ) and artemisinin

H. M. Akala[1], C. N. Waters[1], A. Yenesew[2], C. Wanjala[3] and T. Ayuko Akenga[4]*

[1]Kenya Medical Research Institute, Walter-Reed Laboratories, P. O. Box 54840 - 00100 G. P.O, Nairobi, Kenya.
[2]Department of Chemistry, University of Nairobi, P. O. Box 30197 - 00100 G. P. O. Nairobi, Kenya.
[3]Department of Physical Sciences South Eastern University College (SEUCO) P. O. Box 170-90200, Kitui, Kenya.
[4]Office of the Deputy Principal (Academic Affairs), Bondo University College (BUC) P. O. Box 210-40601, Bondo, Kenya.

In this study, we report *in vitro* chloroquine (CQ) and artemisinin combination studies of eight flavonoids against *Plasmodium falciparum* strains. The flavonoids were previously isolated from *Erythrina sp.* (Family Leguminosae) growing in Kenya. Synergism was observed for chloroquine/ Sigmoidin E (5) combination at ratios of 5:1 and 3:1 respectively, while other chloroquine/flavonoids combinations showed variable response; either additive or even antagonistic effects. The artemisinin/abyssynone IV (1) combination also showed synergistic interaction at a ratio of 5:1. Further investigations revealed that Abyssinone IV (1) and Abyssinone V (2) were effective inhibitors of plasmodial growth and differentiation regulatory enzyme, pfmrk.

Key words: Combination studies, CQ, artemisinin, flavonoids, sigmoid E, synergism, antagonism, pfmrk.

INTRODUCTION

The theory underlying combination drug management of tuberculosis, leprosy, and HIV infection is well known and is now generally accepted for malaria. Combination of drugs greatly lowers the probability of emergence of resistance (Nicholas, 2004; Bell, 2005). The change from monotherapy to combination therapy for malaria was effected and enforced before the year 2000 in most malaria endemic countries by government policies. Several drug combinations for treatment of malaria are now in use. They include pyronaridine/artemisinin; chlor-proguanil/dapsone; chlorproguanil/dapsone/artesunate and artemether /lumefantrine (Coartem®) combinations.

However, the fast emergence of resistance to the existing cheaply available combinations, like sulfadoxine/ pyrimethamine, is a major threat to the future of malaria treatment and control efforts (Krishna et al., 2006; Nzila

et al., 2000). Consequently, this medication has been replaced with the more effective but costly Coartem® (Mutabingwa et al., 2001). Furthermore, there is an overall lack of chemical diversity among the commercially available antimalarial drug compounds except for artemisinin (Macreadie et al., 2000), a problem that is further compounded by the fact that resistance to artemisinin has been reported in various regions (Taylor and White, 2004; Clark, 1996).

Recent studies have shown *in-vitro* antiplasmodial activities of extracts from plants traditionally used as antimalarials (Robert, 2003; Muregi et al., 2004; Brandao et al., 1997; Francois et al., 1996; Freiburghaus et al., 1996). Some of the most interesting results were from a plant called *Erythrina* sp. (Family Leguminosae). The plants in this family are widely used in traditional medicine for treatment of malaria and microbial infections (Kokwaro, 1993). Antiplasmodial activities of flavonoids from the roots and stem bark of these species have been reported (Yenesew et al., 2005; 2004; 2003a, b and c).

Cyclin-dependent protein kinases (CDKs) are attractive

*Corresponding author. E-mail: tezakenga@yahoo.co.uk, takenga@bondo-uni.ac.ke.

targets for drug discovery. Recently efforts have led to the identification of novel CDK selective inhibitors in the development of treatments for cancers, neurological disorders, and infectious diseases and CDKs have now become the focus of rational drug design programs for the development of new antimalarial agents. CDKs are valid drug targets as they function as essential regulators of cell growth and differentiation.

To date, several CDKs, pfmrk and PfPK5, have been characterized from the genome of the malaria-causing protozoan *Plasmodium falciparum* (Canduri et al., 2005; Keenan et al., 2006). Many of the parasitic protein kinases display profound structural and functional divergences from their host counterparts and pfmrk and PfPK5, most likely play an essential role in cell cycle control and differentiation in *P. falciparum*. This, therefore, makes them an attractive target for antimalarial drug development (Geyer et al., 2009). Various 1,3-diaryl-2-propenones (chalcone derivatives) which selectivity inhibit pfmrk in the low micromolar range (over PfPK5) have been reported. It is believed that kinase inhibition could be an additional mechanism of antimalarial activity for this class of compounds.

In this study, potencies of chloroquine (CQ)/flavonoid and artemisinin/flavonoid combinations were evaluated against CQ sensitive (D6) and CQ resistant (W2) strains of *P. falciparum*. The anti-*P. falciparum*, M015 Related Kinase (*pfmrk*), of selected flavonoids has been evaluated, in an attempt to contribute to the discovery of new anti-malarial drugs.

MATERIALS AND METHODS

Flavonoids assayed

Flavonoids 1 - 8 were assayed in this study. These compounds were from the library of compounds isolated, characterized and reported by Yenesew et al., in their studies of 2003, 2004 and 2005.

1: R_1 =OH, R_2 =H
2: R_1 =R_2 =H
3: R_1 =OH, R_2 =Me
4
5
6
7
8

Antiplasmodial activity assay

Antiplasmodial activity test was based on the procedure previously described by Desjardins et al. (1979). *P. falciparum* parasites were maintained by standard culture method (Chulay et al., 1983; Trager and Jansen, 1997). A two-fold serial drug dilution on 96-well plates was done using the Berkmann 1000 TM automated laboratory workstation with 50 µg/ml as starting concentration for all test compounds. The reference drugs had varied preset starting dose. Out of the eight rows on each plate, two were reference antimalarials drugs - chloroquine and quinine- while six were the different test samples.

For combination assays, a 96-well plate had first rows containing the particular reference drug, and row two, the test sample. The remaining six rows contained reference drug to sample drug concentration ratios of 1:1, 3:1, 1:3, 4:1, 1:4 and 5:1 respectively. The proportions were volume/volume parts of the combining components at the preset working doses such that reference drugs were at either 1000 mg/ml for chloroquine sulphate or 100 mg/ml for artemisinin and 50 µg /ml for the sample drugs. For the assay, 25 µl aliquots of the drug were pipetted into each of the microtitre wells on the plates. *P. falciparum* parasites were kept in continuous culture to adapt and attain a parasitemia of 3 - 6% trophozoite stages as proof to successful adaptation to *in-vitro* growth.

Aliquots of 200 µl of a 0.9% (v/v) suspension of parasitized erythrocytes in culture medium were added to all test wells except the three negative control wells. The plates were incubated at 37°C in a gas mixture of 3% CO_2–5% O_2–92% N_2. After 24 h, each well was pulsed with 25 µl of culture medium containing 0.5 µCi of [^{3}H] hypoxanthine and incubated for a further 18 h.

The contents of each well were harvested onto glass fiber filters, washed thoroughly with distilled water, dried, and the radioactivity (in counts per minute) measured by liquid scintillation counting. These tests were carried out in triplicates. The concentration causing 50% inhibition of radioisotope incorporation (IC_{50}) was determined by interpolation as described by Desjardins et al. (1979).

The highest concentrations of drugs were placed in the first column and subjected to a two-fold serial dilution across the row. Each plate had two control drugs, that is, the first two drugs (row A- chloroquine sulphate, and row B- quinine sulphate).

Data analysis

Oracle database software (Data Aspects Corporation, California USA, 1996) was employed in analysis of data to give 50% inhibitory concentration (IC_{50}). It is based on the inhibition of uptake of a radioactive nucleic precursor (hypoxanthine) by parasites as a measure of antiplasmodial activity. This program compares the individual counts to the background and the positive control, and plots a dose response curve (Frederich et al., 1999).
IC_{50} was calculated using Equation 1:

$$\% \text{ inhibition} = 100 - \frac{(\text{cpm test} - \text{mean cpm UC})}{(\text{mean cpm infected cells} - \text{mean cpm UC})} \times 100$$

(1)

where cpm = counts per minute, UC = uninfected cells

Exclusion was considered for all assays that showed: Bacterial contaminations, IC_{50} incorrectly aligned (failure to converge), low counts in the control wells, and inability to fit a logistic dose-response equation as shown by the analysis program. For

Table 1. *In vitro* IC$_{50}$ values of flavonoids isolated from *Erythrina sp.* against W2 and D6 strains of *P. falciparum*.

Category of activity	Compound	IC$_{50}$ (µMl)	
		D6	W2
A	Abyssinone IV (1)	5.4 ± 1.5	5.9 ± 1.8
	Abyssinone V (2)	2.4 ± 0.2	3.6 ± 0.2
	Sigmoidin E (5)	9.1 ± 2.3	11.8 ± 2.5
	5'-Prenylpratensein (7)	6.3 ± 0.3	8.7 ± 1.5
	Shinpterocarpin (8)	6.6 ± 1.2	8.3 ± 1.1
	Sigmoidin A (4)	5.8 ± 0.6	5.9 ± 1.1
B	Abyssinone V-4'-methyl ether (3)	11.3 ± 2.1	11.1 ± 2.4
	Abyssinone 4'-methyl ether diacetate (6)	12.3 ± 3.1	12.4 ± 0.1
	Reference drugs		
	Chloroquine	0.008 ± 0.0	0.075 ± 0.0
	Quinine	0.050 ± 0.02	0.28 ± 0.02

combination assays, it gave 50% fractional inhibition concentration (FIC$_{50}$) plot for every set of combination depicting synergistic, additive and antagonistic effects. Scatter plots were generated from the FIC$_{50}$ to explain the potency of a given combination by putting all the triplicate assays on one plane. Proguanil/artovaquone combination was used as the positive control.

Pfmrk kinase inhibition assays

Expression and purification of pfmrk was performed as described by Li et al., (1996). The kinase assays were performed according to the procedure of Roch et al., (2000). A standard reaction (30 µl) contained 25 mM Tris-HCl, pH 7.5, 15 mM MgCl$_2$, 2 mM MnCl$_2$ 15 µM ATP/0.05 µCi of [γ-^{32}P] ATP, and 5 µg of histone H1 (Life Technologies, Inc.). Reactions were initiated by the addition of 0.5 µg each of the recombinant protein kinase and cyclin H as a partner. Both proteins were allowed to form a complex at 30 °C for 30 min in kinase assay buffer.

The respective flavonoids were then added and incubated at 30 °C for 30 min; the negative controls were reaction mixtures containing only the relevant concentration of solvent. The reaction was stopped by the addition of Laemmli buffer. A fixed volume (25 µl) of each reaction was then spotted onto a small piece of Whatman P81 phosphocellulose paper. The paper was washed five times in 1% orthophosphoric acid, and the amount of acid-precipitable radiolabel incorporated in histone H1 was quantified by scintillation counting (Roch et al., 2000). From the differential counts, 50% inhibitions (IC$_{50}$) were established.

RESULTS AND DISCUSSION

Flavonoids 1-8 were selected based on their reported antiplasmodial activity, which is either in category A or category B (Yenesew et al., 2005; 2004a; 2003a, b and c). These activities were confirmed during this study (Table 1). It was necessary to re-evaluate the antiplasmodial activities of the above compounds. This is because these compounds had been stored for a long time and their activity could have been affected.

All the flavonoids tested showed activities within IC$_{50}$ of 10 - 20 µM. Growth inhibition of the chloroquine-sensitive (D6) strain by chalcones was better than that of the chloroquine-resistant (W2) strain.

Chalcone, abyssinone V-4'-methyl ether (6) was prepared by acetylation of abyssinone V-4'-methyl ether (3) under reflux condition in an attempt to prepare abyssinone V-4'-methyl ether diacetate. However, the product formed a chalcone 6 where ring C has opened. Interestingly, the chalcone showed comparable antiplasmodial activity with that of the flavanone 3.

From this study, the tested compounds can be identified as lead antimalarial structures since they had activities in the same range as the lead antimalarial compound licochalcone A (Ziegler et al., 2004). Structure–activity relationship studies on the antimalarial activity of chalcones have emphasized the importance of ring B for activity (Ziegler et al., 2004). In particular, parasubstitution of ring B with oxygen and non-bulky substituents like hydrogen has been reported to be desirable (Liu et al., 2003). All tested chalcones had an oxygen group in this position and showed antiplasmodial activity in the range of category B. Notably, antiplasmodial activity among these chalcones was comparable in spite of the changes in size, type and position of substituents on ring A.

Combination studies

The potency of flavonoids in combination with either artemisinin or CQ was evaluated in assay against two strains of *P. falciparum*. The flavonoids 1 - 8 being natural products, were in short supply. The number of assays carried out was limited by the availability of these compounds.

Each of flavonoids 1 and 3 was used in combination

Table 2. FIC_{50} for atovaquone/Proguanil combinations activity on D6 strain of *P. falciparum*.

Combining ratio	Mean sum FIC_{50}s ±SD
1:1	0.9 ± 0.1
3:1	0.9 ± 0.1
1:3	1.2 ± 0.2
4:1	0.9 ± 0.1
1:4	0.7 ± 0.2
5:1	1.4 ± 0.2

Number of replicates, n = 3, D6 = CQ sensitive strain of *P. falciparum*.

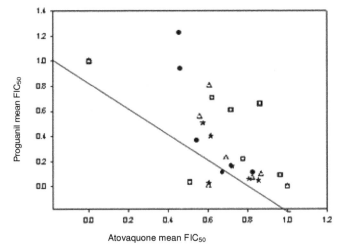

- ● Proguanil vs atovaquone plot 1
- ⚲ Proguanil vs atovaquone plot 1
- ★ Proguanil vs atovaquone plot 1
- □ Proguanil vs atovaquone plot 1

Figure 1. Scatter plot for proguanil/atoquone combination against D6 strain *p. falciparum*. Proguanil vs. atoquone plot 1; Proguanil vs. atoquone plot 2; Proguanil vs. atoquone plot 3; Proguanil vs. atoquone plot 4.

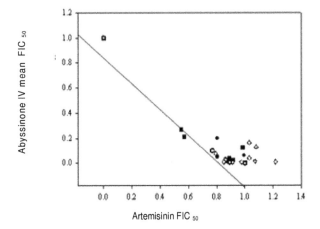

Figure 2. Scatter plot for artemisinin/1 combination.

with artemisinin. The results obtained are summarized in Table 2 and Figures 1 and 3. On the other hand, the results for combination studies of flavonoids 1 - 8 with CQ are summarized in Tables 3 and 5, and Figures 4 - 8.

Activities were evaluated as mean sum of fifty-percent fractional inhibition concentration (FIC_{50}) and grouped into three categories (Ohrt et al., 2002). Those showing synergism ($FIC_{50}<1$), those showing additive effect ($FIC_{50} =1$) and those showing antagonism ($FIC_{50}>1$). The results obtained illustrate activities ranging from having an additive to antagonistic or synergistic effect in combination, against the chloroquine-sensitive (D6) and chloroquine-resistant (W2) strains of *P. falciparum*. Both strains of plasmodium had comparable FIC_{50} values irrespective of the flavonoid used.

The control drug combination atovaquone/proguanil (Table 3) displayed a range of responses across the varying combinations ratios (Fivelman et al., 2004; White and Olliaro, 1996). The ratios 1:1, 3:1 and 1:4 showed activity with FIC_{50} values <1 to symbolize synergistic response.

Artemisinin/flavanoids combinations

The activity of the combination of artemisinin and abyssinone IV (1) was diverse, but the two compounds predominantly showed additive activity (Table 3, Figure 2). This was observed at the artemisinin/1 combination ratios of 1:1, 3:1, 4:1 and 5:1 with FIC_{50} values <1. Synergism was most evident at combination ratio 5:1. This ratio caused the highest reduction in amount of individual component required to attain the 100% inhibition of the chloroquine-sensitive (D6) strain of *P. falciparum* (Table 3). The rest of the combination ratios were either additive (1:3) or antagonistic (1:4).

At artemisinin/abyssinone 4' -methyl ether (3) combination ratios of 3:1, 1:3 and 5:1, the drugs showed additive activities (Table 3) against chloroquine-sensitive (D6) strain of *P. falciparum*. Best activity for this combination was at ratio of 5:1 with the lowest mean FIC_{50} across the set of combinations tested. The other combination ratios had mean FIC_{50} >1 showing antagonism.

Artemisinin is the only antimalarial drug with a notably unique molecular structure (Macreadie et al., 2000). Its mode of action has been described (Giao et al., 2004).

The tenacity of finding new molecules have bred the need to reinforce existing ones through combining them to reduce rate at which parasites develop resistance to these drugs. Indeed, artemisinin has been successfully combined with other antimalarial drugs, and the artemether/lumefantrine combination (Coartem®) is currently a first line antimalarial drug (Bukirwa et al., 2006). Interactions of two phytochemicals, artemisinin and licochalcone A, has been studied against synchronized erythrocytic stages of chloroquine-sensitive 3D7 and chloroquine-resistant RKL 303 strains of *P. falciparum*. These two compounds in combination

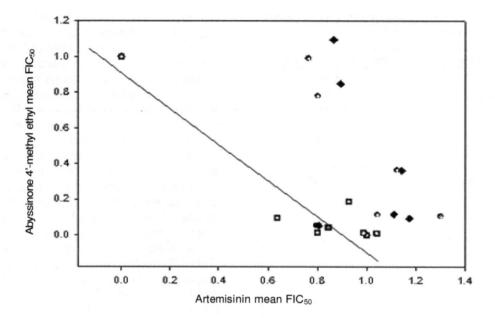

Figure 3. Scatter plots for artemisinin/3 combination activity against W2 strain of *P. falcinarum.*

Legend:
- Artemisinin vs abyssinone 4'-methyl ether plot 1
- Artemisinin vs abyssinone 4'-methyl ether plot 1
- Artemisinin vs abyssinone 4'-methyl ether plot 1

Table 3. FIC$_{50}$ values for selected artemisinin/flavonoid combinations against D6 strain of *P. falciparum.*

Combining ratio	Mean sum FIC$_{50}$s ±SD, number of replicates = 3.	
	Artemisinin/1 combination	Artemisinin/3 combination
1:1	0.9 ±0.1	1.1 ± 0.0
3:1	1.0 ± 0.1	1.0 ± 0.1
1:3	1.2 ±0.2	1.0 ± 0.2
4:1	1.0 ± 0.0	1.0 ± 0.2
1:4	1.3 ±0.2	1.0 ± 0.2
5:1	0.6 ± 0.0	1.0 ± 0.1

Number of replicates, n = 3, D6 = chloroquine sensitive strain of *P. falciparum.*

Table 4. Mean sum fractional inhibition concentration (FIC$_{50}$) for chloroquine/flavonoid combinations activity on D6 strain of *P. falciparum.*

Combining ratio	Mean sum FIC$_{50}$s ±SD				
	CQ / 2	CQ / 3	CQ / 5	CQ / 7	CQ / 4
1:1	1.6 ± 0.3	1.3 ± 0.4	1.2 ± 0.1	1.2 ± 0.1	3.2 ± 1.8
3:1	1.7 ± 0.2	1.1 ± 0.2	0.6 ± 0.8	1.4 ± 0.0	1.7 ± 0.6
1:3	1.3 ± 0.1	1.4 ± 0.5	1.1 ± 0.8	1.3 ± 0.1	4.6 ± 3.0
4:1	1.4 ± 0.2	1.2 ± 0.2	1.0 ± 0.1	1.4 ± 0.3	1.5 ± 0.3
1:4	1.4 ± 0.1	1.6 ± 0.4	1.2 ± 0.2	1.0 ±0.2	3.6 ± 2.2
5:1	1.3 ± 0.2	1.0 ± 0.1	0.8 ± 0.0	0.7 ± 0.2	0.80 ± 0.1

Number of replicates, n =3, D6 = chloroquine sensitive strain.

Table 5. Mean sum fractional inhibition concentration (FIC_{50}) for chloroquine/flavonoid combinations activity on W2 strain of *P. falciparum*.

Combining ratio	Mean sum FIC_{50}s ±SD					
	CQ / 2	CQ / 3	CQ /5	CQ/6	CQ / 7	CQ / 8
1:1	1.8 ± 0.1	1.3 ± 0.1	1.8 ± 0.5	1.3 ± 0.4	2.4 ± 0.3	2.6 ± 0.3
3:1	1.9 ± 0.1	1.2 ± 0.1	1.7 ± 0.4	1.3 ± 0.2	1.9 ± 0.6	2.1 ± 0.1
1:3	1.7 ± 0.4	1.4 ± 0.1	2.1 ± 0.7	1.4 ± 0.5	1.7 ± 0.1	1.6 ± 0.6
4:1	1.8 ± 0.1	1.1 ± 0.1	1.7 ± 0.1	1.2 ± 0.2	1.7 ± 0.4	1.4 ± 0.1
1:4	1.2 ± 0.0	1.3 ± 0.1	2.1 ± 0.7	1.6 ± 0.4	1.3 ± 0.4	1.2 ± 0.1
5:1	1.4 ± 0.5	0.9 ± 0.2	1.0 ± 0.1	1.0 ± 0.1	1.4 ± 0.2	2.2 ± 0.8

Number of replicates, n=3, W= chloroquine resistant strain.

showed synergistic antiplasmodial activity *in vitro* on these strains (Mishra et al., 2008). However, the present results show potent antagonistic activity for the tested artemesinin/flavonoid combinations against *P. falciparum*, with synergistic and additive effects only being observed at higher artemisinin ratios.

Emergence of drug-resistant *P. falciparum* strains to conventional first-line antimalarial drugs has compelled many countries to reorient their drug policies to adopt artemisinin-based combination therapies (ACTs) for treatment of uncomplicated malaria. This has increased the demand of artemisinin, already a scarce commodity. Extensive use of available ACTs will invariably lead to emergence of resistance to these combinations. Thus, there is need to search for new artemisinin-based, inexpensive, synergistic combinations to reduce dependence on artemisinin. The current study indicates that the tested flavonoids do not act synergistically with artemisinin at low ratios. Notably these favonoids have either category A or B activities antiplasmodial activities.

Chloroquine/flavonoid combinations

The results of CQ/ flavonoid combination studies are presented in Tables 4 - 5, and some of the isobolagrams in Figures 4 - 7. Compound 5 in combination with chloroquine yielded additive to synergistic response (Figure 7), while the other flavonoids with chloroquine combinations were mainly antagonistic against the strains of *P. falciparum*. Synergistic response was seen at chloroquine/ 5 ratios of 5:1 and 3:1 with the latter being the best overall chloroquine/flavonoid combination activity observed in this study (Table 4), against CQ D6. Interestingly, 2 singly showed the best activity, among all the flavonoids tested in this study (Table 1), against both strains of *P. falciparum* yet 2 exhibited antagonistic interactions with CQ. This raises questions on the interaction and mechanism of action of these compounds. Chloroquine mechanism of action is mainly through oxidative stress (Domarle et al., 1998) while flavonoids are antioxidants (Liu et al., 2003). Notably,

abyssinone 4'-methyl ether (3) had category B activity against both *P. falciparum* strains; yet again it showed antagonistic interactions. The interaction of chloroquine with shinpterocarpan (8) against chloroquine-resistant (W2) strains of *P. falciparum* was indifferent but tended more towards antagonism (mean sum FIC_{50}s >1). Ironically, compound 8 singly, showed category A but did not augment the activity of chloroquine. Such antagonistic responses have been shown in mefloquine/artemisinin combinations, which are singly very effective against *P. falciparum* but antagonistic in combination (Gupta et al., 2002).

Studies on the binding affinity of chalcones to ferriprotoporphyrin IX (FP) versus antiplasmodial activity have revealed a negative correlation (Elena, 2003). Although the activity patterns portrayed by chalcones in this study against the various strains of *P. falciparum* were similar to that of reference drugs that act by impairing binding of (FP) to haemozoin, it is likely that antiplasmodial activities of chalcones may be mediated by other means.

Activity of selected flavonoid against *P. falciparum* MO15-related protein kinase (pfmrk)

In addition to antiplasmodial activity, selected flavonoids were screened against cyclin dependent Kinase (CDK) pfmrk. Protein kinases are a family of enzymes whose key function is involvement in signal transduction for all organisms. This makes it a very attractive target for therapeutic interventions. This enzyme has been targeted in many diseases such as cancer, diabetes, inflammation, arthritis (Vieth et al., 2004) and lately protozoan parasites, specifically *P. falciparum* (Doerig, 2004). Recently several highly specific cdk inhibitors have been described. Olomoucine has been tested on a wide range of protein kinases, and shown to act very specifically on most members of the CDK family with IC_{50} values in the range of 3 - 50 uM (Vesely et al., 1994). Also, 0.2 µM flavopiridol arrests the cell cycle of breast carcinoma cells at the G/M transition and inhibits purified sea star cdc2

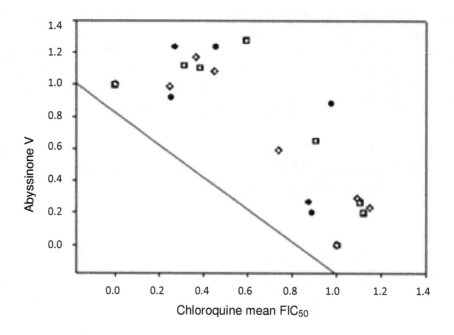

Figure 4. Scatter plot for chloroqine/2 combination against D6 strain *P. falciparum.*

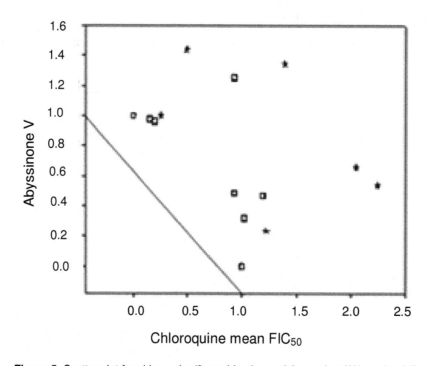

Figure 5. Scatter plot for chloroquine/2 combination activity against W2 strain of *P. falciparum.*

kinase with an IC$_{50}$ of 0.5 µM (Worland et al., 1993). Both drugs: Olomoucine and flavopiridol, act as CDK-specific

ATP-analogues (Vesely et al., 1994). These two compounds have shown inhibition of kinase activity of PfPK5

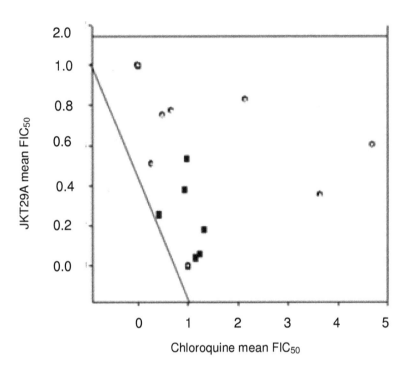

Figure 6. Scatter plot for chloroquine/6 combination against D6 strain *P. falciparum*. JKT 29A = Abyssinone-4'-methyl ether diacetate.

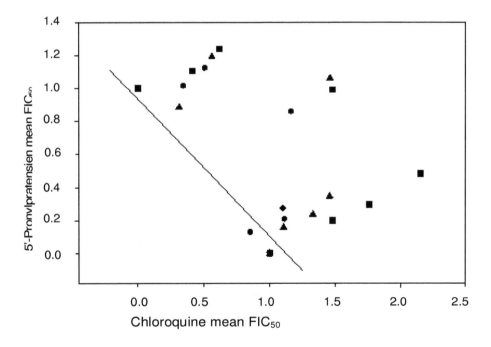

• Chloroquine vs 5'-prenylpratensein FIC$_{50}$ plot 1

▲ Chloroquine vs 5'-prenylpratensein FIC$_{50}$ plot 2

■ Chloroquine vs 5'-prenylpratensein FIC$_{50}$ plot 3

Figure 7. Scatter plot for chloroquine / 5 combinations against W2 strain of *P. falciparum*

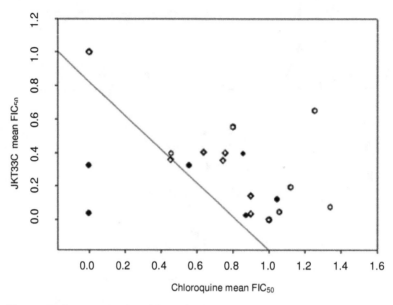

Figure 8. Scatter plot for chloroquine/5 combination against D6 strain *P. falciparum*. JKT 33C = 5 = Sigmoid E.

Table 6. *In vitro* IC$_{50}$ of flavonoid activity against CDK-pfmrk.

Test compound	Anti-pfmrk IC$_{50}$ μM
Abyssinone IV (1)	0.05
Abyssinone V (2)	0.04
Abyssinone V-4' - methylether (3)	>0.24

(IC$_{50}$ values flavopiridol 0.06 μM, olomoucine 0.000015 μM [15 PM]), as well as inhibition of growth of parasite cultures (IC$_{50}$ values flavopiridol 2 μM, olomoucine 0.000015 μM [15 PM]) (Graeser et al., 1996). In this study, compounds that have very good antiplasmodial activities of category A (26, 27, 69), were screened against CDK Pfmrk.

Interestingly in this study, many compounds that have good *in vitro* activity against the *P. falciparum* parasites are effective inhibitors of the *pf*mrk. Notably, abyssinone V (27) that had the best antiplasmodial activity also showed the best inhibition potency. It is interesting to note that when the 4' -OH in abyssinone IV (26) is methylated (abyssinone V-4'-methyl ether 28) the pfmrk IC$_{50}$ increased more than five-fold showing the importance of free -OH at C-4'.

Compounds 1 - 3, with category A antiplasmodial activity, were tested for their pfmrk activities. The results of the pfmrk assays are listed in Table 6.

Flavonoids 1 and 2 have good *in vitro* activity against the *P. falciparum* parasites and were found to be effective

inhibitors of the pfmrk (Table 5). Notably, abyssinone V (2) that had the best antiplasmodial activity also showed the best inhibition (IC$_{50}$ of 0.038 μM), while chalcone (3), did not show anti-pfmrk activity within the range of concentration (highest ≈ 0.3 μM). It is important to note that when the 4' -OH in abyssinone IV (1) is methylated (abyssinone V-4'-methyl ether 3) the pfmrk IC$_{50}$ increases more than five-fold and hence indicates the importance of free -OH at C-4'.

Conclusion

The flavonoids tested in this study probably have a mechanism of action similar to chloroquine since they have better activity against the chloroquine-sensitive (D6) than the chloroquine-resistant (W2) strain of *P. falciparum*. In addition, the most active flavonoid (2) in combination with chloroquine was antagonistic across most ratios. In addition, the most active flavonoid in combination with chloroquine showed antagonistic activity across all ratios. Since flavonoids are antioxidants, it is possible that as strong oxidants, they may scavenge the chloroquine that is needed to inhibit heme binding thus leading to the observed antagonism. The chloroquine, flavonoid and artemisinin/flavonoid combination ratio of 5:1 was the best combination giving synergistic response in most of the tested combinations. It is therefore possible that antiplasmodial activity of flavornoids could also be mediated by pfmrk inhibition since the molecules with the best antiplasmodial activity proved to be effective pfmrk inhibitors.

ACKNOWLEDGEMENTS

The authors are grateful to Institute of Tropical Medicine and Infectious Diseases (ITROMID-JKUAT), University of Nairobi (Chemistry department), The authors are also grateful to Bondo University College and South Eastern University College for their support and lastly the Walter Reed Project /Kenya Medical Research Institute (KEMRI) and Kigali Institute of Science and Technology (KIST) for providing the funds for the study.

REFERENCES

Bell A (2005). Antimalarial drugs synergism and antagonism: Mechanistic and clinical significance. Microb. Lett., 253: 171-184.

Brandao MG, Krettli AU, Soares LS, Nery CG, Marinuzzi HC (1997). Antimalarial activity of extracts and fractions from Bidens pilosa and other Bidens species (Asteraceae) correlated with the presence of acetylene and flavonoid compounds J. Ethnopharmacol., 57: 131-138.

Bukirwa H, Yeka A, Kamya MR, Talisuna A, Banek K, Bakyaita N, Rwakimari JB, Rosentha PJ, Wabwire-Mangen F, Dorsey G, Staedke S (2006). Artemisinin Combination Therapies for Treatment of Uncomplicated Malaria in Uganda. PLoS Clin. Trials. 1.

Canduri F, Perez PC, Caceres RA, Filgueira de Azevedo W (2005). CDK9 a potential target for drug development. Comb Chem. High Throughput Screen, 8: 27-38.

Chulay JD, Haynes JD, Diggs CL (1983). Plasmodium falciparum: Assessment of in vitro Growth by [3H] hypoxanthine Incorporation. Expt. Parasit., 55: 138-146.

Clark AM (1996). Natural products as a resource for new drugs. Pharm. Res., 13: 8.

Desjardins ER, Canfield CJ, Haynes JD, Chulay JD (1979). Quantitative Assessment of Antimalarial Activity In Vitro by a Semiautomated Microdilution Technique, Antimicrob. Agents Chemother., 16: 710-718.

Doerig C (2004). Protein kinases as targets for anti-parasitic chemotherapy Biochim. Biophy. Acta, 1697: 155-168.

Domarle O, Blampain G, Agnaniet H, Nzadiyabi T, Lebibi J, Brocard J, (1998). In Vitro Antimalarial Activity of a New Organometallic Analog, Ferrocene-Chloroquine. Antimicrob. Agents Chemother., 42: 540-544.

Elena LMS (2003). Interaction of Chalcones with Ferriprotoporphyrin IX Department of Pharmacy, National University of Singapore. http://www.ntu.edu.sg/eee/urop/congress2003/Proceedings/abstract/

Fivelman QL, Adagu IS, Warhurst DC (2004). Modified fixed-ratio isobologram method for studying in vitro interactions between atovaquone and proguanil or dihydroartemisinin against drug-resistant strains of Plasmodium falciparum. Antimicrob. Agents Chemother., 48: 4097-4102.

Francois G, Ake AL, Holenz, J, Bringmann G (1996). Constituents of Picralima nitida display pronounced inhibitory activities against asexual erythrocytic forms of Plasmodium falciparum in vitro. J. Ethnopharmacol., 54: 113-117.

Freiburghaus F, Kaminsky R, Nkunya MHH, Brun R (1996). Evaluation of African medicinal plants for their in vitro trypanocidal activity; J Ethnopharmacol., 55: 1-11.

Geyer JA, Keenan SM, Woodard CL, Thompson PL, Gerena L, Nichols DA, GutteridgeEG, Waters NC (2009). Selective inhibition of Pfmrk, a Plasmodium falciparum CDK, by antimalarial 1,3-diaryl-2-propenones Bioorgan. Med. Chem. Lett., 19: 1982-1985.

Giao PT, de Vries PJ, Hung LQ, Binh TQ, Nam NV, Kager PA (2004). CV8, a new combination of dihydroartemisinin, piperaquine, trimethoprim and primaquine, compared with atovaquone–proguanil against falciparum malaria in Vietnam. Trop. Med. Inte. Health, 9: 209-216.

Gupta S, Thapar MM, Wernsdorfer WH, Björkman A (2002). In vitro interactions of artemisinin with atovaquone, quinine and mefloquine against Plasmodium falciparum. Antimicrob. Agents Chemother., 1510-1515.

Keenan SM, Geyer JA, Welsh WJ, Prigge ST, Waters NC (2006). Rational inhibitor design and iterative screening in the identification of selective plasmodial cyclin dependent kinase inhibitors. Biochimica Biophysica acta, 1754: 160-170.

Kokwaro JO (1993). Medicinal plants of East Africa, second Edition; Kenya Literature bureau, p. 56.

Krishna S, Woodrow CJ, Staines HM, Haynes RK, Mercereau-Puijalon O (2006). Re-evaluation of how artemisinins work in light of emerging evidence of in vitro resistance. Trends Mol. Med., 12(5): 200-2005.

Li JL, Robson KJ, Chen JL, Targett GA, Baker DA (1996). Pfmrk, a MO15-related protein kinase from Plasmodium falciparum. Gene cloning, sequence, stage-specific expression and chromosome localization. Eur. J. Biochem., 241: 805-813.

Liu M, Wilairat P, Croft SL, Tan AL, Go M (2003). Structure–Activity Relationships of Antileishmanial and Antimalarial Chalcones. Bio. Med. Chem., 11: 2729-2738.

Macreadie I, Ginsburg H, Sirawaraporn W, Tilley L (2000). Antimalarial Drug Development and New Targets, Parasit. Today, 16: 10-15.

Mishra LC, Bhattacharya A, Bhasin VK (2008). Phytochemical licochalcone A enhances antimalarial activity of artemisinin in vitro. Acta tropica, 109(3): 194-198.

Muregi FW, Chhabra SC, Njagi EN, Lang'at-Thoruwa CC, Njue WM, Orago AS, Omar SA, Ndiege IO (2004). Anti-plasmodial activity of some Kenyan medicinal plant extracts singly and in combination with chloroquine. Phytother. Res., 18: 379-384.

Mutabingwa T, Nzila A, Mberu E, Nduati E, Winstanley P, Hills E, Watkins W (2001). Chlorproguanil-dapsone for treatment of drug-resistant falciparum malaria in Tanzania. Lancet, 358: 1218-1223.

Nicholas JW (2004). Antimalarial drug resistance. J. Clin. Invest., 113: 1084-1092.

Nzila AM, Nduati E, Mberu EK, Hopkins SC, Monks SA, Winstanley PA Watkins WM (2000). Molecular evidence of greater selective pressure for drug resistance exerted by the long-acting antifolate Pyrimethamine/Sulfadoxine compared with the shorter-acting chlorproguanil/dapsone on Kenyan Plasmodium falciparum. J. Infect. Dis., 181: 2023-2028.

Ohrt C, Willingmyre GD, Lee P, Knirsch C, Milhous W (2002). Assessment of Azithromycin in Combination with other Antimalarial Drugs Against plasmodium falciparum In Vitro, Antim. Agents Chemother., 46: 2518-2524.

Robert GR (2003). Twenty-seven years of WHO/TDR experience with public–private partnerships in Product R&D for neglected diseases. EMBO reports, 4: 43-46.

Roch KL, Sestier C, Dorin D, Waters N, Kappesi B, Chakrabarti D, Meijer L, Doerig C (2000). Activation of a Plasmodium falciparum cdc2-related Kinase by Heterologous p25 and Cyclin H. J. Biol. Chem., 275: 8952-8958.

Taylor WR, White NJ (2004). Antimalarial drug toxicity: a review; Drug Saf., 27(1): 25-61.

Trager W, Jansen BJ (1997). Continuous culture of plasmodium falciparum: Its impact on malaria research. Int. J. Parasit., 29: 989-1006.

Vieth M, Higgs RE, Robertson DH, Shapiro M, Gragg EA, Hemmerle H (2004). Kinomics-structural biology and chemogenomics of kinase inhibitors and targets. Biochim. Biophys. Acta, 11: 243-257.

White N, Olliaro P (1996). Strategies for the prevention of antimalarial drug resistance: rationale for combination chemotherapy for malaria. Parasitol. Today, 12: 399-401.

Yenesew A, Derese S, Irungu B, Midiwo JO, Waters NC, Liyala P, Akala H, Heydenreich M, Peter MG (2003a). Flavonoids and isoflavonoids with anti-plasmodial activities from the roots of Erythrina abyssinica. Planta Medica, 69: 658-661.

Yenesew A, Derese S, Midiwo JO, Bii CC, Heydenreich M, Peter MG (2005). Antimicrobial flavonoids from the stem bark of Erythrina burttii. Fitoterapia, 76(5): 469-472

Yenesew A, Derese S, Midiwo OJ, Oketch-Rabah HA, Lisgarten J, Palmer R, Heydenreich M, Peter MG, Akala H, Wangui J, Liyala P Waters NC (2003c). Anti-Plasmodial Activities and X-Ray Crystal Structures of Rotenoids from Millettia Usaramensis Subspecies Usaramensis. Phytochem., 64: 773-779

Yenesew A, Induli M, Derese S, Midiwo JO, Heydenreich M, Peter M G, Akala H, Wangui J, Liyala P, Waters NC (2004). Anti-plasmodial flavonoids from the stem bark of *Erythrina abyssinica*. Phytochemistry, 65: 3029-3032.

Yenesew A, Irungu B, Derese S, Midiwo JO, Heydenreich M, Peter MG (2003b). Two prenylated flavonoids from the stem bark of *Erythrina burttii*. Phytochemistry, 63: 445-448.

Ziegler HL, Hansen HS, Staerk D, Christensen SB, Ha¨gerstrand H Jaroszewski1 JW (2004). The Antiparasitic Compound Licochalcone A is a Potent Echinocytogenic Agent that Modifies the Erythrocyt Membrane in the Concentration Range where Antiplasmodial activit is observed. Antim. Agents Chemother., 48: 4067-4071.

11

Potential therapeutic interventions on toll like receptors for clinical applications

Zhengwu Lu

1006 S De Anza Blvd#K104, San Jose, CA 95129, USA. E-mail address: Zhengwu.Lu@ieee.org.

Toll like receptors (TLRs) function as pattern-recognition receptors (PRRs) and play key roles in the recognition of microbial components or endogenous ligands induced during inflammatory response. Studies on TLR-deficient mice have indicated TLRs' involvement in multiple pathologic conditions, and targeting of either the TLRs themselves or the signals they generate is proving to be of great interest to researchers as evidenced by increased research findings among immunologists, pharmacologist, and pharmaceutical scientists on TLRs. As animal models, cellular and molecular mechanisms on TLR mediated disease pathogenesis are made available, drug intervention strategies and early stage clinical studies can be planned and initiated to seek clinical proof for justifying TLRs and their associated signaling pathway/molecules as therapeutic targets. Moreover, a key functional output from TLRs is the generation of inflammatory cytokines such as tumor necrosis factor (TNF) and IL-6, which are excellent targets for inflammatory diseases such as rheumatoid arthritis.

Key words: TLR, PRR, NF-κB, agonist, antagonist, drug discovery.

INTRODUCTION

It is well established that the innate immune system is essential to human survival, offering the first line of defense by recognizing and responding to pathogenic threats when microorganisms invade an organism's barriers. Recent research using positional cloning and knockout animal models has provided us with insight of the powerful Toll like receptors (TLRs) involved in innate immunity. TLRs are pattern-recognition receptors (PRRs) and play a key role in the innate immune system (Akira and Hemmi, 2003). Once microbes have breached physical barriers such as the skin or intestinal tract mucosa, TLRs recognize specific components of microbial invaders and activate an immune response to these pathogens. A downstream signaling cascade is activated to stimulate the release of inflammatory cytokines and chemokines as well as to upregulate the expression of immune cells. All TLRs have a Toll-IL-1 receptor (TIR) domain that initiates the signaling cascade through TIR adapters. Adapters are platforms that organize downstream signaling cascades leading to a specific cellular response after exposure to a given pathogen (Guo and Cheng, 2007).

There are ten TLRs in humans; and they recognize different microbial ligands during infection (Janssens and Beyaert, 2003). It is recognized that TLRs bind and become activated by different ligands located on different types of organisms or structures. They also have different adapters to respond to activation located either at the cell surface or in internal cell compartments. Additionally, TLRs are expressed by different types of leucocytes or other cell types (Waltenbaugh et al., 2008). Also of great interest are the different signaling pathways activated by TLRs. These pathways lead to the activation of the respective transcription factors, nuclear factor kB (NF-kB) and interferon regulatory factor 3 (IRF3), which in turn induce various immune and inflammatory genes. A greater understanding of the TLRs and their roles in immunity holds potential for the development of therapeutics for bacterial and viral infections, allergies and cancer, and also to limit the damage caused by autoimmune disorders. Moreover, the role of TLRs in tissue repair and regeneration provides a further avenue for drug targeting (Coyne, 2008). However, the fine balance of cell signaling these receptors participate in has wide-ranging and powerful effects on phenotype expression owing to the impact on thousands of individual genes; clearly, the issue of adverse effects could be quite a challenge to address. It is recognized that TLRs bind to specific ligands, distribute on different cell types, and play key roles in the pathophysiology of various disorders involving both the innate and adaptive immunity (O'Neill et al., 2009). Additionally, NF-kB governs the expression of numerous genes that are important for various cellular responses. Its activation is induced by a wide variety of stimuli including stress, cigarette smoke, viral and bacterial products, cytokines, free radicals, carcinogens and tumor promoters (Li et al., 2005). Deregulation of the NF-kB pathway has been observed in and attributed to the development of a variety of human ailments including cancers, autoimmune disorders, pulmonary, cardiovascular, neurodegenerative and skin diseases. Efforts to develop modulators of NF-kB have yielded several candidates, some of which are currently in Phase I/II of clinical trials such as NF-kB inhibitors CH828 from Leo Pharma to treat solid tumors and AS602868 from Serono International to treat acute myeloid leukemia (Sethi and Tergaonkar, 2009). On pharmacokinetic perspective, the wide tissue distribution of TLRs indicates complexity in deciding whether an agonist or an antagonist will be most effective therapeutically in humans for specified indications and disease types. This will need both pre-clinical and clinical data support to push any drug candidates further in the study phases. In this review, we focus on recent development of novel therapeutics that target TLRs or their pathways in various diseases.

Drugs/candidates stimulating toll like receptors

Therapeutic development targeting TLRs is at early clinical stages. There are currently approximately twenty drugs in pre-clinical development, with a further dozen or so in clinical trials (Coyne, 2008). Innate Pharma is developing IPH-3201, a series of TLR7/8 modulators to treat cancer, autoimmune and infectious diseases. Also in Innate's pipeline is IPH-3102, a double-stranded RNA and natural ligand of TLR3. Activation of the TLR3 pathway leads to the activation of NF-kB and the production of type I interferons to elicit antiviral defenses, and it is hoped that this may be an effective method of destroying cancerous cells. TLR3 detects virus invasion and initiates the antiviral immune response via TRIF/IKK signaling in the activation and maturation of dendritic cells (DCs) and monocytes, allowing for the regulated processing and presentation of antigens, the up-regulation of major histocompatibility complex, and co-stimulatory molecules and secretion of pro-inflammatory chemokines and cytokines (Kawai & Akira, 2009). These events then mediate the activation of antigen-specific T- and B-cell responses. Both of Innate's TLR candidates are in the early stages of development, it remains to be seen how they perform in the clinical subjects.

Similarly, the development of safe and efficacious vaccines remains a major challenging goal in global public health. For these reasons, TLR ligands have become a focus for their potential use as adjuvants in vaccine formulations (Pulendran, 2007). By physically linking the TLR ligand and antigen, each antigen would be delivered to a vesicle with an activated TLR in a host antigen-presenting cell, potentially achieving optimal antigen processing and presentation (Blander, 2007). Monophosphoryl lipid A (MPL) derived from detoxifying Salmonella minnesota lipid A, produced its adjuvant effect through the stimulation of the TRAM/TRIF signal transduction pathway of TLR4 and deactivation of Mal/MyD88 signaling (Mata-Haro et al., 2007), thereby acting as a partial rather than full agonist at the receptor and has been licensed for use as a vaccine adjuvant (Casella and Mitchell, 2008). It is also recognized that the major use for compounds that activate TLR2 are as adjuvant. The synthetic compounds, such as Pam3CSK4 and mycoplasma-derived lipopeptide (MALP)-2, may be developed for adjuvant usage (Lombardi et al., 2008; Ishii and Akira, 2007).

TLR5 is the receptor for bacterial flagellin monomers and is the only TLR that recognizes a protein ligand (Andersen-Nissen et al., 2007). CBLB502, an engineered flagellin derivative was found to have potent NF_κB activation and reduced immunogenic characteristics. A single injection of CBLB502 before lethal total body irradiation protected mice and rhesus monkeys from both gastrointestinal (GI) and hematopoietic acute radiation symptoms and resulted in improved survival and yet, importantly, did not decrease tumor radio sensitivity (Burdelya et al., 2008). These results imply that TLR5 agonists may be valuable as adjuvants for cancer radiotherapy. The activation of TLR5 has also been recently reported to be an efficient adjuvant for influenza A vaccine. A recombinant protein containing a consensus extracellular domain of M2 protein (M2e) sequence linked to the TLR5 ligand provides an effective approach to developing vaccines against wide-spread epidemic and pandemic influenza (Huleatt et al., 2008). The findings suggest that TLR5 agonist may have broad therapeutic applications, not only in its role as a linker adjuvant for vaccines, but also as a stopper of excessive apoptosis in acute radiation syndromes, degenerative diseases, or myocardial infarction as well (O'Neill, 2009). Such potential application needs to be verified and confirmed by animal models, preclinical, and clinical studies.

Investigators have focused on developing TLR7/8 agonists as antiviral agents against virus such as human papillomavirus (HPV). Imidazoquinolines were originally developed as such antiviral agents, and many such small molecule compounds have been tested for their ability to induce TLR7/TLR8-mediated cytokine induction. Imiquimod is the first approved topically active TLR7 agonist. It is prescribed for treatment of external virus induced skin lesions, such as the genital and perianal warts resulting from papillomavirus infections (Gupta et al., 2004). There is also a growing evidence to indicate therapeutic interest in TLR7/TLR8 agonists for cancer treatment. As such, imiquimod is now also used as a treatment for cancer and has shown itself to be efficacious against primary skin tumors and cutaneous metastases (Schon and

Schon, 2008). In fact, imiquimod has been approved for the treatment of external genital and perianal warts, but has also been found to be effective for a host of other virus-associated dermatologic lesions, including common and flat warts, molluscum contagiosum and herpes simplex. Oncological lesions showing improvement with the use of imiquimod include basal cell carcinoma, actinic keratosis, squamous cell carcinoma in situ, malignant melanoma, cutaneous T-cell lymphoma, and cutaneous extramammary Paget's disease (Berman et al., 2002; Miller et al., 2008). A number of studies suggest that activation of TLR7 would be beneficial in patients infected with hepatitis C virus (HCV). One study has shown that TLR7 is expressed in normal and HCV infected hepatocytes; and, activation of TLR7 alone reduces HCV mRNA and protein levels (Lee et al., 2006). An oral prodrug of isatoribine, ANA975 was developed as an antiviral HCV treatment but clinical studies for this TLR7 agonist were discontinued by Anadys Pharmaceuticals due to indicated unacceptable toxicity via long term animal studies (Fletcher et al., 2006). Though the drug candidate produced intense immune stimulation, its chronic administration would have been inadvisable. Further studies with different dosing strategy are necessary to determine whether there will be any advantage of TLR therapy over the current option.

Cytosine-phosphate-guanosine oligodinucleotide (CpG-ODN), the common TLR9 agonist has shown substantial potential as vaccine adjuvants, and as mono- or combination therapies for the treatment of cancer, infectious and allergic diseases (Vollmer and Krieg, 2009). Phase I and II clinical trials have indicated that CpG-ODNs have antitumor activity as single agents and enhance the development of antitumor T-cell responses when used as therapeutic vaccine adjuvants. CpG-ODNs have shown benefit in multiple rodent and primate models of asthma and other allergic diseases, with encouraging results in some early human clinical trials. Though their potential clinical contributions are enormous, the safety and efficacy of these TLR9 agonists in humans remain to be determined. Chikh et al. (2009) reported that both methylated and unmethylated CpG ODN acts through a common receptor signaling pathway, specifically via TLR9 to initiate potent immune responses. It seems that CpG ODN holds great potential in further clinical development. Pfizer's agatolimod, a CpG oligonucleotide, selectively targets TLR9, thereby activating dendritic and B cells and stimulating cytotoxic T cell and antibody responses against tumor cells bearing tumor antigens. This product is in Phase II trials in breast and renal cancers, asthma, allergies and hepatitis-B virus infection. One of the Phase II trials "Agatolimod and Trastuzumab in Treating Patients With Locally Advanced or Metastatic Breast Cancer" registered through the http://clinicaltrials.gov website is currently in enrollment stage and will evaluate if monoclonal antibodies, such as trastuzumab, can block tumor growth and kill more tumor

cells via concurrent administration of agatolimod for the locally advanced or metastatic breast cancer. However, the drug's clinical development for advanced non-small cell lung carcinoma (NSCLC) was discontinued after an independent Data Safety Monitoring Board (DSMB) found that trial data did not show increased efficacy over standard chemotherapy alone. This is not the only CpG oligonucleotide targeting TLR9 that has failed to live up to expectations for Pfizer; CpG-10101 was suspended at Phase II, when it failed to show efficacy in treating hepatitis C (Coyne, 2008). It seems important to realize that TLR agonist may not work equally well on different clinical indications. Pfizer has had more success using oligonucleotide TLR9 agonists as vaccine adjuvants; its vaccine adjuvant CpGTLR9 is currently in Phase III trials with GlaxoSmithKline's MAGE-A3 cancer vaccine. It is therefore proposed that use as adjuvants is the most promising avenue for TLR agonists due to low dosing requirement.

Drugs or antibodies inhibiting toll like receptors

Antagonists of lipid A have been under clinical development before the discovery of TLRs as treatments for Gram-negative sepsis and endotoxemia (Leon et al., 2008). The following analogs or natural molecules E5564 (eritoran), curcumin, auranofin (an antirheumatic gold compound), cinnamaldehyde, and acrolein are just a few of the sample candidates currently under investigation. For instance, Acrolein with an alpha, beta-unsaturated carbonyl group inhibits LPS-induced homodimerization of TLR4 (Lee et al., 2008). Small molecules that inhibit MyD88 binding to TLR4 are also emerging. Cell-penetrating peptides fused with the BB loop (a highly conserved sequence in the TIR that is situated between the second -strand and the second helix) sequences of TLR2 and TLR4 also inhibit LPS-induced signaling, probably by interfering with either receptor dimerization or adapter recruitment (Toshchakov et al., 2007). Treatment of patients with sepsis with anti-inflammatory therapies has so far not been beneficial (Rittirsch et al., 2008); therefore, it will be of interest to ascertain the clinical efficacy of inhibiting TLR4/MD-2 activity in sepsis. Numerous diseases such as sepsis, diabetes, rheumatoid arthritis, and cardiovascular diseases, seem to be associated with both TLR2 and TLR4; therefore, Mal seems to be an attractive therapeutic target for these diseases (O'Neill et al., 2009). Blocking TLR2 or TLR4 with a neutralizing antibody seems to be another promising route of drug discoveries. One such antibody, T2.5, has been shown to prevent sepsis induced by TLR2 ligands (Meng et al., 2004); furthermore, when T2.5 is used in combination with an anti-TLR4/MD-2 antibody, it protects mice against sepsis induced by Salmonella enterica or *Escherichia coli* when given with antibiotics (Spiller et al., 2008). This latter finding suggests that a combination approach involving anti-TLR4 and anti-TLR2 might be an effective adjunct to antibiotics in the prevention or treatment of sepsis. It is well known that combination medication in clinical practice is not an uncommon application. Another TLR4 antagonist, Eisai's eritoran tetrasodium, has reached Phase III trials for the treatment of sepsis and septic shock. In Phase I trials it proved its ability to dose-dependently inhibit TNFα production. Though the results from Phase II trials were not outstanding, it remains to be seen how the drug will perform in the larger scale Phase III trial (Coyne, 2008).

TLR3 antagonist may be beneficial in treating West Nile virus (WNV) infection. Infection of macrophages or DCs by WNV in peripheral lymphoid tissue induces TLR3-dependent secretion of TNFα and results in a transient increase in the permeability of the blood-brain barrier (BBB), facilitating the penetration of WNV across the BBB and into the CNS. It is clear that TLR3 activation is vital to the passage of the virus into the CNS (Wang et al., 2004). Therefore, inhibition of TLR3 signaling and the subsequent reduction in TNFα may be effective treating persons infected with WNV. However, this needs to be confirmed by further animal model, pre-clinical, or clinical studies.

Current therapies for systemic lupus erythematosus (SLE) are general immunosuppressants often leading to a host of serious adverse effects. TLR-targeted therapy may represent a more targeted approach. TLR9 and/or TLR7 antagonist may provide therapeutic benefits to SLE by inhibiting the production of anti-nuclear immune complex, interferon-α, and TLR activation (Kim et al., 2009; Kalia and Dutz, 2007). Recent data supports that several suppressive oligodeoxynucleotides (ODNs) block IFNα and reduce symptoms in SLE murine models, therefore representing a promising therapeutic agent for SLE (Barrat et al., 2007). Dynavax Technologies' TLR7/9 antagonist, IRS954, has shown early signs of efficacy; in a murine model of lupus, it reduced serum levels of nucleic acid-specific antibodies and decreased proteinurea, glomerularnephritis and end-organ damage, demonstrating an overall survival benefit.

Asthma is a human disease characterized by a massive accumulation of eosinophils that release an array of tissue-damaging mediators. Respiratory viral infections are thought to be a leading cause of exacerbations of asthma. One possible explanation might be a direct activation of viral components through TLRs. The virus-recognizing TLRs are TLR3, TLR7/8 and TLR9, which respond to viral dsRNA, ssRNA and CpG-DNA. Mansson and Cardell (2008) investigated the expression of these TLRs and their functions in human eosinophils and showed that Poly (I:C), R-837 and CpG directly activate eosinophils through their TLRs pointing this system represents a clinical target for the resolution of asthmatic disease. A recent interesting finding in relation to TLR4 and disease concerns allergy caused by airborne allergens. Derp2, the key allergen from the

house dust mite, has been shown to be structurally similar to MD-2 and acts to deliver LPS to TLR4 in airways, thereby provoking inflammation (Trompette et al., 2009). This might be a common mechanism, because several airborne allergens are lipid-binding proteins and might act analogously. This makes TLR4 an interesting target for allergy in the airways. Any potential interventional success in this area will generate huge benefits to the allergic population.

Inhibitors of NF-kB function

Given that hyperactivation of NF-kB has a central role in the development and progression of cancer and chronic inflammatory disorders, a substantial amount of effort has been put in to developing strategies that block NF-kB signaling (Sethi and Tergaonkar, 2009). More than 700 compounds have been reported to inhibit NF-kB activation (Gilmore and Herscovitch, 2006). These NF-kB inhibitors include small molecules, biologics, inhibitory peptides, antisense RNAs, and natural agents blocking various steps leading to NF-kB activation. They may be classified further depending where in the signaling steps the inhibitory effect is exerted.

One of the drugs currently used for the treatment of chronic myelogenous leukemia is arsenic trioxide (ATO) as Fowler's solution. A multicenter trial in the USA in patients with relapsed acute promyelocytic leukemia found a complete response rate of 85% (Niu et al., 1999); and, ATO has been approved by the FDA for the indication since 2001. ATO is being evaluated in ongoing clinical trials in patients with other hematological and solid tumors. Preliminary evidence of some activity in patients with multiple myeloma has been reported (Hussein et al., 2004). Several newer classes of chemotherapeutics have been developed that were intended, at least in part, to target NF-kB. The best example is the proteasome inhibitor bortezomib (Velcade, Millenium Pharmaceuticals), approved by the USA-FDA for clinical use in 2003 for relapsed multiple myeloma refractory to conventional therapy (Kane et al., 2003). Because proteasome inhibition impacts many signaling pathways, it is not clear whether the therapeutic effects of bortezomib are mediated by inhibition of NF-kB activation. However, numerous preclinical studies with bortezomib have shown that proteasome inhibition blocks activation of NF-kB and enhances the effects of chemotherapeutic drugs, including Camptothecin-11 (Adams, 2002). Bortezomib is currently undergoing further clinical development in hematological malignancies and solid tumors, as a single agent and in combination with conventional chemotherapeutic drugs and new agents. Anti-TNF antibodies (e.g. Humira) and a soluble TNF receptor (e.g. Enbrel), approved by the FDA, have also been shown to suppress NF-kB activation in patients with arthritis and inflammatory bowel disease

(Gaddy and Robbins, 2008). Drugs like Humira have helped many arthritis patients by relieving pain, improving joint function, and slowing disease progression. Humira is a fully human monoclonal antibody, meaning it is manufactured in a laboratory using human proteins, and no animal proteins thus pointing another drug targeting strategies in TLRs. Because NF-kB is an important target in the IL-1β signal transduction pathway, inhibition of IL-1β also inhibits NF-kB activation. Additionally, ongoing research has also prompted new signal pathways and furthered our understanding in disease pathogenesis, pharmacotherapeutic targeting, and systematic balancing mechanisms. A study by Koga et al (2008) shows that *Streptococcus pneumoniae* (*S. pneumoniae*) activates nuclear factor of activated T cells (NFAT) transcription factor independently of TLR2 and 4, brings new insights into the molecular pathogenesis of *S. pneumoniae* infections through the NFAT-dependent mechanism and further identify gene tumor suppressor cylindromatosis as a negative regulator for NFAT signaling, thereby opening up new therapeutic targets for these diseases.

Directions in TLRs therapeutic development

Many attempts to use TLR manipulation for the treatment of infectious, allergic and autoimmune diseases, as well as cancer, are in the early clinical phases, and results have not been always positive. One successful TLR candidate is Ampligen, a mismatched, double-stranded RNA which activates TLR3 and is currently awaiting registration in the US for the treatment of chronic fatigue syndrome (CFS), an illness that is not fully understood, but often seems to be associated with viral infection (Gowen et al., 2007). Ampligen new drug application (NDA) was filed, but marketing for the treatment of CFS has not yet been approved. Ampligen is received intravenously. It is generally administered twice weekly for periods of one year or greater. Two toxicology studies were recently completed that establish the safety of intranasal and intramucosal methods of Ampligen administration. Hemispherx Biopharma reports that it is currently researching an oral drug that uses nucleic acid technology related to Ampligen (Hemispherx Biopharma Inc R&D. Drug candidates - Ampligen®). Aditionally, Ampligen is in Phase II development for HIV and hepatitis infections, as well as for cancer treatment indicating the sponsor company's active development interest for multiple challenging indications.

While TLRs are able to recognize viral PAMPs, the exact action mechanism is complex and involves multiple key signal pathways and participant molecules/genes. Moreover, an increasing number of host breakdown products from the extracellular matrix such as hyaluron, intracellular components released when cells rupture, and products of proteolytic cascades are all able to stimulate TLRs, suggesting TLRs' function in sensing

tissue damage signals caused by disease, stimuli or injury. Recognition of these products by TLRs leads to the activation/recruitment of immune cells and cytokines that repair the tissue damage. There are already drugs in the pipeline for tissue regeneration applications, such as Clinquest's TLR3 agonist CQ-07001, an endogenous human protein, currently in clinical development for anti-inflammatory and tissue regeneration applications (Clinquest Group BV openPR. Clinquest obtains exclusive worldwide rights to clinical development and commercialization - Amsterdam, the Netherlands, 06-03-2007). Progress in this relative new area may provide hint on developing new treatment strategies for several challenging diseases such as coronary myocardial infarction. Great strides are being made worldwide in our ability to synthesize and assemble nanoscale building blocks to create advanced materials with novel properties and functionalities. The novel properties of nanostructures are derived from their confined sizes and their very large surface-to-volume ratios. A fundamental issue in much of nanomedicine, and especially tissue regeneration, is to understand and to eventually control nanostructure-biomolecule interactions (Nuffer and Siegel, 2009).

Accumulating evidence indicates that TLRs seem to be implicated in many unmet medical conditions due to the fact that many TLR induced cytokines are well manifested in these diseases. A number of strategies may be considered to alter TLRs, including agonists, antagonists, neutralizing antibodies, and signal transduction inhibitors or regulators. Neutralizing antibodies to TLRs may be possible, but only for those on the cell surface, such as TLR2, TLR4, and TLR5. TLRs typically initiate pathologic conditions in the event of microbe invasion or stimuli with the ensuing inflammation leading to the production of endogenous ligands, further propagating inflammation. The two discreet signaling pathways (Mal/MyD88 and TRAM/TRIF) offer targets for selective modulation of TLR activity. The precise clinical goal of modifying TLR activity remains a challenging question (Beutler, 2004). We may have a partial agonist or a drug identified *in vitro* that selectively stimulates TRAM/TRIF signaling. But, such results are hard to be expected *in vivo* or in clinical studies when multiple other factors must be considered. Species differences in the response to different agonists at TLR4 suggest that caution needs to be exercised in developing safe new drugs with well planned preclinical and early stage clinical studies. It is critical to select objective study outcomes, analyze clinical end points, and drug safety from a contextual systems approach. It is imperative to run controlled randomized studies to minimize bias. Drug safety seems to cause a lot more damages in later study stages; and, it must be emphasized to conduct a full toxicity analysis in preclinical and phase 1 studies and ensure proper safety data monitoring, data collection, and independent adverse event adjudication. Other notable pointers for running a clinical study such as therapeutic indication for the selected patient population, dosing (exposure), the measurable indicators (molecular, cellular, and *in vivo*), assessment of patients' prior medical history, baseline characteristics, functional modalities, and even patient reported outcome and quality of life, must all be considered to conduct evaluation of the efficacy and adverse effects associated with the medical regimens. All these details must be clearly planned, reviewed, defined, and deemed feasible in the clinical protocol prior to seeking institutional review board (IRB) approval to conduct a clinical study. In conducting clinical studies, the will to initiate and be creative will be primary, the study design secondary, and collecting and analyzing data critical to accept or reject the research hypothesis. The goal is to achieve the expected efficacy with acceptable adverse event profile.

Small-molecule antagonists seem to present a promising prospect, though these are not traditional "drug-like" molecules. One concern, however, is that such inhibitors might block multiple TLRs and therefore gives rise to unwanted immunosuppression. In addition, adjuvancy study seems to yield new agents. More adjuvants may be expected to improve vaccine efficacy or have antitumor effects. In terms of antagonism, we have data beyond phase II for only one TLR inhibitor - eritoran. As described, its effects were significant but somewhat marginal (Parkinson, 2008). Based on the literature reviewed, it reasons to state that manipulating the activity of TLRs to modulate immune responses for therapeutic intervention has created strong interest in the pharmaceutical industry. The focus has been largely in the areas of infectious diseases, cancer, allergic diseases and vaccine adjuvants. Though initial clinical trials for infectious diseases and cancer showed early promise, longer-term trials have not always been positive and more research is required to find dosing regimes that balance efficacy with acceptable side-effect profiles and suitable indications. So far, the clinical data indicates that TLR agonists as vaccine adjuvants seem to hold greater potential and have less safety concerns than for other applications.

Though it is hard to predict where therapeutic targeting TLRs is going, we have some promising data and late phase trials on the horizon, where the fundamental research and development have never been stopped. To further develop more effective TLR therapeutic targeting strategy, there are a few more tasks: further identifying and determining the pathogenesis of challenging medical conditions such as virus infection, allergy, cancer, and SLE; analysis of genetic sequence, molecular structure, epigenetic observations, and functional activities on both animal model and human clinical studies; design of clinical study based on study indication, dosing regimens, drug delivery route or format consideration, and pharmacokinetics; timely and objective assessment of adverse events with details. With the insights of all these revealed, disease occurring mechanisms on genetic, molecular,

functional and *in vivo* levels for challenging pathologic conditions may be defined (Chen et al., 2009). Target driven molecular, drug or biological interventions may further be designed and developed to act on specific receptor or sub-unit, cellular signaling or metabolic pathways to induce therapeutic cure.

REFERENCES

Adams J (2002). Proteasome inhibition: A novel approach to cancer therapy. Trends Mol. Med. 8: S49–S54.

Akira S, Hemmi H (2003). Recognition of pathogen-associated molecular patterns by TLR family. Immunol. Lett. 85: 85-95.

Andersen-Nissen E, Smith KD, Bonneau R, Strong RK, Aderem A (2007). A conserved surface on Toll-like receptor 5 recognizes bacterial flagellin. J. Exp. Med. 204: 393–403.

Barrat FJ, Meeker T, Chan JH, Guiducci C, Coffman RL (2007). Treatment of lupus-prone mice with a dual inhibitor of TLR7 and TLR9 leads to reduction of autoantibody production and amelioration of disease symptoms. Eur. J. Immunol. 37: 3582–3586.

Berman B, Poochareon VN, Villa AM (2002). Novel Dermatologic Uses of the Immune Response Modifier Imiquimod 5% Cream. Skin Ther. Lett. 7: 1-6.

Beutler B (2004). Inferences, questions and possibilities in Toll-like receptor signaling. Nature 430: 257-263.

Blander JM (2007). Coupling Toll like receptor signaling with phagocytosis: potentiation of antigen presentation. Trends Immunol. 28: 19–25.

Burdelya LG, Krivokrysenko VI, Tallant TC (2008). An agonist of Toll like receptor 5 has radioprotective activity in mouse and primate models. Science 320: 226–230.

Casella CR, Mitchell TC (2008). Putting endotoxin to work for us: monophosphoryl lipid A as a safe and effective vaccine adjuvant. Cell. Mol. Life Sci. 65: 3231–3340.

Chen XC, Zhang MX, Zhu XY (2009). Engagement of Toll-like receptor 2 on CD4+ T cells facilitates local immune responses in patients with tuberculous pleurisy. J. Infect. Dis. 200: 399–408.

Chikh G, de Jong SD, Sekirov L (2009). Synthetic methylated CpG ODNs are potent *in vivo* adjuvants when delivered in liposomal nanoparticles. Int. Immunol. 21: 757-767.

Coyne L (2008). Target Analysis - Toll-like Receptors. Pharmaprojects. 29: 1-4.

Fletcher S, Steffy K, Averett D (2006). Masked oral prodrugs of Toll like receptor 7 agonists: A new approach for the treatment of infectious disease. Curr Opin Inv. Drugs. 7: 702–708.

Gaddy DF, Robbins PD (2008). Current status of gene therapy for rheumatoid arthritis. Curr. Rheumatol. Rpt. 10: 398-404.

Gilmore TD, Herscovitch M (2006). Inhibitors of NF-kB signaling: 785 and counting. Oncogene 25: 6887–6899.

Gowen BB, Wong MH, Jung KH (2007). TLR3 is essential for the induction of protective immunity against Punta Toro virus infection by the double-stranded RNA (dsRNA), poly(I:C12U), but not poly(I:C) Differential recognition of synthetic dsRNA molecules. J. Immunol. 178: 5200-5208.

Guo BC, Cheng GH (2007). Modulation of the interferon antiviral response by the TBK1/IKKi adaptor protein TANK. J. Biol. Chem 282: 11817-11826.

Gupta AK, Cherman AM, Tyring SK (2004). Viral and nonviral uses of imiquimod: a review. J. Cutan. Med. Surg. 8: 338–352.

Huleatt JW, Nakaar V, Desai P (2008). Potent immunogenicity and efficacy of a universal influenza vaccine candidate comprising a recombinant fusion protein linking influenza M2e to the TLR5 ligand flagellin. Vaccine 26: 201–214.

Hussein MA, Saleh M, Ravandi F, Mason J, Rifkin RM, Ellison R (2004). Phase 2 study of arsenic trioxide in patients with relapsed or refractory multiple myeloma. Br. J. Haematol. 125: 470–476.

Ishii KJ, Akira S (2007). Toll or Toll-Free Adjuvant Path Toward the Optimal Vaccine Development. J. Clin. Immunol. 27: 363-371.

Janssens S, Beyaert R (2003). Role of Toll-Like Receptors in Pathogen

Recognition. Clin. Microbiol. Rev. 16: 637–646.

Kalia S, Dutz JP (2007). New concepts in antimalarial use and mode of action in dermatology. Dermatol. Ther. 20: 160–174.

Kane RC, Bross PR, Farrell AT, Pazdur R (2003). Velcade®: U.S. FDA approval for the treatment of multiple myeloma progressing on prior therapy. Oncologist 8: 508–513.

Kawai T, Akira S (2009). The roles of TLRs, RLRs and NLRs in pathogen recognition. Int. Immunol. 21: 317-337.

Kim WU, Sreih A, Bucala R (2009). Toll-like receptors in systemic lupus erythematosus; prospects for therapeutic intervention. Autoimmun. Rev. 8: 204-208.

Koga T, Lim JH, Jono H (2008). Tumor Suppressor Cylindromatosis Acts as a Negative Regulator for Streptococcus pneumoniae-induced NFAT Signaling. J. Biol. Chem. 283: 12546–12554.

Lee J, Wu CC, Lee KJ (2006). Activation of anti-hepatitis C virus responses via Toll like receptor 7. Proc. Natl. Acad. Sci. USA 103: 1828–1833.

Lee JS, Lee JY, Lee MY, Hwang DH, Youn HS (2008). Acrolein with an alpha, beta-unsaturated carbonyl group inhibits LPS-induced homodimerization of toll like receptor 4. Mol. Cells 25: 253–257.

Leon CG, Tory R, Jia J, Sivak O, Wasan KM (2008). Discovery and Development of Toll-Like Receptor 4 (TLR4) Antagonists: A New Paradigm for Treating Sepsis and Other Diseases. Pharm. Res. 25: 1751–1761.

Li QT, Withoff S, Verma IM (2005). Inflammation-associated cancer: NF-ᴋB is the lynchpin. Trends Immunol. 26: 318-325.

Lombardi V, Van Overtvelt L, Horiot S, Moussu H, Chabre H, Louise A, Balazuc AM, Mascarell L, Moingeon P (2008). Toll-like receptor 2 agonist Pam3CSK4 enhances the induction of antigen-specific tolerance via the sublingual route. Clin. Exp. Allergy 38: 1705-1706.

Mansson A, Cardell LO (2008). Activation of eosinophils via Toll like receptor (TLR)3, TLR7 and TLR9: link between viral infection and asthma? Eur. Resp. Rev. 17: 46-48.

Mata-Haro V, Cekic C, Martin M, Chilton PM, Casella CR, Mitchell TC (2007). The vaccine adjuvant monophosphoryl lipid A as a TRIF-biased agonist of TLR4. Science 316: 1628–1632.

Meng G, Rutz M, Schiemann M (2004). Antagonistic antibody prevents toll like receptor 2- driven lethal shock-like syndromes. J. Clin. Inv. 113: 1473–1481.

Miller RL, Meng TC, Tomai MA (2008). The antiviral activity of Toll like receptor 7 and 7/8 agonists. Drug News Perspect. 21: 69–87.

Niu C, Yan H, Yu T (1999). Studies on treatment of acute promyelocytic leukemia with arsenic trioxide: remission induction, follow-up, and molecular monitoring in 11 newly diagnosed and 47 relapsed acute promyelocytic leukemia patients. Blood 94: 3315-3324.

Nuffer J, Siegel R (2009). Nanostructure–Biomolecule Interactions: Implications for Tissue Regeneration and Nanomedicine. Tissue Engineering Part A. (in press).

O'Neill LA, Bryant CE, Doyle SL (2009). Therapeutic Targeting of Toll-Like Receptors for Infectious and Inflammatory Diseases and Cancer. Pharmacol. Rev. 61: 177-197.

Parkinson T (2008). The future of toll-like receptor therapeutics. Curr. Opin. Mol. Ther. 10: 21-31.

Pulendran B (2007). Tolls and Beyond - Many Roads to Vaccine Immunity. NEJM. 356: 1776- 1778.

Rittirsch D, Flierl MA, Ward PA (2008). Harmful molecular mechanisms in sepsis. Nat. Rev. Immunol. 10: 776–787.

Schon MP, Schon M (2008). TLR7 and TLR8 as targets in cancer therapy. Oncogene 27: 190–199.

Sethi G, Tergaonkar V (2009). Potential pharmacological control of the NF-kB pathway. Trends Pharmacol. Sci. 30: 313-321.

Spiller S, Elson G, Ferstl R (2008). TLR4-induced IFN-gamma production increases TLR2 sensitivity and drives Gram-negative sepsis in mice. J. Exp. Med. 205: 1747–1754.

Toshchakov VY, Fenton MJ, Vogel SN (2007). Cutting Edge: Differential inhibition of TLR signaling pathways by cell-permeable peptides representing BB loops of TLRs. J. Immunol. 178: 2655–2660.

Trompette A, Divanovic S, Visintin A (2009). Allergenicity resulting from functional mimicry of a Toll like receptor complex protein. Nature 457: 585–588.

Vollmer J, Krieg AM (2009). Immunotherapeutic applications of CpG oligodeoxynucleotide TLR9 agonists. Adv. Drug. Deliv. Rev. 61: 195-204.

Wang T, Town T, Alexopoulou L, Anderson JF, Fikrig E, Flavell RA (2004). Toll like receptor 3 mediates West Nile virus entry into the brain causing lethal encephalitis. Nat. Med.10: 1366–1373.

Waltenbaugh C, Doan T, Melvold R, Viselli S (2008). Immunology. Lippincott's Illustrated reviews. Philadelphia: Wolters Kluwer Health/Lippincott Williams & Wilkins pp. 17.

12

Antifungal activity of aqueous and ethanolic extracts of *Picralima nitida* seeds on *Aspergillus flavus, Candida albicans* and *Microsporum canis*

Peace Ubulom[1]*, Ekaete Akpabio[1], Chinweizu Ejikeme udobi[2] and Ruth Mbon[1]

[1]Faculty of Pharmacy, University of Uyo, Akwa Ibom State, Nigeria.
[2]College of Science and Technology, Kaduna Polytechnic, Kaduna, Nigeria.

Aqueous and ethanolic extracts of *Picralima nitida seeds* were tested for their antifungal activities using *Aspergillus flavus, Candida albicans* and *Microsporum canis* as test organisms. Phytochemical analysis revealed the presence of some plant metabolites which have been reported to have antimicrobial effects. Assays were performed using extract concentrations of 25, 50, 100 and 200 mg/ml and the agar well diffusion technique was employed. Results obtained, revealed a significant difference ($P<0.05$) in inhibition zone diameter between *A. flavus,* and *C. albicans* and between *C. albicans* and *M. canis.* However, there was no significant difference ($P>0.05$) in inhibition zone diameter between *A. flavus* and *M. canis.* With the aqueous seed extract, a significant difference ($P<0.05$) in inhibition zone diameter was observed between *A. flavus* and *C. albicans* and between *A. flavus* and *M. canis* but there was no significant difference ($P>0.05$) in inhibition zone diameter between *C. albicans* and *M. canis.* The inhibitory activity of the ethanolic extract on each test organism was compared with that of the aqueous extract and in all cases the observed difference was significant ($P<0.05$). These findings indicate the potentials of the seeds of *P. nitida* as panacea for some fungal infections.

Key words: Antifungal activity, aqueous extract, ethanolic extract, *Picralima nitida* seeds.

INTRODUCTION

Humans everywhere in the world are still plagued by a myriad of ailments and infections with microorganisms (including fungi) causing a good number of them. Inspite of the availability of drugs for treatment, diseases of microbial origin remain a scourge. The use of herbal medicine in the treatment of infection with microorganisms predates the introduction of antibiotics (Owoyale et al., 2005). Herbalists have claimed that certain ailments and infections which have defied western medicine can be cured with local herbs. As such they have used different plant parts in the treatment of various infections. Discovery of active principles in plants have given credence to the idea that integration of traditional medicine into the health care delivery would be very promising and should therefore be encouraged. Several medicinal plants have been screened for their activity on different species of microorganisms. Ibrahim and Osman (1995) screened *Cassia alata* from Malaysia for antimicrobial activity. Their report indicated that the plant demonstrated high activity against dermatophytic fungi, including *Microsporum canis* (MIC: 25 mg/ml). Owoyale et al. (2005) evaluated the antifungal and antibacterial activities of alcoholic extracts of *Senna alata* leaves. Wokoma et al. (2007) reported on the *in vitro* antifungal activity of *Allium sativum* and *Allium cepa* extracts against dermatophytes and yeast. The antimicrobial activity of ethanolic and aqueous extracts of *Sida acuta* on microorganisms from skin infections has been documented by Ekpo and Etim (2009).

Picralima comprises a single specie-*Picralima nitida* and belongs to the family Apocynaceae. It is a tree that grows up to 35 m tall with white latex in all parts. The leaves are opposite, simple and entire. It is restricted to Africa and throughout its distribution area, the seeds, stem bark and roots have a reputation as a febrifuge and remedy for malaria. They are also extensively used for

*Corresponding author. E-mail: upema84@yahoo.com.

pain relief and to treat chest and stomach problems, pneumonia and intestinal worms. The biological activities of the plant, *P. nitida* have been reported by researchers such as Nkere and Iroegbu (2005) and Okokon et al. (2007). Although as aforementioned, so much has been documented on the biological activities of the different parts of *P. nitida*, but there is a paucity of information on its activity against *Aspergillus flavus* (one of the causative agents of aspergillosis), *Candida albicans* (the most common cause of candidiasis) and *Microsporum canis*, a tinea causal organism.

This study was therefore designed to evaluate the inhibitory effect of crude ethanolic and aqueous extracts of the seeds of *P. nitida* on *A. flavus*, *C. albicans* and *M. canis*.

EXPERIMENTAL

Collection of plant materials

The seeds of *P. nitida* used in this study were obtained from Anua Obio in Uyo Local Government Area of Akwa Ibom State. The plant was authenticated at the Department of Botany and Ecological Studies, University of Uyo and a voucher specimen with herbarium number Ubulom UUH 875 (Uyo) was deposited in the herbarium of the same department for further referencing.

Preparation of extracts

The plant parts were first of all dried on laboratory tables at room temperature (27 ± 2°C). They were later pulverized using the crusher machine in the pilot plant unit of National Institute for Pharmaceutical Research and Development (NIPRD) Abuja. 100 g each of the pulverized seeds were macerated separately in distilled water and 50% ethanol, for 72 h, with periodic stirring. Each extract was filtered repeatedly using a sterile muslin cloth, cotton wool and filter paper. This was to get rid of the marc. All aqueous filtrates were concentrated using a lyophilizer at the freeze drying unit of NIPRD, Abuja. Ethanolic filtrates were concentrated in vacuo at 40°C, using a rotary evaporator. All extracts were stored in a refrigerator at 4°C until used for the experiments reported in this study. The percentage yield of each extract was also determined.

Phytochemical screening

The extracts of *P. nitida* seeds were screened for their phytochemical components, using the methods described by Harborne (1984), Evans (2002) and Sofowora (2006). The plant metabolites that were tested for were alkaloids, anthraquinones, cardiac glycosides, flavonoids, saponins, phlobatannins, tannins and terpenes.

Test microorganisms

Test organisms *A. flavus*, *C. albicans* and *M. canis* used in this study were laboratory isolates obtained from the Department of Microbiology, University of Uyo. These fungal specimens were separately plated out on sterilized Sabouraud Dextrose Agar (Biomark). They were purified after isolation through repeated subculturing and characterized using the methods of Collins and Lyne (1970) and Cruickshank et al. (1975). They were

subsequently stored in agar slants in the refrigerator at 4°C, until used for the experiments reported in this study.

Antifungal assay

The extracts were screened for antifungal property using the agar well diffusion technique. Standardized inoculum (1×10^6 cfu/ml) of each test fungus was spread on to sterile Sabouraud dextrose agar plate so as to achieve a confluent growth. The plates were allowed to dry and a sterile cork borer of diameter 6 mm was used to bore wells in the agar plates. From a stock solution, different concentrations of the extracts were prepared (200, 100, 50 and 2 5 mg/ml) and were separately introduced into the wells. Each extract concentration was replicated thrice. In all cases of preparation of extract solution, appropriate volumes of the solvent dimethyl sulphoxide (DMSO) were used to achieve solubilisation and required concentrations of the extracts. The plates were allowed to stand for 1 h for diffusion to take place and then were incubated at room temperature (27± 2°C), for 48 h. The external diameters of visible zones of growth inhibition were measured after incubation. A positive control was set up using separate plate. The assay in this case consisted of each test organism and the drug, ketoconazole at a concentration of 30 mg/ml. Negative control consisted of test organism each in separate plate and distilled water. These plates were also incubated at room temperature (27± 2°C) for 48 h. These controls were set up in triplicate too. The mean inhibition zone diameter was determined in each case.

Statistical analysis

Data obtained from this study were statistically analyzed using one way analysis of variance (ANOVA) and t-test.

RESULTS

The yield of the ethanolic and aqueous extracts of *P. nitida* seeds were 8.76 and 11.08% w/w respectively.

Phytochemical analysis of the extract of *P. nitida* seeds revealed the presence of alkaloids, cardiac glycosides, flavonoids, saponins, tannins and terpenes (Table 1).

The inhibitory activities of extracts of P. nitida on the fungal species tested are shown in Figure 1. Generally, the zone of inhibition increased with increase in concentration of extract. The aqueous extract of *P. nitida* seeds inhibited *A. flavus* with inhibition zone diameter ranging from 8 to 15 mm. For *C. albicans* it was 8 to 13 mm, but the least extract concentration (25 mg/ml) did not show any inhibition. For *M. canis*, the zone of inhibition ranged from 6 to 18 mm. The least extract concentration (25 mg/ml) also did not inhibit the growth of *M. canis*. However, significant inhibition was observed in all cases with ethanolic extract of *P.nitida* seeds. The zone of inhibition ranged from 11 to 20, 5 to 15 and 13 to 25 mm for *A. flavus*, *C. albicans* and *M. canis* respectively, but the least extract concentration (25 mg/ml) did not inhibit the growth of *M. canis*. Inhibition of test fungal species was observed in all cases with the use of the standard drug (ketoconazole) as positive control (Figure 1). No inhibition was observed in the negative control. In conclusion, the fungal species used in this study showed

Table 1. Phytochemical constituents of the extract of *P.nitida* seeds.

Phytochemical constituent	Test	Seed extract
Alkaloids	Dragendorff's	+
Anthraquinones		
free Anthraquinones	Borntrager's	-
combined anthraquinones	Borntrager's	-
Cardiac glycosides	Salkowski's	+
Flavonoids	Shinoda's reduction test	+
Saponins	Froth	+
Tannins	Ferric chloride	+
Phlobatannins	Hydrochlonc acid	-
Terpenes	Liebermann – Burchard	+

Legend: + = Detected, - = Not detected.

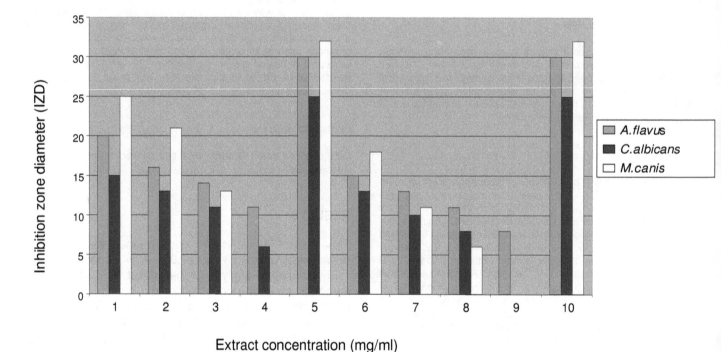

Figure 1. Effect of different concentrations of aqueous and ethanolic extracts of *P. nitida* seeds on test organisms. Key: 1 – 5 show results obtained due to the activity of ethanolic seed extracts. 6 – 10 show results obtained due to the activity of aqueous seed extracts. 1 = 200 mg/ml, 2 = 100 mg/ml, 3 = 50 mg/ml, 4 = 25 mg/ml, 5 = ketoconazole (30 mg/ml), 6 =200 mg/ml, 7 =100 mg/ml, 8 = 50 mg/ml, 9 =25 mg/ml 10 = Ketoconazole (30 mg/ml).

variable sensitivity to extracts of *P. nitida*.

Results obtained from this study were statistically analyzed using one way ANOVA and t-test. ANOVA was used to determine the significance of difference in inhibitory activity of the extracts on the test organisms. T-test was used to compare the effect of the extracts on each test organism. Analysis of results of antifungal assays involving the ethanolic extract revealed that there was significant difference ($P<0.05$) in inhibition zone diameter between *A. flavus* and *C. albicans* and between

C. albicans and M. canis. However, there was no significant difference ($P>0.05$) in inhibition zone diameter between *A. flavus* and *M. canis*. With the aqueous extract significant difference ($P<0.05$) in inhibition zone diameter IZD was observed between *A. flavus* and *C. albicans* and between *A. flavus* and *M. canis*. However, there was no significant difference ($P>0.05$) in inhibition zone diameter IZD between *C. albicans* and *M. canis*. Also the inhibitory activity of the ethanolic extract was compared with that of the aqueous extract, using t-test. For *A.*

flavus, the difference in activity between the ethanolic and aqueous extract was very significant (P<0.05). The difference between the inhibitory activity of the ethanolic and aqueous extracts was also significant (P<0.05), for *C. albicans* and *M. canis*.

DISCUSSION

The use of water and alcohol for extraction in this research is in consonance with folkloric practice. The percentage yield of extracts used in this study varied with the solvent used for extraction. However, the yield was low when compared with the amount of pulverized plant part used for extraction. This is attributable to the method of extraction employed (maceration). Maceration has been reported to result in low extract yield compared to soxhlet and other methods of extraction (Ibrahim et al., 1997), but it was preferred in this research because it does not require heating, thus preserving thermolabile components. The aqueous extract had higher yield than the ethanolic extract, suggesting a higher proportion of water-soluble components in the seeds of *P. nitida*.

Phytochemical screening revealed the presence of certain plant metabolites (Table 1), which have been reported in other studies to elicit inhibitory effect on microorganisms (Leven et al., 1979). These phytochemicals may have caused the observed inhibitory effect either singly or in synergy with each other. This requires further investigation. Also, Reyes–Chilpa et al. (2009), reported that flavonoids possess antifungal pro-perty. Earlier, Baba-Moussa et al. (1999) reported that tannins present in some plant species possess antifungal property. It is hoped that the elucidation of the structure of the active principle(s) and its/their subsequent use in antifungal investigations would give better results.

In this study, the ethanolic extract demonstrated higher activity on the test organisms than the aqueous extract. This suggests that the active principle(s) were more soluble in ethanol than in the aqueous medium.

It was observed that the fungal isolates used in this research exhibited varying degrees of susceptibility to the extracts. Thus, the values obtained for the zones of inhibition differed, for each test organism (Figure 1). These results corroborate the findings of Anani et al. (2000) and Rajakaruna et al. (2002). Results of this study also agree with the report of Karou et al. (2007). The difference in susceptibility observed in this study could be attributed to the inherent resistance factor of the test organisms among other factors (Ekpo and Etim, 2009). The significant difference (P<0.05) observed bet-ween the inhibitory activity of the ethanolic and aqueous extracts agrees with the research findings of Nkere and Iroegbu (2005) and Ekpo and Etim (2009).

This study has revealed that the extracts of *P. nitida* seeds hold antifungal potential, which can be further explored in the treatment and control of some fungal infections.

ACKNOWLEDGEMENT

The authors are thankful to the technical staff of the Department of Medicinal Plant Research and Traditional Medicine, NIPRD, Abuja.

REFERENCES

Anani K, Hudson JB, Desouza C, Akpagana K, Lower GHN, Amason J T, Gabeassor M (2000). Investigation on Medicinal Plants of Togo for Antiviral and Antimicrobial Activities. Pharm. Biol., 38: 40-45.

Baba-Moussa F, Akpagana K, Bouchet P (1999). Antifungal Activities of Seven West African Combretaceae used in Traditional Medicine. J. Ethnopharm., 66(3): 335-338.

Collins CH, Lyne PM (1970). Microbiological Methods (3rd Ed.). Butterworth and Co. Ltd., pp. 414 -427.

Cruickshank R, Duguid JP, Marmion BP, Swain RH (1975). Medical Microbiology (12th ed.) Longman Group Ltd. Edinburgh London, pp. 180-188.

Ekpo MA, Etim PC (2009). Antimicrobial activity of ethanolic and aqueous extracts of *Sida acuta* on microorganisms from skin infections. J. Med. Plants Res., 3(9): 621-64.

Evans WC (2002). Trease and Evans Pharmacology. 15th edition W. B. Saunders Company Ltd. pp. 135 -150.

Harborne JB (1984). Phytochemical Methods. Chapman and Hall, London, pp. 166-226.

Ibrahim D, Osman H (1995). Antimicrobial Activity of *Cassia alata* from Malaysia. J. Ethnopharm., 45(3): 151-156.

Ibrahim MB, Owonubi MO, Onaolapo JA (1997). Antimicrobial effects of extracts of leaf, stem and root bark of *Anogiessus leicarpus* on *Staphylococcus aureus* NCTC 8190, *Escherischia coli* NCTC 10418 and *Proteus vulgaris* NCTC 4636. J. Pharm. Res. Dev., 2: 20-26.

Karou SD, Nadembeg WMC, Ilboudo DP, Ouermi D, Gbeassor MDC, Souze C, Simpore J (2007). Sida acuta Burm, F. A. Medicinal Plant with numerous potencies. Afr. J. Biotech., 6: 2953 – 2959.

Leven M, Vanden Berghe DA, Mertens F, Vlictinck A, Lammers E (1979). Screening of Higher Plants for Biological Activities/ Antimicrobial Activity. Planta Medica, 36: 311-321.

Nkere CK, Iroegbu CU (2005). Antibacterial screening of the root, seed and stem bark extracts of *Picralima nitida*. Afr. J. Biotech., 4(6): 522-526.

Okokon JE, Antia BS, Igboasoiyi AC, Essien EE, Mbagwu HOC (2007). Evaluation of Antiplasmodial activity of ethanolic seed extract of *Picralima nitida*. J. Ethnopharmacol., 4514: 1-4.

Owoyale JA, Olatunji GA, Oguntoye SO (2005). Antifungal and Antibacterial Activities of an Alcoholic Extract of *Senna alata* leaves. J. Appl. Sci. Environ. Man., 9(3): 105-107.

Rajakaruna N, Haris CS, Towers GHN (2002). Antimicrobal activity of plants collected from serpentine outcrops in Sri Lanka. Pharm. Biol., 40: 235-244.

Reyes-chilpa, Garibay, Moreno-torres, Jimenez-Estrada and Quiroz-Vasquez (2009). Flavonoids and Isoflavonoids with Antifungal properties from *Platymiscium yucatanum* heartwood Holzforschuna. Inter. J. Biol. Chem. Phys. Tech. Wood., p. 52.

Sofowora A (2006). Medicinal Plants and Traditional Medicine in Africa. Spectrum Books Ltd. Ibadan, pp. 150 -183.

Wokoma EC, Essien IE, Agwa OK (2007). The invitro antifungal activity of garlic (*Allium sativum*) and onion (*Allium cepa*) extracts against dermatophytes and yeast. Nig. J. Microbiol., 21: 1478 – 1484.

13

Ethnobotanical importance of halophytes of Noshpho salt mine, District Karak, Pakistan

Musharaf Khan[1]*, Shahana Musharaf[2] and Zabta Khan Shinwari[3]

[1]Department of Botany, University of Peshawar, Pakistan.
[2]Government Girls Degree College S. Malton, Mardan, Pakistan.
[3]Department of Plant Sciences, Quaid-i-Azam University, Islamabad- 45320, Pakistan.

The present study documents the traditional knowledge of medicinal halophytes of Noshpho Salt Mine District Karak, Khyber Pakhton Khwa (KPK), Pakistan. These medicinal halophytes are wide spread and are common in Noshpho Salt Mine. We have documented the use of 33 species belonging to 18 families. The dominant families are Asteraceae with 6 species, followed by Chenopodiaceae and Poaceae with 3 species, Asclepiadaceae, Capparidaceae, Mimosaceae, Rhamnaceae, Solanaceae and Zygophyllaceae with 2 species each. These medicinal plants are used to cure about 30 to 35 types of diseases. The main diseases in this area were cough, diabetes, stomach problem, headache, jaundice, toothache and skin diseases. Leaves are the most frequently used plant part against diseases. The area was investigated for the first time ever and information about the traditional remedies were collected and documented before they are lost. With a little support, the cultivation and conservation of such natural resources may result in sustainable maintenance and utilization of this plant wealth and uplift the socio-economic status of the people. It is also recommended that both the public and private sector should be encouraged to invest in these plants which have potential to become an economically viable industry.

Key words: Medicinal halophyte, conservation, Noshpho salt mine, Pakistan.

INTRODUCTION

Soil salinization is one of the most important constraints for plant growth and crop production all over the world. Around 800 million hectares of land (about 6% of the world's total land area) are salt affected (Munns and Tester, 2008). Menzel and Lieth (1999) indicated that halophytes or salt tolerant plants have multiple uses for the local inhabitants and are an underutilized resource. In Pakistan about 26% of total irrigated land is saline (Anonymous, 2008). Even now days most of the population of the area of district Karak is still depend on the folk medicines as they live in far flung areas where the facilities of the medical treatment are scarcely available. In view of the wide spread usage of medicinal plants in Unani, Greeco-Arabic systems, it seems worth while to carry out a study on the medicinal flora of Pakistan and particularly on halophytes and delineates important and persistent usage of these remedies in different countries. Such a study will bear out a very fruitful evidence for their authenticity in a particular disease and hence it will provide a very interesting and rewarding prepharmacological ground for undertaking its investigation on scientific basis (Farooq, 1990). Ethnobotanical studies in various areas of Pakistan have also been carried out (Shinwari, 2010; Shinwari and Khan, 2000; Shinwari and Gilani, 2003; Hussain et al., 2006; Qureshi and Bhatti, 2008) including those of the northern mountainous regions (Adnan et al., 2010) which include a considerable number of halophytes.

The present research was aimed to collect and document traditional local information about the uses of some halophytes plants of district Karak in KPK. Pakistan.

Study area

The district Karak is situated at 32° 47 to 33° 28 N and 70° 30 to 71° 30 E. The total population of district Karak is about 536000. The total area of district is 264,775 ha. I

*Corresponding author. E-mail: k.musharaf@gmail.com

is the only district of KPK Province of Pakistan having the salt mine (Figures 1 and 2). Majority of the study area consists of curved dry hills and rough fields areas. Although the hills are very dry, but it is a fact that it contains precious minerals like salt, gypsum and gas etc. There is shortage of drinking water, so the people bring water from remote area (Figures 3 and 4). The Rainfall is scanty in the area. In the year 2005, 300 to 400 mm of rainfall per annum recorded on district level (Table 1). The area is very hot in summer and very cold in winter. In the year 2005 the mean maximum temperature was 42°C, in the month of the June, where as the mean minimum temperature was as low as 4°C, in the month of December and January, recorded on district level (Table 1).

The salt quarries are at Noshpho where the hills present great amount of exposed rocks salt (Khan, 2007).

MATERIALS AND METHODS

The study was conducted by frequently surveying in winter, spring and summer during 2006 to 2007. Information on demographic (age, gender) and ethnobotanical information was gathered from each site by using a semi-structured questionnaire. During survey personal observation was also recorded. Information about the local uses of the species as medicinal, fuel wood, timber and fodder etc were obtained through random sampling by interviewing 300 respondents from different walks of life because different age group and gender use these plant for different purposes. Individual questionnaire was filled from plant collectors, housewives, shopkeepers, elders, plant traders, those working in salt mines and local healers (Hakims), who are the actual users and have a lot of indigenous knowledge about the plants and their traditional uses. Analysis of data was made with the help of group discussions among different age classes of district Karak that include genders, village people and medicine men (Hakims) of the society. The data was classified, tabulated, analyzed and concluded for final report. The plants were collected, dried and preserved for identification. Plants were identified with the help of available literature (Stewart, 1972; Nasir and Ali, 1971 to 1995) and voucher specimens have been deposited in herbarium, Department of Botany, University of Science and Technology, Kohat, KPK. Pakistan.

The information about the medicinal uses of the plants was obtained from local experienced people through personal interview.

RESULTS

The present study includes indigenous knowledge of medicinal wild halophytes of Noshpho salt mine district Karak. All plant species are alphabetically arranged mentioning botanical name; voucher number; family; local name; parts used; method of preparation and application. A total of 33 species belonging to 18 families are reportedfrom the study area. The dominant families are steraceae with 6 species, followed by Chenopodiaceae and Poaceae with 3 species, Asclepiadaceae, Capparidaceae, Mimosaceae, Rhamnaceae, Solanaceae and Zygophyllaceae with 2 species each. This study is mainly focused on traditional uses of plants of the area

used by the local people. The local inhabitants use 50 species of plants for treating various ailments. Most species had multi uses. The plants were mostly used in the crude form. The main diseases in this area were cough, diabetes, stomach problem, headache, jaundice, toothache and skin diseases. The most common plants used by the locals for multiple purposes are; *Zizyphus maurtiana* Lam., *Withania coagulans* Dunal., *Rhazya stricta* Dcne., *Fagonia cretica* L., *Kochia prostrate* (L) Schrad, *Peganum harmala* L. and *Solanum surratens* Burm. f. (Figure 5)

The ethnobotanical inventory is presented in Tables 2, 3 and 4.

DISCUSSION

These medicinal plants which are growing naturally in different seasons of year in this area are used for different purposes. The benefits of about 33 wild medicinal halophyte were studied and described by local people and habitants. All these species are the main source of medicine and other requirements of the local communities, because of the shortage of trained manpower and resources. Health authorities in Pakistan are not able to provide services to greater part of the rural population. Therefore, the wide spread use of folk herbal remedies appears to be not only a case of preference but also a situation without other native choices. Such a system of medical treatment on which the majority of the population has been relying upon for generations with considerable success, should not be overlooked for further medical investigation, specially on those plants which have not been looked at for medical research, although the same have been in use by local inhabitants over hundreds of years.

So the indigenous knowledge, accordingly, continue to provide the building blocks for development in rural communities because the medicinal plants are the precious economic resources of the area and wild are used in the crude form locally or collected and transported into the drug markets inside the area and country. The people depend upon the local resources around them particularly on plants. 300 Individual questionnaires were filled from plant collectors, housewives, shop-keepers, elders, plant traders, those working in salt mines and local healers (Hakims) (Figure 6). It was observed that 75% among men and 25% among women were knowledgeable about plants. It was noted that elderly people had more knowledge about the folk uses of medicinal plants than younger generation. In the remote areas like Charpara, modern health care facilities are lacking.

The present study indicated that the leaves and fruit are the most common parts of plant used against diseases. Similar finding were also reported from other areas of Pakistan (Shinwari and Khan, 2000; Shinwari

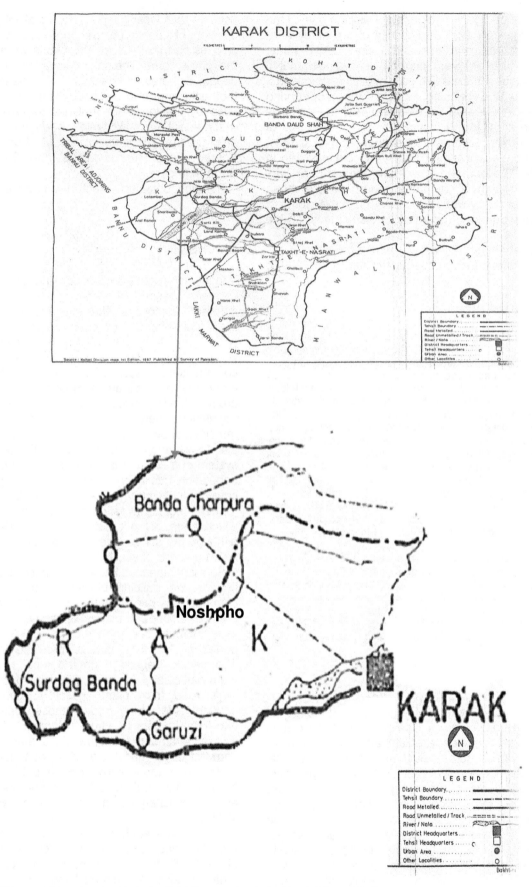

Figure 1. Map showing Noshpho Salt Mine area in district Karak (Khan, 2004).

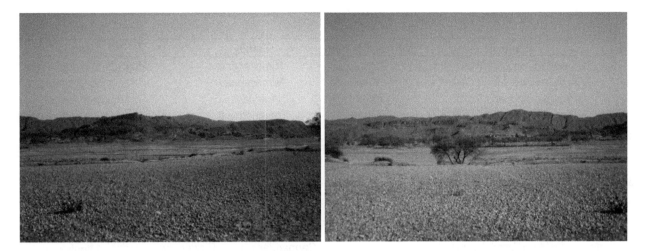

Figure 2. Study area site.

Table 1. Climatic data of district Karak for the year 2005.

Months	Temperature (°C)				Rainfall (mm)	Relative humidity (%)		Soil temperature (°C) average	Wind speed (km per hour)
	Mean maximum	Highest recorded	Mean minimum	Lowest recorded		5 A.M	5 P.M		
January	16.9	20	4	0	64.8	83.1	37.2	4.6	2.4
February	16.8	24	7	2	95.1	82.6	42.7	6.8	2.7
March	24.38	29	12.6	10	80.6	85	39	13.2	3.3
April	32	38	16	10	14.6	65.9	24.3	22.1	3.4
May	33.2	39	20.8	16	34.8	58.7	28	15.4	6.2
June	42	49	26	19	19.8	47.2	22	22	5.3
July	36.7	41	26.1	22	19.8	77.4	38.6	22.7	4.6
August	37	41	26.1	21	73.40	79.6	40.5	23.22	4.2
September	35.9	40	24.7	19	82.2	75.6	39.5	23.1	3.1
October	33.1	37	18.3	10	54	65.3	28.4	17.7	4.2
November	26	29	10	9	Nil	62	35	11.2	3.8
December	22.9	26	4	1	Nil	60	30.3	5.8	3.6

Source: Agricultural Research Farm Ahmadwala Karak. Economically important halophytes of district Karak.

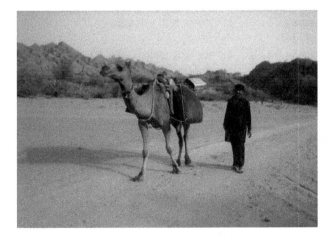

Figure 3. In search of water that become extinct due to salinity.

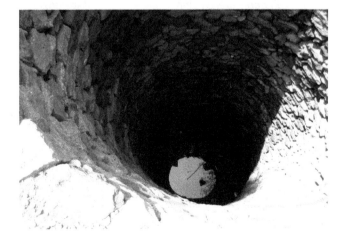

Figure 4. Brackish water in well.

Table 2. Tree. Economically important halophytes of district Karak.

S/N	Plants	Vernacular name	Family	Uses
1	*Acacia modesta* Wall	Palosa	Mimosaceae	Emollient and demulcent .
2	*Acacia nilotica* (Linn.) Delile	Kiker	Mimosaceae	Diarrhea and tonic.
3	*Phoenix sylvestris* Roxb.	Kajoor	Arecaceae	Tonic and fodder.
4	*Tamarix articulata* Vahl	Ghaz	Tamaricaceae	Hair colouration and pain killer.
5	*Zizyphus maurtiana* Lam	Bare	Rhamnaceae	Fodder, hedge plant and scabies, honey.

Table 3. Shrub. Economically important halophytes of district Karak.

S/N	Plants	Vernacular name	Family	Uses
1	*Calotropis procera* (Willd.) R. Br.	Spalmi	Asclepiadaceae	Hand pain, stomach ulcer and fever.
2	*Capparis decidua* (Forssk.) Edgew	Tap	Capparidaceae	Pickles, fuel wood, bird hunting and white ants.
3	*Capparis spinosa* L.	Berri	Capparidaceae.	Pickles, diuretic and tonic.
4	*Periploca aphylla* Dcne.	Barara	Asclepiadaceae	Swollen joints, cough and flu.
5	*Rhazya stricta* Dcne.	Ganderi	Apocynaceae	Cooling agent, skin rashes, blood purifier and sore eyes.
6	*Saccharum griffithii* Munro ex Boiss.	Sormal	Poaceae	Fodder, making kites and fuel.
7	*Withania coagulans* Dunal	Shopyanga	Solanaceae	Stomach ulcer, skin rashes and blood purifier.
8	*Zizyphus nummularia* (Burm. f.) Wight and Arn.	Kerkana	Rhamnaceae	Fodder, hedge plant, laxative, bird hunting and Haney bee spp.

Table 4. Herb. Economically important halophytes of district Karak.

S/N	Plants	Vernacular name	Family	Uses
1	*Arabis nova* Vill	Ger Beta	Brassicaceae	Fodder and forage.
2	*Asparagus capitatus* Baker	beta	Liliaceae	Chronic gout and insomnia.
3	*Blumea lacera* (Burm.f.)DC.	Beta	Asteraceae	Disinfectant.
4	*Chenopodium murale* Linn.	Tor Soba	Chenopodiaceae	Decoction and fodder
5	*Cynodon dactylon* (Linn.) Pers.	Barawa	Poaceae	Fodder, diuretic and fuel wood.
6	*Fagonia cretica* Linn	Aspalagzia	Zygophyllaceae	Laxative, constipation and blood purifier.
7	*Gnaphalium luteo-album* Linn.	Tetesi gul	Asteraceae	Astringent and vulnerary.
8	*Hertia intermedia* (Boiss.) O. Ktze.	Unknown	Asteraceae	Painkiller.
9	*Inula grantioides* Boiss.	Zir gul	Asteraceae	Asthma and tonic.
10	*Kickxia incana* (Wall.) Penn.	Shen beta	Scrophulariaceae	Antidiabetic, laxative and tonic.
11	*Kochia prostrate* (L) Schrad	Tanoba	Chenopodiaceae.	Used as a soap for washing utensils.
12	*Lactuca auriculata* Wall. ex DC.	Warhora	Asteraceae	Increase lactation and laxative.
13	*Launea procumbens* (Roxb.) Amin	Tariza	Asteraceae	Fodder for birds and tonic.
14	*Medicago polymorpha* Linn.	Karushka	Papilionaceae	Fodder and forage.
15	*Peganum harmala* Linn.	Sponda	Zygophyllaceae	Tonic, asthma, blood purifier and joint pain.
16	*Plantago psyllium* Linn.	Beta	Plantaginaceae	Dysentery.
17	*Solanum surratens* Burm. f.	Zyara marana	Solanaceae	Laxative, fodder and rheumatism.
18	*Stipa capensis* Thunb.	Her beta	Poaceae	Poisonous to sheep.
19	*Suaeda monoica* Forssk.	Babara	Chenopodiaceae	Ophthalmia...
20	*Teucrium stocksianum* Boiss.	Ger Beta	Lamiaceae	Expectorant, fever and sour throat.

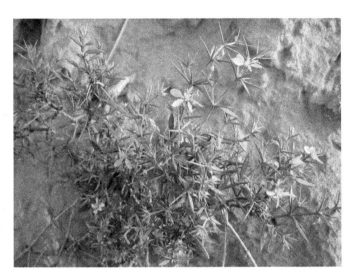

Figure 5. *Fagonia cretica* L. (Spelaghzai).

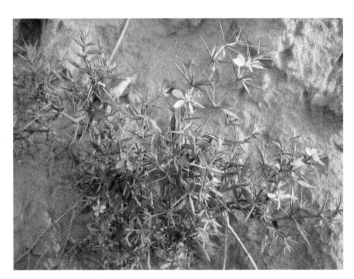

Figure 6. *Fagonia cretica* L. (Spelaghzai).

and Gilani, 2003; Hussain et al., 2006; Shinwari et al., 2006; Shinwari, 2010). The local people depend on fuel wood and other needs on these halophytes. Overgrazing and up rooting of medicinal plants for fuel wood and commercial exploitation has resulted in poor vegetation cover, promoted soil erosion and deterioration of habitat. There is an urgent need of conserving the medicinal plants that are over harvested so that in future the coming generations could be benefited from these precious plants that are a real gift of nature for the mankind. It is a collaborative venture between people in local communities and various scientists and specialists. It is therefore necessary to find the ways of promoting the local people towards conservation as Shenji (1994) suggested that ethnobotany is the science of documenting the traditional knowledge on the use of plants by the indigenous people and for further assessing human interactions with the natural environment. A chief goal of present study is to ensure that local natural history becomes a living tradition in communities used with great interests and are active participants in the trade and economy of the country.

According to WHO reports more than 80% of Asia's population cannot afford formal health care facilities and therefore relies on wild medicinal plant species owing to their cultural familiarity, easy access, simple use and effectiveness (Anon, 2009). In China as many as 2394 traditional Tibetan medicines are used all from plants (1106), animals (448) and natural minerals (840) (Rizwana et al., 2009). Many of the important medicinal plants are sold at higher prices in the market. Most of the plants used by the local people are not conserved but are over exploited.

Conclusion

The present study show that the people of the area

possessing good knowledge of herbal drugs but as people are going to modernization; their knowledge of traditional uses of plants may be lost in due course. The investigated area has a rich diversity of medicinal halophytes and provides a conductive habitat and ideal conditions for their growth. It is suggested that local people should be encourage to use the knowledge of their indigenous medicinal halophytes because of the shortage of trained manpower, resources and the health authorities in Pakistan are not able to provide services to greater part of the rural population. Such studies may also provide some information to biochemist and pharmacologist in screening of individual species and in rapid assessing of phyto-chemical constituent and bioanalysis for authentic treatment of various diseases.

ACKNOWLEDGEMENTS

Authors are grateful to the local people and salt mine workers who have revealed the precious information of medicinal plant species.

REFERENCES

Adnan M, Hussain J, Shah MT, Ullah F, Shinwari ZK, Bahadar A, Khan AL (2010). Proximate and nutrient composition of medicinal plants of humid and sub-humid regions in northwest Pakistan. J. Med. Pl. Res., 4: 339-345.
Anonymous (2008). Balochistan fisheries development studies: Options for Balochistan coastal fisheries and aquaculture. *In*: Competitiveness support fund. p. 17
Farooq S (1990). A review of medicinal plants of Pakistan. Sci. Khyber, 3(1): 23-31.
Hussain F, Badshah L, Dastigar G (2006). Folk medicinal uses of some plants of South Waziristan, Pakistan. Pak. J. Pl. Sci., 12: 27-40..
Khan M (2004). A Fraction of Angiosperm of Tehsil B.D Shah. Karak. MSc Thesis. Gomal University D.I.Khan, Khyber Pakhton Khawa, Pakistan.
Khan M (2007). Ethnobotany of Tehsil Karak NWFP PAKISTAN. M.Phil

Thesis. Kohat University of Science and Technology, Kohat, Khyber Pakhton Khawa, Pakistan.

Menzel U, Lieth H (1999). Halophyte Database Vers. 2.0. Halophyte Uses in different climates I: Ecological and Ecophysiological Studies. In: Progress in Biometeriology. (Eds.): H. Lieth, M. Moschenko, M. Lohman, H.–W. Koyro and A. Hamdy. Backhuys Publishers. The Netherlands. pp: 77-88.

Munns R, Tester M (2008). Mechanisms of Salinity Tolerance. Ann. Rev. Plant Biol., 59: 651--81.

Nasir E, Ali SI (1971-1995). Flora of West Pakistan Department of Botany, University of Karachi, Karachi.

Qureshi R, Bhatti GR (2008). Ethnobotany of plants used by the Thari people of Nara Desert, Pakistan. *Fitoterapia*, 79: 468-473.

Rizwana AQ, Muhammad AG, Syed AG, Zaheer YGA, Aniqa B (2009). Indigenous medicinal plants used by local women in Southern Himalayan Regions of Pakistan. Pak. J. Bot., 41(1): 19-25.

Shinwari ZK, Watanabe T, Rehman M, Youshikawa T (2006). A Pictorial Guide to medicinal plants of Pakistan.

Shinwari MI, Khan MA (2000). Folk use of medicinal herbs of Margalla Hills National Park, Islamabad. J. Ethnopharmacol., 69: 45-56.

Shinwari ZK (2010). Medicinal plants research in Pakistan. J. Med. Pl Res., 4: 161-176.

Shinwari ZK, Gilani SS (2003). Sustainable harvest of medicinal plants at Bulashbar Nullah, Astore (Northern Pakistan). J. Ethnopharmacol, 84: 289-298.

14

Disposition of quinine and its major metabolite, 3-hydroxyquinine in patients with liver diseases

Chinedum P. Babalola[1]*, Olayinka A. Kotila[1], Patrick A. F. Dixon[2] and Adefemi E. Oyewo[3]

[1]Department of Pharmaceutical Chemistry, Faculty of Pharmacy, University of Ibadan, Nigeria.
[2]Department of Pharmacology, Faculty of Pharmacy, Obafemi Awolowo University, Ile-Ife, Nigeria.
[3]Department of Clinical Pharmacology, Faculty of Pharmacy, Obafemi Awolowo University, Ile-Ife, Nigeria.

Quinine, extensively metabolized by CYP 3A4, has 3-hydroxyquinine as the major metabolite which also contributes to its antimalarial activity. This study assessed the impact of various liver diseases on the disposition of quinine and 3-hydroxyquinine. Ten adult patients with liver diseases ranging from cirrhosis, primary liver carcinoma, hepatitis, ascites, and amoebic liver disease as well as six healthy subjects received single oral dose of 600 mg quinine sulphate tablets. Venous blood and urine were collected over 48 h. Quinine and 3-hydroxyquinine were determined from the matrices by a validated high performance liquid chromatography (HPLC) method. Wide inter-individual variations were observed in the subjects especially those with liver diseases. Cmax (4.47 vs 2.41mcg/ml) and AUC (73 vs 51mcg.h/ml) values were significantly increased in liver disease patients. Clearance was reduced by 30% from 3.27 to 2.31 (p = 0.009). Metabolic ratio of quinine/3-hydroxyquinine in plasma decreased from 5.5 to 1.42 over 4 to 48 h. Cumulative amount of quinine and 3-hydroxyquinine produced in urine were 38 mg (8%) and 32 mg (7%) respectively. Compromised metabolism of quinine in liver disease patients suggests the necessity of reviewing the dosage of quinine in liver disease patients who come up with malaria, a situation that further reduces liver function.

Key words: Quinine, 3-hydroxyquinine, liver diseases, CYP3A4.

INTRODUCTION

The cinchona alkaloids has been an important antimalarial drugs for more than 350 years and its principal constituent, quinine (QN), still remains effective against chloroquine-resistant falciparum malaria. It is still widely used for the treatment of cerebral and complicated malaria as well as leg cramps (Roy et al., 2002). Development of quinine resistance in *Plasmodium falciparum* has been relatively slow and incomplete by comparison with those of the other notable antimalarial drugs such as chloroquine, mefloquine, and sulphadoxine-pyrimethamine (Pukrittayakamee et al., 2003). In areas with multidrug-resistant strains, 7 day regimens of quinine and tetracycline still provide cure rates well over 90% in patients with uncomplicated falciparum malaria (Looareesuwan et al., 1992). Reports

show that the pharmacokinetic properties of and therapeutic responses to quinine vary with age, pregnancy, immunity, and disease severity (Pukrittayakamee et al., 1997; White, 1997). Approximately 80% of QN is systemically cleared by hepatic biotransformation and the major metabolite 3-hydroxyquinine (3-OHQN), which contributes 5 to 12% of antimalarial activity is formed by cytochrome P450 3A4 (Muralidharan et al., 1991; Zhang, 1997; Wilairatana, 1994).

The clearance of QN is reported to be significantly reduced during malaria, liver and renal diseases (Purkrittayakamee et al., 1997; Auprayoon, 1995; Newton, 1999). Its reduction in liver disease condition has been shown to be predominantly as a result of disease-induced dysfunction in hepatic mixed-function oxidase activity (majorly CYP3A) which impairs the conversion of quinine to its major metabolite, 3-OHQN, but the effect on 3-OHQN disposition is unknown.

QN is a low clearance drug with a narrow therapeutic index therefore changes in disposition due to liver lesions

---

*Corresponding author. E-mail: peacebab2001@yahoo.com.

Table 1. Pharmacokinetics of quinine in patients with liver disease and healthy subjects.

Parameter	Liver disease (n=10)	Healthy (n=6)	P value	Significance
C_{max} (mcg/ml)	4.47 ± 2.81 (2.22 -11.06)	2.41 ± 0.76 (1.45 – 3.16)	$p<0.05$	Significant
t_{max} (h)	3.60 ± 0.84 (2.0 – 4.0)	2.67 ± 0.51 (2.0 – 3.0)	$p<0.05$	Significant
AUC (mcg.h/ml)	73.39 ± 35.98 (35.63 – 39.70)	50.82 ± 24.27 (29.37 – 93.64)	$p<0.05$	Significant
$t_{1/2}$ (h)	15.00 ± 6.03 (8.77 – 28.06)	13.64 ± 4.01 (7.00 – 17.32)	$p>0.05$	Not significant
Cl/F (ml/min/kg)	2.31 ± 0.92 (1.02 – 3.84)	3.27 ± 1.46 (1.31 – 4.72)	$p<0.05$	Significant
V_d/F (l/kg)	3.01 ± 1.43 (0.89 – 5.00)	3.55 ± 1.63 (1.96 – 6.30)	$p>0.05$	Not significant

may have implications in treatment outcome. Liver diseases or lesions are varied and tend to contribute differently to the disposition of drugs. Previous animal studies show that liver lesions affect clearance of QN and its metabolite differently and it is been reported that *in vivo* function of CYP3A is relatively disease sensitive in human malaria (Purkrittayakamee et al., 1997). Previous studies on QN disposition in liver disease did not monitor the parent active metabolites therefore in this study we have carried out disposition of QN and its major metabolite, 3-OHQN in patients with various kinds of liver diseases.

Objectives

(i) To determine the pharmacokinetics (PK) of QN in patients with various liver diseases.
(ii) To compare the PK of QN in liver disease patients with data from healthy subjects.
(iii) To determine the disposition of the major and active metabolite of quinine, 3-OHQN in patients with liver diseases.

METHODS

Subjects

Ten adult patients with different liver diseases aged between 31 and 65 years and weighing 43 to 89 kg plus six healthy adult subjects aged 20 to 30 years and weighing 53 to 68 kg were recruited into the study. Liver diseases were diagnosed by clinical and pathological findings. Diseases were classified as liver cirrhosis, primary liver carcinoma, hepatitis, ascites and amoebic liver disease. The study was approved by Ethics Committees of Obafemi Awolowo University Teaching Hospital, Ile-Ife and UI/UCH, and informed consent was obtained from each participant.

Treatment and sample collection

Following an overnight fast, subjects were given a single dose of 600 mg QN sulphate (equivalent to 500 mg QN base) tablet (acf Chemiafarma, Maarsen, Holland) with a glass of water. Venous blood (5 ml) was collected from the forearm vein at predetermined times: 0, 1, 2, 3, 4, 6, 12, 24, and 48 h. Total urine voided were collected at time intervals from 0 to 24 h in patients with liver diseases.

Drug analysis

QN and 3-OHQN concentrations in plasma and urine were analysed by a validated high performance liquid chromatography (HPLC) method developed in our laboratory with retention times of 7.8 and 3.4 min respectively (Babalola et al., 1993). A reversed-phase C18 column was used with an UV detector at a wavelenght of 254 nm. Primaquine was employed as internal standard. The mobile phase was a mixture of 0.02 M potassium dihydrogenphosphate, methanol and acetonitrile (75:15:10 v/v/v) containing 74 mM perchloric acid as the counter ion. Blank plasma collected prior to QN administration showed no endogenous sources of interference with the assay. 3-OHQN was not assessed in healthy subjects.

Pharmacokinetic analysis

Pharmacokinetic parameters of QN (such as tmax, Cmax, $t_{1/2}$, AUC, CL/F and Vd) in both groups were analyzed by model-independent method (Gibaldi, 1991). Cmax and tmax were noted directly from concentration-time data. $t_{1/2}$ was calculated from terminal plasma drug concentrations. [AUC] $0 \rightarrow \infty$ was calculated from linear trapezoidal method. Apparent oral clearance (Cl/F) was estimated from dose/AUC while apparent Vd/F was calculated from clearance (Cl $\times$ $t_{1/2}$/0.693). Comparison of pharmacokinetic parameters obtained from patients with liver disease and healthy subjects was made by using student t-test and F-test and a $p<0.05$ was regarded as significant.

RESULTS

Quinine sulphate at a single oral dose was well tolerated by both patients and healthy subjects. Plots of mean plasma concentration calculated in microgram per milliliter (mcg/ml) vs time (h) for QN in both groups are shown in Figure 1, indicating higher levels of QN in patients than volunteers. The plasma profiles of QN and 3-OHQN are shown in Figure 2. Pharmacokinetic parameters are summarized in Table 1.

Wide inter-individual and inter-disease variations were observed especially in liver disease patients. In comparison with healthy subjects, there were four significant changes in pharmacokinetic parameters of QN in patients with liver disease. Cmax and AUC were significantly larger: 4.47 ± 2.81 vs 2.41 ± 0.76 mcg/ml and 73.4 ± 36.0 vs 50.82 ± 24.27 mg.h/ml respectively ($p<0.05$). tmax was prolonged: 3.6 ± 0.84 vs 2.67 ± 0.51 h, while

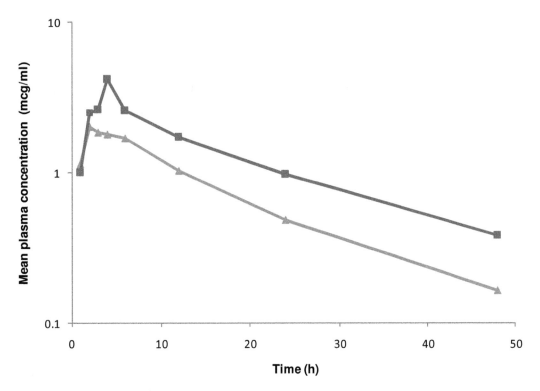

Figure 1. Plot of mean plasma concentrations of quinine after a single oral dose of 600 mg in patients with liver disease (■) and healthy subjects (▲).

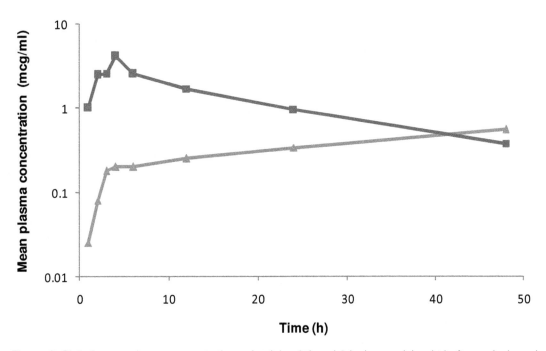

Figure 2. Plot of mean plasma concentrations of quinine (■) and 3-hydroxy quinine (▲) after a single oral dose of 600mg in patients with liver disease.

clearance was reduced (2.31 ± 0.92 vs 3.27 ± 1.46 ml/min/kg (p<0.05). Metabolite ratio (QN/3-OHQN) in plasma decreased in patients from 4 to 48 h ranging from 5.5 to 1.42. Cumulative QN and 3-OHQN excreted in urine in the patients were 37.69 ± 27.05 mg (7.5%) and 32.90 ± 20.96 mg (6.6%) respectively (Table 2). The limit

Table 2. Quinine/3-hydroxyquinine plasma and urine profile in varied liver disease conditions.

Disease	Subject	QN/3-OHQN plasma ratio		Urine analysis			
		4 h	48 h	Cumulative amount of QN (mg)	%	Cumulative amount of metabolite (mg)	%
Liver cirrhosis	1	0	2.13	60.45	12.09	65.89	13.18
	2	6.25	0	6.09	1.22	6.51	1.30
Primary cell carcinoma	3	6.67	1.27	49.44	9.89	31.7	6.34
	4	2.63	0	19.4	3.88	29.8	5.96
Hepatitis	5	7.14	1.82	42.75	8.55	12.92	2.58
	6	6.67	0	20.8	4.16	31.6	6.32
Ascites	7	3.23	1.52	98.46	19.69	66.78	13.36
	8	12.5	2.63	34.72	6.94	17.22	3.44
	9	6.25	0	14.76	2.95	19.8	3.96
Amoebic liver disease	10	3.57	1.96	30.03	6.01	46.8	9.36
Mean		5.49	1.42	37.69	7.5	32.9	6.6
SD		3.38	0.96	27.05	5.41	20.96	4.19
Data range		(2.63-12.5)	(0-2.63)	(6.09-98.46)		(6.51-66.78)	

Mean quinine/3-hydroxyquine ratio from 4hr to 48 h = 5.49 ± 3.38 to 1.42 ± 0.96, Mean cumulative quinine excreted = 37.69 ± 27.05 (~ 8%), Mean cumulative 3-hydroxyquinine excreted = 32.9 ± 20.96 (~ 7%).

of detection was 10 ng/ml. The between-day precision for this method averaged between 1.4 and 6% over the concentration range of 0.4 to 10 µg/ml while the recovery ranged between 91 and 98%.

DISCUSSION

The results obtained exhibited wide intra and inter individual variations especially in liver disease patients. Out of the 10 patients with liver diseases, 2 had liver cirrhosis, primary liver cell carcinoma (2), hepatitis (2), ascites (3) and 1 with amoebic liver disease. There was no correlation between the type of liver disease and the pharmacokinetic parameters obtained, rather there was wide intra and inter disease variation. Liver function and mixed function oxidase activities including the activity of CYP3A4 and liver blood flow are all compromised during hepatitis and malaria, (Wilairatana et al., 1994) and therefore can alter the disposition of drugs such as QN, which are majorly cleared by the liver. In the presence of malaria, patients with liver disease may experience more reduction in QN clearance and metabolism of its major metabolite, 3-OHQN, although this can be counteracted in the presence of higher levels of QN and longer half-life. As a result of impaired hepatic biotransformation, plasma levels of QN were higher than levels observed in healthy

subjects – with AUC and Cmax of patients being 44 and 86% higher respectively than healthy subjects.

Profile of 3-OHQN in plasma shows a steady increase with time compared to the decline of the parent drug QN (Figure 2). Considering the varied hepatic dysfunction, it will be expected that the profile of the metabolite be at most similar in pattern to the parent compound. Reason for this deviation may likely be the high protein binding property of QN (to α–acid glycoprotein AAG) as compared to its major metabolite, 3-OHQN, which is ~ 50% bound to plasma proteins thereby leading to reduced amount of free QN. Plasma protein binding is established as an important determinant of QN clearance (Orlando, 2009). In all of the patients there was a continuous increase in the metabolite level with time with a value as high as 62% of that of the parent compound (median 30%, range 22 to 62%) at 24 h post dose. A similar result was observed by Newton et al. (1999) in a study of 3-OHQN in patients having severe malaria coupled with acute renal failure. This incremental observation of 3-OHQN can be advantageous during malaria treatment with the metabolite adding to the antimalarial activity of the parent drug and this contribution could be greater in conditions of renal failure as it is seen in severe malaria (Purkrittayakamee et al. 1997; Newton et al., 1999). On the other hand it can also be contributory to adverse effects that occur with QN intake if it contributes to parent drug activity like 3-hydroxyquinidine (the diastereomer) does to quinindine and as noted by Newton et al. (1999) 3-OHQN should be monitored routinely when QN is administered for malaria treatment in liver compromised patients (Newton et al., 1999).

From its disposition profile (Figure 2) we assume that the elimination pattern of 3-OHQN is completely different from that of QN and therefore follows another pathway but the results obtained by Orlando et al. (2009) differs with a formation rate-elimination that virtually mimics that of the parent compound both in the presence as well as absence of a CYP3A4 inhibitor – erythromycin. The diversity of liver disease conditions could account for this difference as there was wide intra and inter individual variations in this study and the results reflected are a mean of these variations.

Mean percentage of QN excreted unchanged in patients' urine (8%) observed in this study (Table 2), is higher than earlier reports of 5% obtained for healthy subjects (Babalola et al., 1998) and further confirms compromised clearance. Although QN is majorly cleared by the liver, the percentage contribution of 3-OHQN to this amount is unknown; approximately 7% was reported in this study in patients with liver disease (Table 2). The clearance of QN is intrinsically low and appears sensitive to disease. These data are consistent with earlier observations suggesting impaired metabolic clearance of QN in patients with liver diseases and malaria (Auprayoon et al., 1995; Karbwang et al., 1993); the difference being that in the present study, the major and active metabolite, 3-OHQN was monitored. Although other hydroxylated metabolites (e.g, 2-OHQN) are also eliminated but 3-OHQN has approximately one tenth (1/10) antimalarial activity of the parent compound and is also indicative of the activity of the hepatic metabolizing enzyme CYP3A4 (Mirghani et al., 2003).

Conclusion

The apparent reduction in QN clearance and its major metabolite in liver disease patients is from disease-induced dysfunction in hepatic mixed function oxidase activity especially CYP3A. Such conditions will impair the biotransformation of QN to its major and active metabolite 3-OHQN and at the same time will have benefits in the combined antimalarial activity of both parent drug and metabolite. There will therefore be the need for routine monitoring of both quinine and 3-hydroxyquinine to ensure that the administered dose of quinine is such that will not lead to pronounced adverse effects should it be assumed that 3-hydroxyquinine exhibits similar adverse effects as quinine just as its diastereomer, 3-hydroxyquinidine does to its own parent drug, quinindine.

This data suggests the necessity to review current dosage regimen of QN when used in treatment of falciparum malaria in patients with most forms of liver diseases especially since the activity of the liver and kidney are reported to be compromised during falciparum malaria.

REFERENCES

Auprayoon P, Sukontason K, Na-Bangchang K, Banmairuroi V, Molunto P, Karbwang J (1995). Pharmacokinetics of quinine in chronic liver disease. Br. J. Pharmacol., 40: 494-497.

Babalola CP, Bolaji OO, Dixon PAF, Ogunbona FA (1993). Column liquid chromatographic analysis of QN in human plasma, saliva and urine. J. Chromatogr. 616: 151-154

Babalola CP, Oyewo EA, Bolaji OO, Dixon PAF (1998). Quinine pharmacokinetics and toxicity in Nigerian subjects. West African J. Pharmacol. Drug Res. 14: 1-5.

Gibaldi M (1991). Biopharmaceutics and Clinical Pharmacokinetics, 4th edition, Lea & Febiger Ltd, pp: 14-23.

Karbwang J, Thanavibul A, Molunto P, Na Bangchang K (1993). The pharmacokinetics of quinine in patients with hepatitis. Br. J. Clin. Pharmacol., 35: 444 – 446.

Looareesuwan S, Wilairatana P, Vanijanonta S, Kyle D, Webster K (1992). Efficacy of quinine-tetracycline for acute uncomplicated falciparum malaria in Thailand. Lancet I. pp: 367-370.

Mirghani RA, Ericsson O, Tybring G, Gustafsson LL, Bertilsson L (2003). Quinine 3-hydroxylation as a biomarker reaction for the activity of CYP3A4 in man. Eur. J. Clin. Pharmacol. 59: 23-28.

Muralidharan G, Hawes EM, McKay G, Korchinski ED, Midha KK (1991). Quinidine but not quinine inhibits in man the oxidative metabolic routes of methoxyphenamine which involve debrisoquine 4-hydroxylase. Eur. J. Clin. Pharmacol. 41: 471-474.

Newton P, Keeratithakul D, Teja-Isavaham P, Pukrittayakamee S, Kyle D, White N (1999). Pharmacokinetics of quinine and 3-hydroxyquinine in severe falciparum malaria with acute renal failure. Trans. R. Soc. Trop. Med. Hyg., 93: 69-72.

Orlando R, De Martin S, Pegoraro P, Quintieri L, Palatini P (2009). Irreversible CYP3A inhibition accompanied by plasma protein-binding displacement: A comparative analysis in subjects with normal and impaired liver function. Clin. Pharmacol. Ther., 85(3): 319-326.

Pukrittayakamee S, Wanwimolruk S, Stepniewska K, Jantra A, Huyakorn S, Looareesuwan S, White NJ (2003). Quinine pharmacokinetic-pharmacodynamic relationships in uncomplicated falciparum malaria. Antimicrob. Agents Chemother., 47: 3458-3463.

Purkrittayakamee S, Looareesuwan S, Keeratithakul D, Davis TME, Teja-Isavadharm P, Nagachinta B, Weber A, Smith AL, Kyle D, White NJ (1997). A study of the factors affecting the metabolic clearance of quinine in malaria. Eur. J. Clin. Pharmacol., 52: 487-493.

Roy L, Leblanc M, Bannon P, Villeneuve JP (2002). Quinine pharmacokinetics in chronic haemodialysis patients. Br. J. Clin. Pharmacol., 54: 604-609.

White NJ (1997). Assessment of the pharmacodynamic properties of antimalarial drugs in vivo. Antimicrob. Agents Chemother., 41: 1413-1422.

Wilairatana P, Looareesuwan S, Vanijanonta S, Charoenlarp P, Wittayalertpanya S (1994). Hepatic metabolism in severe falciparum malaria: caffeine clearance study. Ann. Trop. Med. Parasitol., 88: 13-19.

Zhang H, Coville PF, Walker RJ, Miners JO, Birkett DJ, Wanwimolruk S (1997). Evidence for involvement of human CYP3A in 3-hydroxylation of quinine. Br. J. Clin. Pharmacol., 43: b245-252.

15

Antinociceptive potential of the methanolic extract of *Microdermis puberula* (Hook. F. Ex. Planch)

Clement Jackson[1]*, Herbert Mbagwu[1], Chidinma Okany[2], Emmanuel Bassey[2] and Iniunwana Udonkang[3]

[1]Department of Pharmacology and Toxicology, Faculty of Pharmacy, University of Uyo, Nigeria.
[2]Department of Pharmacology, College of Medicine University of Lagos, Nigeria.
[3]Department of pharmaceutics and Pharmaceutical Technology, Faculty of Pharmacy, University of Uyo, Nigeria.

This study investigated the antinociceptive effects of the methanolic extract of the stem wood of *Microdermis puberula* (Hook. F. Ex. Planch) in Swiss albino mice of either sex with weights ranging from 17 to 25 g. Acetylsalicylic acid and morphine were used as standards for the antinociceptive tests while distilled water was used as control. Acetic acid - induced mouse writhing reflex test and hot plate test were used to determine peripheral and central pain inhibition respectively, using five groups of five animals for each model. The extract was administered in three dosages: 600, 1200 and 2400 mg/kg orally. Acetylsalicylic acid was administered at 100 mg/kg p.o., morphine at 10 mg/kg intraperitoneally and distilled water at 1 ml/kg p.o. Results showed that the extract of. *Microdermis puberula,* at 1200 and 2400 mg/kg significantly inhibited peripheral pain, compared with acetylsalicylic acid ($p<0.05$). The extract of *Microdermis puberula,* at a dose of 2400 mg/kg inhibited pain by increasing the pain threshold in the hot plate test 58.83%. These, therefore, suggest that the methanolic extract of *Microdermis puberula* possesses mild antinociceptive property. The phytochemical analyses of the extract showed the presence of flavonoids, saponins and cardiac glycosides. Results from the LD_{50} determination showed that a dose of 1412.5 mg/kg i.p. produced 50% death in mice.

Key words: Antinociceptive, *Microdemis puberula*, phytochemical analysis, LD_{50}, acetylsalicylic acid.

INTRODUCTION

In the last decades, there has been a renewed interest in research and utilization of medicinal plants, particularly flora of the tropical rainforest. The revived interest in plant-derived drugs is attributed to the current wide-spread belief that "green medicine" is cheap, safe, more dependable and accessible than the costly synthetic drugs many of which are associated with intolerable effects (Adeneye and Benebo, 2007). According to the World Health Organization (WHO), about 80% of the world's population depends wholly or partly on plant-derived pharmaceuticals (WHO, 1996). Correspondingly, in most developing countries, including Nigeria, there is a heavy dependence on herbal preparations for the treatment of human and animal diseases despite the availability of conventional pharmaceuticals.

Microdermis puberula belongs to the family Pandaceae (Hook.f.ex Planch). It is a shrub of about 60 m in height. In Igboland of Southern Nigeria, it is called "Mgbugbo", while in Yorubaland in same southern Nigeria; it is called "Apata". *M. puberula* contains 57.73% DL- methionine, 17.32% crude protein, 9.6% ash, 15.05% crude fibre (Esonu et al., 2004). Previous studies on the roots showed that it has significant hypotensive and vasorelaxing properties (Zamble et al., 2006). The plant has been evaluated as a leaf- meal feed in laying hen diets, improving egg output production and size (Esonu et al., 2004). The aqueous extracts and alkaloids of *Microdermis* have been shown to stimulate sexual parameters in male rats' sexual behaviour (Zamble et al. 2008).

Whereas much work has been done on this plant as stated above, there is no documented record on its pain relieving activity. The objective of the present study was

*Corresponding author. E-mail: clementjackson1@yahoo.com.

to evaluate the antinociceptive effects of *M. puberula*.

MATERIALS AND METHODS

Drugs

Acetylsalicylic acid, morphine and acetic acid were purchased from Sigma Aldrich, U.S.A. Distilled water of pH 6.62 was obtained from the Department of Biochemistry, Nigerian Institute of Medical Research (NIMR), Yaba and was used as the control test substance.

Animals

Swiss albino mice weighing 17 to 25 g were employed for this study. All the animals were obtained from the Animal House of the College of Medicine, University of Lagos. They were kept in a hygienic, well-ventilated environment and had free access to food and water *ad-libitum*. All animal experiments were conducted in compliance with NIH Guidelines for care and use of laboratory animals (Zimmermann, 1983).

Plant material

The dried stem wood of *M. puberula* was purchased from Mushin market, Lagos. The voucher specimen of the plant was deposited in the herbarium of the Department of Pharmacognosy, College of Medicine, University of Lagos with Number FHI109038, where it was identified and authenticated   by the Chief Laboratory Technologist of the Department of Pharmacognosy, Faculty of Pharmacy, College of Medicine, University of Lagos—Mr. T. I. Adeleke.

Preparation of extract

The dried stem wood of *M. puberula* weighing about 100 g was cleaned, air-dried, chopped into smaller bits and dried in the oven at 60°C for at least 5 days. This was then milled into fine powder using the warring blending machine. An 80 g quantity of the powder obtained was extracted with methanol using the Soxhlet extraction apparatus and 83 ml of the extract was obtained. The extract obtained was concentrated to a light brown residue in an oven at 38°C. The yield of the extract was 8.1% w/w (15.2 g)–of dry matter reference to the powdered stem.

Phytochemical screening

The methanolic extract of *M. puberula* stem wood was screened for the presence of its active compounds using different phytochemical analysis procedures (Trease and Evans, 2000).

Chromatography

The methanolic extract of *M. puberula* stem wood was weighed and dissolved in 20 ml distilled water to obtain 200 mg/ml concentration of the herbal preparation. The pH of the resulting solution was determined at 26.8°C ambient temperature. The extract was thereafter subjected to thin layer chromatographic separation.

Acute toxicity study

Fifteen mice were randomly divided into three groups of five mice each. Mice in Group 1 received 5000 mg/kg of the extract while the mice in Groups 2 and 3 received 10,000 and 15,000 mg/kg respectively, orally. Toxic signs and mortality were observed for 24 h (Jayasekar et al., 1997). No mortality was recorded at the end of this time, for up to 15 g/kg body weight p.o.

The methanolic extract was also administered to another 3 groups of five mice each in graded doses of 1875, 3750 and 7500 mg/kg respectively, intraperitoneally. The highest oral dose was half the value of i.p dose. Signs and symptoms of toxicity and mortality were observed for 24 h. At the end of this period, different degrees of mortality were observed in each of the groups of mice. Probit analysis using SPSS software was used to determine the LD_{50} of the methanolic extract.

Evaluation of antinociceptive potential

Pharmacological investigation was carried out on the extract of the test plant to evaluate its antinociceptive potential. Two experimental models (acetic acid - induced mice writhing reflex test and Hot-plate test) were employed, using acetylsalicylic acid and morphine as the standard reference drugs and distilled water as the test control.

Rotarod test in mice

Potential central nervous system effects, including sedation or nonspecific motor effects, were evaluated by measuring the ability of mice to maintain balance on an accelerating and rotating rod (rate of rotation was 4 to 40 rpm over a 5-min period) after s.c. administration of normal saline vehicle. Mice were conditioned before the experiment (at least five trials), and animals were selected as those remaining on the Rotarod for 300 s. On the day of experiment, three trials were consecutively performed to establish baseline values. Mice were tested at 30, 60, 90, and 120 min after administration.

Acetic acid induced mouse writhing reflex

The acetic acid induced mouse writhing reflex test was performed based on the method described by Koster et al. (1959). The mice were divided into 5 groups of 5 animals each, A 200 mg/ml concentration of the extract of *M. puberula* at 600, 1200 and 2400 mg/kg and distilled water (1 ml/kg) were administered orally to the mice 30 min before the intraperitoneal injection of 0.6% acetic acid solution (at the dose of 10 ml/kg). The animals were observed for writhing or stretching for 15 min. A reduction in the number of writhings as compared to the control group was considered an evidence of analgesia, which was expressed as the percentage inhibition of writhing.

Hot plate test

The mice were divided into 5 groups of 5 animals. The surface of the hot plate was maintained as 55 ±0.5°C. The mice were individually placed one at a time onto the heated plate and time required for the animal to begin to lick its paw or attempt to escape from the heated surface was taken as the end point for the initial response of the animal to avoid tissue damage. The cut-off time for latency response was 15 s. This was determined before the administration of the different concentrations of the extract (9600, 1200 and 2400 mg/kg) p.o., acetylsalicylic acid (100 mg/kg p.o.), morphine (10 mg/kg i.p) and distilled water (100 ml/kg) at 0, 30, 60, 90 and 120 min intervals, and after the administration of the drug.

Table 1. Effect of *Microdermis puberula* on writhing reflex in mice.

Group	Dose (mg/kg)	Number of Writhes	Percentage Inhibition (%)
Distilled water	-	85.5	-
Microdermis puberula extract	600	60.5	29.23
	1200	46.0	46.20*
	2400	35.2	58.83*
Acetylsalicylic acid	100	15.7	81.60*

n=5, 'n' represents the number of animals in each group. Duration of test =15 min. Values are expressed as percentage inhibition
*P<0.05 is statistically significant.

Data analysis

In the writhing test, the degree of antinociception was expressed as the percentage decrease in the number of writhings and was calculated according to the formula:

Percentage inhibition of writhing (%) = $(C - T)/C \times 100$

where C is the mean number of writhings in saline-treated mice and T is the number of writhings in drug-treated mice. In the radiant tail-flick test, the data were expressed as percentage antinociception, which was calculated using the equation:

Percentage antinoception (%) = $[(TL - BL)/(7 - BL)] \times 100$

where TL is test latency and BL is baseline tail-flick latency. All values were expressed as mean ± SEM. Comparisons of the means of two groups were performed with Student's t-test for non-paired and paired data. Several treatment groups were compared with the control group by using analysis of variance followed by the Duncan test. The differences between means were considered significant when the value of P was < 0.05 and results obtained were recorded as Mean ± SEM (Standard error of the mean). Statistical comparisons were made using the student's 't' test. P values less than 0.05 (p<0.05) were considered statistically significant.

RESULTS

Antinociceptive tests

Acetic acid induced writhing reflex test

Table 1 shows the effect of the extract of *M. puberula* on mouse writhing reflex as an evaluation of the antinociceptive property of the extract. In this assay, the extract at 600 to 2400 mg/kg p.o produced dose–dependent reduction in the numbers of writhes. The mice given distilled water produced the greatest number of writhes. Acetylsalicylic acid (100 mg/kg) reduced the number of writhes considerably and acted as a good inhibitor of peripheral pain. The extract at 1200 and 2400 mg/kg p.o produced reduction in the number of writhes, comparable with acetylsalicylic acid.

Hot plate test

The antinociceptive effects of the methanolic extract of *M. puberula* are presented in Table 2. The extract (600 to 2400 mg/kg p.o) increased the pain threshold in a dose-related manner. At 600, 1200, and 2400 mg/kg, the extract inhibited pain stimuli by 3.15, 3.5 and 11.90% respectively, comparable with the control group. Acetylsalicylic acid, however, inhibited pain stimuli but could not prolong the reaction time. In contrast, morphine (10 mg/kg i.p) significantly (p <0.05) prolonged the reaction time to pain to almost 10 s and inhibited pain by 61%. The extract at the dose of 2400 mg/kg significantly (p< 0.05) increased the pain threshold, in comparison with the control, and produced antinociceptive effect higher than that of acetylsalicylic acid.

Phytochemical analysis

Previous works have reported the vasorelaxing hypotensive and antioxidant properties of the root extract of *M. puberula*. These properties could be attributed to the active constituents of *M. puberula*. Phytochemical analyses reported the presence of flavonoids, saponins and cardiac glycosides (Trease and Evans, 2000).

Acute toxicity test

Results obtained from the intraperitoneal administration of graded doses up to 7.5 kg/mg of the extract of *M. puberula* indicated a lethal dose of 1412.5 mg/kg, after 24 h.

DISCUSSION AND CONCLUSION

The rationale behind the antinociceptive evaluation of the methanolic extract of *M. puberula* was to scientifically establish the claim of its effectiveness in peripheral pain management. A dose-dependent antinociceptive effect

Table 2. Effects of *M. puberula* on hot-plate test in mice.

Group	Dose (mg/kg)	Time for licking paw(Pre treatment) (s)	Time for licking paw (Post treatment) (s)	Percentage inhibition (%)
Distilled water	-	1.50±0.21	1.57±0.19	0.52
Microdermis	600	1.67±0.22*	2.09±0.25	3.15
puberula	1200	1.96±0.17	2.41±0.34	3.45
extract	2400	2.01±0.32	3.56±0.56	11.90*
Acetylsalicylic acid	100	1.39±0.17	2.15±0.05	5.58
Morphine	10	1.99±0.31	9.90±0.25	60.79*

n=8, Values are expressed as mean ± SEM,*p<0.05 is statistically significant.

was exerted by the extract on acetic acid induced mouse-writhing reflex. The analgesic action of NSAIDs has been explained by their inhibition of cyclooxygenase, which synthesizes prostaglandins at the peripheral cell-damage sites (Vain, 1971). It is possible that prostanoids released from cyclooxygenase are involved in the processing of acetic acid-induced visceral nociception. The extract (2400 and 1200 mg/kg p.o) produced a slight inhibition of pain stimuli similar to NSAIDs. This suggests that the extract possesses mild antinociceptive activity that may be peripherally mediated.

This effect may be attributed to its ability to prevent some pain mediators such as prostaglandins from sensitizing nociceptors that induce writhes in response to chemical substances injected intraperitoneally.

The hot-plate test is referred to as an acute test of nociception. It is considered selective for centrally acting or opioid-like antinociceptive compounds. Centrally acting antinociceptive drugs elevate pain threshold of animals towards heat. The extract at higher doses elevated pain threshold in hot plate model.

Previous studies have reported that *M. puberula* possessed vasorelaxing, hypotensive and antioxidant activities (Zamble et al., 2006) and these may perhaps account for its resistance to some level of stress and pain.

In conclusion, the extract produced mild antinociceptive actions.

REFERENCES

Adeneye AA, Benebo AS (2007). Pharmacological Evaluation of a Nigerian Polyherbal Health Tonic Tea in Rat. Afr. J. Biomed. Res., 10: 249-255.

Esonu BO, Iheukwumere FC, Iwuji TC, Akanu N, Nwugo OH (2004) Evaluation of *Microdemis puberula* leaf meal as feed ingredient in broiler starters' diet. Nig. J. Anim. Prod., 30: 3-8

Esonu BO, Azubuike JC, Ukwu HO (2004). Evaluation of *microdermis puberula* leaf meal as feed ingredient in laying hen diets. Int. J. Poult. Sci., 3(2): 96-99.

Jayasekar P, Mohanan PV, Rathinam K (1997). Hepatoprotective activity of ethyl acetate extract of Acacia catechu. Ind. J. Pharmacol., 29: 426.

Koster R, Anderson M, Debeer EJ (1959). Acetic and Antinociceptive Screenings. Fed. Proc., 18: 418-420

Trease GE, Evans MCT (2000). Textbook of Pharmacognosy. 20th Edition, Billiere Tindall, London. pp. 179-280

Vain JR (1971). Inhibition of prostaglandin synthesis as a mechanism of action for aspirin-like drugs. Nat. New Biol., 231: 232–235.

World Health Organisation (1996); WHO guidelines for the assessment of herbal medicines. WHO Expert Committee on Specification for Pharmaceutical Preparations. Technical Report Series No. 863. Geneva.

Zamble A, Yao D, Martin-Nizard F, Shapaz S, Offoumou M, Bordet R, Duriez P, Brunet C, Bailleul F (2006). Vasoactivity and antioxidant properties of *microdermis keayana* roots. J. Ethnopharmacol., 104(1-2): 263-269.

Zamble A, Sahpaz S, Brunet C, Bailleul F (2008). Effects of *Microdermis keayana* roots on sexual behaviour of male rats. Phytomedicine, 15(8): 625 -629

Zimmermann M (1983). Ethical guidelines for investigations of experimental pain in conscious animals. Pain, 16: 109-110.

16

Neuropharmacological effects of *Sorghum bicolor* leaf base extract

F. C. Nwinyi* and H. O. Kwanashie

Department of Pharmacology and Clinical Pharmacy, Ahmadu Bello University Main Campus, P. M. B. 1045, Zaria 810271, Kaduna State, Nigeria.

The neuropharmacological effects of aqueous methanolic extract of leaf base of *Sorghum bicolor* were studied on Wistar rats and Swiss albino mice; evaluations were done on spontaneous motor activity, exploratory behaviour, apomorphine-induced stereotypic behaviour, pentobarbitone sleeping time and rota-rod performance for motor coordination. The results showed a significant ($P < 0.05$) reduction in the spontaneous motor activity. The treated animals exhibited: (i) A reduction in the exploratory behaviour as did diazepam (1 mg/kg i.p.); (ii) No change in Apomorphine-induced stereotypic behaviour; (iii) Prolonged pentobarbitone-induced sleep as did diazepam (1 mg/kg i.p.) and cimetidine (100 mg/kg p.o) and no significant ($P < 0.05$) effect on rota-rod performance for motor coordination. These findings suggest that leaf base extracts of *S. bicolor* contains sedative substances that act via centrally-mediated actions rather than peripheral neuromuscular blockade and may also be microsomal enzyme inhibitor like cimetidine.

Key words: *Sorghum bicolor*, spontaneous motor activity, exploratory behaviour, stereotype behaviour, pentobarbitone sleep, motor coordination.

INTRODUCTION

Medicinal herbs are used as traditional medicine worldwide as these are cheaper, easily available and their use depends on ancestral experience (Marin-Bettolo, 1980). *Sorghum bicolor* (Linn.) Pers. (Family: Poaceae) is a cultivated annual plant with widely reported ethnomedicinal uses in different parts of the world (Grieve, 1931; Watt and Breyer-Brandwijk, 1962; Perry, 1980; Duke and Wain, 1981; Morton, 1981; Chiej, 1984; Grieve, 1984; Okokoh, 1999). This plant is used as a remedy for epilepsy (a central nervous system related condition). The World Health Organisation encourages the inclusion of herbal medicines proven safe and efficacious in the health care programs of developing countries because of the great potential they have in combating various diseases. Evaluation of the effects of medicines on different body systems constitutes safety evaluation of these medicines. Presently, there is paucity of information about the neuropharmacological effects of this widely used plant.

The present study was therefore aimed at evaluation of the neuropharmacological effect of *S. bicolor* leaf base extract.

MATERIALS AND METHODS

Plant preparation and extraction

The dry mature leaves of *S. bicolor* were collected from Maganawa town, Sokoto State, Nigeria between November and January, 2006. The plant was authenticated by a plant taxonomist, Mr. Ibrahim Muazzam of Herbarium Unit, Department of Medicinal Plant Research and Traditional Medicine, National Institute for Pharmaceutical Research and Development (NIPRD), Abuja, Nigeria. The specimen was deposited at NIPRD's Herbarium with voucher specimen number 3815. The dark red portions of the leaves attached to the suckers of the plants were cut out from the entire leaves (the portion of the leaves especially claimed to be used ethnomedicinally). They were then pulverized in a mortar. Two hundred grams (200 g) of the pulverized sample was cold macerated successively in 5 litres of 70% v/v methanol over 96 h period on a shaker (GFL D 3006 mgH, Germany) to ensure maximum extraction. The extract was then filtered using clean cotton wool. The filtrate was placed on water bath to allow evaporation of the solvents and consequent concentration of the extract for subsequent studies. A yield of 23.6% w/w extract was obtained.

The aqueous-methanolic extract was further partitioned into non-

---

*Corresponding author. E-mail: fchyme@yahoo.co.uk.

polar, medium polar and polar components using the solvents; hexane, ethylacetate and water (aqueous). 10.15 g of the 70% methanolic extract was dissolved in distilled water and then gently mixed separately with each of the solvents in a separating funnel and allowed to stand for about 30 min to produce two immiscible layers that were then separated. The process was repeated until the upper partitioning solvent became clear. All the portions (hexane, ethylacetate and aqueous portions) were concentrated to small volumes in a rota vapour and finally concentrated on water bath for subsequent use.

The hexane portion of the crude extract was greenish, fatty/oily and very small with a yield of 0.5% w/w (a probable indication of presence of only very small quantities of non-polar components in the crude extract). Ethylacetate portion appeared shinny, deep brownish-black in colour, clumped up but not sticky. It had a yield of 95.9% w/w (constituting the major component) while the aqueous component appeared deep brownish, clumped up but sticky. It gave a yield of 3.6% w/w.

Animals

Wistar rats (81.0 - 172.3 g), Swiss albino mice (15.3 - 35.6 g) of both sexes were used for the studies. They were obtained from the Animal Facility Centre, Department of Pharmacology and Toxicology, National Institute for Pharmaceutical Research and Development (NIPRD), Abuja, Nigeria. The experimental animals were separated for two weeks in the experimental room for acclimatization. They were housed in appropriately designed cages. The animals were maintained under normal environmental temperature (26 - 28°C), approximately normal 12 h day and night illumination cycle. The animals were fed *ad libitum* with standard NIPRD formulated feed and had free access to water from Abuja Municipal water supply. Cleanliness was ensured throughout the study.

In the experimental grouping of the animals, the body weights and sex of the animals were taken into consideration to achieve approximately equal conditions among the groups. The animals were identified using small cards stuck to different cages indicating the study number, group number, animal number and dose levels. The 'principles of laboratory animal care' (NIH Publication # 85 - 23, 1985) were followed in the study.

Drugs and Chemicals

Some of the drugs and chemicals used for carrying out the studies included: Diazepam (Calmpose®; Ranbaxy, India), Apomorphine (Sigma, USA), Pentobarbitone sodium (Sigma, USA), Phenobarbitone (Vitabiotics, England), Cimetidine (Smithkline and French, England), Methanol (Fluka Chemie, Switzerland), Hexane (BDH Chemicals Ltd., Poole, England), Ethylacetate (BDH Chemicals Ltd., Poole, England).

Acute toxicity study (LD$_{50}$)

The modified method of Lorke (1983) was adopted for the studies. The estimation of the median lethal dose (LD$_{50}$) values for the aqueous-methanolic extract, its ethylacetate and aqueous fractions was done using adult Swiss albino mice and Wistar rats of both sexes. The test routes were intraperitoneal (i.p.) and oral (p.o.) for the aqueous-methanolic extract and only intraperitoneal route for the fractions. The extract administration was done in biphasic manner using doses ranging from 100 - 2000 mg/kg. The animals were observed for 72 h for behavioural effects such as nervousness, ataxia, excitement, alertness, dullness and death.

The LD$_{50}$ was calculated as the geometric mean of the dose that caused 100% mortality and that which caused 0% mortality.

Studies on spontaneous motor activity (SMA)

The spontaneous motor activity of mice were recorded using ventilated activity cages (LE 886) connected to multi-counter (LE 3806) obtained from LETICA (Spain) and by employing the procedure described by Gamaniel et al. (1998).

Adult Swiss albino mice of both sexes were divided into four groups (n = 6). Normal saline (20 ml/kg i.p.) was administered to the first group to serve as the control. Graded doses of the aqueous methanolic extract (100, 200 and 400 mg/kg i.p.) were administered to mice in groups two, three and four, respectively. After 30 min of treatment, the animals were transferred individually into the LETICA activity cages. The activity counts were recorded for 6 min after 1 min latency period, at intervals of 30 min for 2 h (120 min). Baseline activity counts were recorded prior to the treatment.

Test for exploratory behaviour in mice

The hole-board test of Perez et al. (1998) was adopted in this test. The LETICA board (Signo 720; Printer LE 3333) of 60 cm × 30 cm with 16 evenly spaced holes with in-built infra-red sensors was used for the study. Adult Swiss albino mice of either sex used for the investigation were placed individually in the arena of the LETICA hole board. The number of times an animal dipped its head into the holes during a 5 min period was automatically counted and recorded by the instrument (Wolfman et al., 1994). A baseline count was taken for each mouse. The mice were then divided into five groups (of 5 mice each). Mice in group one received normal saline (20 ml/kg i.p.) to serve as the negative control. The aqueous methanolic extract (100, 200 and 400 mg/kg) was given intraperitoneally to mice in groups two, three and four, respectively while diazepam (1 mg/kg i.p.) was given to mice in group five to serve as a reference standard. Recording was repeated as described above at 30, 60 and 90 min post treatment.

Studies on apomorphine-induced stereotypic behaviour

The effect of the aqueous methanolic extract on apomorphine-induced stereotypic behaviour was investigated as described by Kenneth and Kenneth (1984). Adult Swiss albino mice of both sexes were divided into four groups (n = 5). Normal saline (20 ml/kg i.p.) was administered to mice in group one to serve as the control while graded doses of the extract (100, 200 and 400 mg/kg i.p.) were given to mice in groups two, three and four, respectively. 30 min post treatment, apomorphine (0.1 mg/kg i.p.) was administered to each mouse. Signs of stereotypic behaviours, which included mainly sniffing and gnawing were observed and rated. The stereotypic episodes were scored as follows: absence of stereotype (0); occasional sniffing (1); occasional sniffing with occasional gnawing (2); frequent gnawing (3); intense and continuous gnawing (4); intense gnawing and jumping (5). The stereotypic behaviour was measured 1 min post apomorphine administration. They were scored after every minute over 5 min period. The mean of the 5 min period was calculated and recorded.

Studies on pentobarbitone sleeping time

The procedure described by Wambebe (1985) was adopted for the study. The test was carried out on adult Swiss albino mice of either sex divided into five groups (of five mice each). The first group of mice received normal saline (20 ml/kg i.p.) to serve as the control. Groups two, three and four received the aqueous methanolic extract (100, 200, 400 mg/kg i.p.), respectively while the fifth group was given diazepam (1 mg/kg i.p.) to serve as the reference standard. 30 min post treatment, pentobarbitone sodium (30 mg/kg i.p.) was administered to each mouse to induce sleep. The time of onset and duration of sleep observed for each mouse was recorded. The criterion for sleep was loss of righting reflex (Miya et al., 1973; Wambebe, 1985; Ramirez et al., 1998). The interval between loss and recovery of righting reflex was used as the index of hypnotic effect (Fujimori, 1965). This model/test was also adopted as one of the bioassay guides for evaluation of ethylacetate and aqueous fractions of the extract. The study was repeated using 100, 200 and 400 mg/kg i.p. doses of ethylacetate fraction as well as 100, 200 and 400 mg/kg i.p. doses of the aqueous fraction. Diazepam (1 mg/kg i.p.) was used as the reference drug while normal saline (20 ml/kg i.p.) was used as the negative control.

Use of pentobarbitone-induced sleep as a model to test effect of S. bicolor on microsomal enzyme of mice and rats

The study was carried out on adult Swiss albino mice and adult Wistar rats of both sexes. They were divided into six groups of mice and six groups of rats (n = 5). Group one received normal saline (20 ml/kg p.o.) to serve as the control. Phenobarbitone (1 mg/kg p.o.) was given to group two to serve as a reference microsomal enzyme inducer drug. Group three was given cimetidine (100 mg/kg p.o.) to serve as reference microsomal enzyme inhibitory drug. Graded doses of the aqueous methanolic extract (100, 200 and 400 mg/kg p.o.) were administered to groups four, five and six, respectively. The treatment was administered for six (6) consecutive days. 30 min post 6th day treatment, pentobarbitone (30 and 40 mg/kg i.p.) was administered to all the groups of mice and rats respectively to induce sleep. Each experimental animal was observed for the onset and duration of sleep, with the criterion for sleep being loss of righting reflex (Miya et al., 1973; Wambebe, 1985; Ramirez et al., 1998). The index of microsomal enzyme effect was taken as the duration of hypnosis observed in the experimental animals to which it is inversely related.

Test for motor coordination (rota-rod performance)

The test was conducted following the procedure of Ozturk et al. (1996). A rota-rod treadmill device (Ugo Basile No. 7650, Varies, Italy) was used to assess the locomotor activity of mice. Adult Swiss albino mice of either sex were placed on a horizontal rotating rod with diameter of 5 cm set at 16 revolutions per min. Mice that were able to continuously walk on the rotating rod for 3 min (180 s) were selected and grouped into four (of five mice each). Normal saline (20 ml/kg i.p.) was given to group one mice to serve as the control. Graded doses of the aqueous methanolic extract (100, 200 and 400 mg/kg i.p.) were administered to mice in groups two, three and four respectively. After 30 min post-treatment, each mouse was placed back on the rotating rod for 3 min (180 s) at intervals of 30 min up to a period of 3 h (180 min). The time an animal fell from the rod within the 180 s was recorded. Failing of an animal more than once within 180 seconds indicated lack of motor coordination (Fujimori and Cobb, 1965).

Statistical analysis

The results of the studies were expressed as mean ± SEM (standard error of mean). The difference between the control and treated means were analysed using analysis of variance (ANOVA). Student t-test and Least Significant Difference (LSD) were applied where ANOVA showed significant difference. P-values < 0.05 were taken to be statistically significant. Results were presented as Tables and Figure.

Compliance with good laboratory practice (GLP)

The studies were carried out according to Good Laboratory Practice (GLP) Regulations of Organization for Economic Cooperation and Development – OECD (UNDP/World Bank/WHO, 2001).

RESULTS

Acute toxicity studies (LD$_{50}$)

No overt toxicity sign or death was observed in rats and mice during the 72 h post oral treatment with 100 - 2,000 mg/kg doses of S. bicolor leaf base extract. The oral median lethal dose (LD$_{50}$) of the extract in rats and mice was therefore ≥ 2000 mg/kg p.o. The rats treated intraperitoneally (i.p.) with the leaf base extract (100 - 2,000 mg/kg) showed no overt toxicity sign or death in the 24 h post treatment. However, all the rats treated with 2,000 mg/kg i.p. dose became recumbent and died within 48 h of the intraperitoneal treatment while those treated with 100 - 1,000 mg/kg i.p. doses neither showed toxicity signs nor death during 72 h post i.p. treatment. For the estimation of the intraperitoneal median lethal dose (LD$_{50}$ i.p.) in rats, assessment based on 24 h post treatment showed a median lethal dose (LD$_{50}$) ≥ 2,000 mg/kg i.p. since no overt toxicity sign or death was observed in i.p.-treated rats after 24 h. However, an assessment based on 48 h post i.p. treatment observation gave a calculated median lethal dose of 1,414.2 mg/kg i.p. in rats. The mice treated with doses of the extract ≤ 1,200 mg/kg i.p. showed neither toxicity signs nor death during the 24 h post treatment. At the dose of 1,500 mg/kg i.p., the mice were calm, dull, with increased respiratory rate. At this dose, mortality of 66.7 and 100.0% occurred within 24 and 48 h of i.p. treatment respectively.

The mice treated i.p. with 2,000 mg/kg dose were calm, dull and recumbent with increased respiratory rate. A mortality of 100.0% occurred at this dose within 24 h. The calculated intraperitoneal medial lethal dose in mice was 1,248.0 and 1,341.6 mg/kg i.p. for 24 and 48 h post treatment observations, respectively. For the ethylacetate fraction of S. bicolor leaf base extract, 33.3 and 66.7% of 1000 and 2000 mg/kg i.p-treated mice were dull, immobilised with increased respiration within 12 min post administration. All the mice later recovered and no further toxicity signs or death was observed during the 24, 48 and 72 h post intraperitoneal administration. The intraperitoneal LD$_{50}$ of ethylacetate fraction of S. bicolor leaf base extract in mice is therefore ≥ 2000 mg/kg. For the aqueous fraction of S. bicolor leaf base extract, only 33.3% of mice treated intraperitoneally with the dose of 2,000 mg/kg were dull, immobilized with increased respiration within 10 min of administration. The mice observed during the 24, 48 and 72 h post i.p. administration. The intraperitoneal LD$_{50}$ of aqueous fraction of S. bicolor leaf base extract in mice is therefore ≥ 2000 mg/kg.

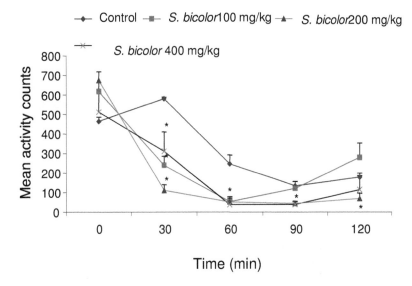

Figure 1. Effect of aqueous methanolic extract of *S. bicolor* leaf base (100, 200 and 400 mg/kg i.p.) on spontaneous motor activity in mice.

Effect on spontaneous motor activity (SMA)

S. bicolor leaf base extract (100, 200 and 400 mg/kg i.p.) produced a significant ($p < 0.05$) reduction of spontaneous motor activity in mice in relation to the control. This effect was time related. Maximum effect was observed at 60th minute for 100 mg/kg dose and at 90th minute for both 200 and 400 mg/kg doses. The SMA of the control group was also observed to have decreased also recovered and no further toxicity sign or death was from the 60th minute of the experiment. The reduction was however, not as the treated groups (Figure 1).

Effect on exploratory behaviour of mice

The study revealed a reduction in the exploratory activity of mice in all the groups. However, the observed reductions were more in the treated groups. The statistical comparisons made for every group with its zero readings showed statistical significance ($p < 0.05$) for the extract (100 mg/kg i.p) at 30, 60 and 90 min, for extract (200 mg/kg i.p.) at 90 min, the extract (400 mg/kg i.p.) at 30, 60 and 90 min and for diazepam (1 mg/kg i.p.) at 30, 60 and 90 min.

The statistical comparisons made between the treated groups and normal saline control group showed significant ($p < 0.05$) reduction for the extract (100 mg/kg i.p.) at 30 min, extract (400 mg/kg i.p. at 90 min and for diazepam (1 mg/kg i.p.) at 30 and 60 min intervals (Table 1).

Effect on apomorphine-induced stereotypic behaviour

The aqueous methanolic extract of *S. bicolor* leaf base

(100 - 400 mg/kg i.p.) did not inhibit apomorphine-induced stereotypic behaviour in mice (Table 2).

Effect on pentobarbitone sleeping time

The aqueous methanolic extract of *S. bicolor* leaf base caused a reduction in the sleep onset of mice dosed once with the extract. This effect was not dose-dependent and was only significant ($p < 0.05$) at the dose of 100 mg/kg i.p. The extract also prolonged the duration of pentobarbitone sleep in a manner that was also not dose-dependent. The prolongation was only significant ($p < 0.05$) at the dose of 100 mg/kg i.p. Diazepam (1 mg/kg i.p.) on the other hand significantly ($p < 0.05$) caused a reduction in the sleep onset and prolongation of the sleep duration (Table 3). However, the aqueous (100 - 400 mg/kg i.p.) and ethylacetate (100 - 400 mg/kg i.p.) fractions of *S. bicolor* leaf extract produced no significant effect on both the onset and duration of pentobarbitone-induced sleep in mice while diazepam (1 mg/kg i.p.) caused a significant ($p < 0.05$) prolongation of the sleep duration (Table 4).

Effect on pentobarbitone-induced sleep for microsomal enzyme of mice and rats

Mice dosed cumulatively for six days with aqueous methanolic extract of *S. bicolor* leaf base had slightly increased onset of pentobarbitone (30 mg/kg i.p.)-induced sleep at 100 mg/kg p.o. dose while the doses of 200 and 400 mg/kg p.o. of the extract produced reduced sleep onset. These observations were however, non-significantly different from the control. The duration of

Table 1. Effect of aqueous methanolic extract of *S. bicolor* leaf base (100, 200, 400 mg/kg i.p.) on exploratory behaviour of mice.

Treatment (i.p.)	Mean Head-dips ± SEM			
	0 min	30 min	60 min	90 min
Normal saline (control; 20 ml/kg) *S. bicolor*	79.8 ± 6.3	70.6 ± 14.1	59.8 ± 13.3	43.2 ± 14.4
100 mg/kg	81.0 ± 11.3	30.4 ± 9.3*@	46.8 ± 9.2*	40.4 ± 4.6*
200 mg/kg	66.4 ± 5.1	78.4 ± 22.5	47.6 ± 10.9	25.4 ± 9.7*
400 mg/kg	91.4 ± 16.8	61.0 ± 12.6*	39.2 ± 10.5*	16.4 ± 4.4*@
Diazepam (1 mg/kg)	70.4 ± 7.6	39.4 ± 14.0*@	17.0 ± 6.3*	16.8 ± 4.7*

SEM= Standard error of mean; 0 min = reading before treatment; * = $p < 0.05$, statically different from zero reading of same group (2-way ANOVA; Least Significant Difference - LSD). @ = $P < 0.05$, statistical difference from normal saline control reading (2-way ANOVA; LSD).

Table 2. Effect of aqueous methanolic extract of *S. bicolor* leaf base (100 - 400 mg/kg i.p.) on apomorphine-induced stereotypic behaviour in mice.

Treatment	Mean score per 5 min ± SEM
Control *S. bicolor*	2.76 ± 0.9
100 mg/kg i.p.	3.10 ± 1.0
200 mg/kg i.p.	4.40 ± 0.7
400 mg/kg i.p.	4.60 ± 0.6

Table 3. Effect of aqueous methanolic extract of *S. bicolor* leaf base (100 - 400 mg/kg i.p.) on pentobarbitone-induced sleep in mice.

Treatment (i.p.)	Onset of sleep (min)	Duration of sleep (min)
Normal saline (control; 20 ml/kg) S. bicolor	5.6 ± 0.51	56.0 ± 5.1
100mg/kg	4.2 ± 0.37*	92.0 ± 9.3*
200 mg/kg	5.4 ± 0.70	69.2 ± 13.2
400 mg/kg	4.0 ± 0.71*	111.3 ± 43.1*
Diazepam (1 mg/kg)	3.2 ± 0.60*	126.0 ± 16.7*

Values are expressed as mean ± SEM (n = 5)= $p < 0.05$; statistical difference between treated and control group (ANOVA, Student t-test)

Table 4. Effects of aqueous and ethylacetate fractions of *S. bicolor* leaf extract (100 - 400 mg/kg i.p.) on pentobarbitone-induced sleep in mice.

Treatment (i.p.)	Onset of sleep (min)	Duration of sleep (min)
Normal saline (control; 20 ml/kg)	6.0 ± 1.5	87.0 ± 22.3
Aqueous fraction		
100 mg/kg	3.8 ± 0.5	109.0 ± 37.3
200 mg/kg	4.0 ± 1.1	94.0 ± 37.4
400 mg/kg	7.3 ± 2.0	89.8 ± 24.2
Ethylacetate fraction		
100 mg/kg	8.5 ± 0.3	80.0 ± 24.7
200 mg/kg	4.3 ± 0.8	101.5 ± 32.4
400 mg/kg	7.0 ± 1.3	88.8 ± 19.1
Diazepam (1 mg/kg)	4.0 ± 0.4	137.0 ± 6.7*

Values are expressed as mean ± SEM. * = $P < 0.05$; statistical difference between treated and control group (ANOVA, Student t-test)

Table 5. Effect of aqueous methanolic extract of *S. bicolor* leaf base (100 - 400 mg/kg p.o.) on microsomal enzyme of mice tested on pentobarbitone-induced sleep model.

Treatment (p.o. x 6 days)	Onset of sleep (min)	Duration of sleep (min)
Control (normal saline; 20 ml/kg)	15.25 ± 7.0	31.25 ± 5.7
S. bicolor		
100 mg/kg	18.42 ± 6.4	28.00 ± 1.2
200 mg/kg	6.83 ± 0.5	38.5 ± 0.4
400 mg/kg	13.00 ± 0.5	72.75 ± 27.0
Phenobarbitone (1 mg/kg)	11.33 ± 2.6	10.00 ± 0.6*
Cimetidine (100 mg/kg)	3.47 ± 0.46*	92.23 ± 16.0*

Values are expressed as mean ± SEM; Pentobarbitone dose = 30 mg/kg i.p. *= $p < 0.05$; statistical difference between treated and control group (ANOVA, Student t-test).

Table 6. Effect of aqueous methanolic extract of *S. bicolor* leaf base (100 – 400 mg/kg p.o.) on microsomal enzyme of rats tested on pentobarbitone-induced sleep model.

Treatment (p.o. X 6 days)	Onset of sleep (min)	Duration of sleep (min)
Normal saline (control; 20 ml/kg)	3.75 ± 0.25	90.5 ± 7.27
S. bicolor		
100 mg/kg	3.33 ± 0.33	105.67 ± 4.33
200 mg/kg	4.25 ± 0.75	128.75 ± 39.1
400 mg/kg	4.50 ± 0.50	128.50 ± 10.0*
Phenobarbitone (1 mg/kg)	3.25 ± 0.25	86.25 ± 3.42
Cimetidine (100 mg/kg)	3.67 ± 0.33	222.0 ± 19.17*

Values are expressed as mean ± SEM; pentobarbitone dose = 40 mg/kg i.p.*= $p < 0.05$; statistical difference between treated and control group (ANOVA, Student t-test).

pentobarbitone sleep was slightly reduced by the leaf base extract at 100 mg/kg p.o. dose while they were prolonged at 200 and 400 mg/kg p.o. doses. These effects were also non-significantly different from the control. Phenobarbitone (1 mg/kg p.o.) produced non-significant reduction of sleep onset but a significant ($p < 0.05$) reduction in the duration of sleep while cimetidine (100 mg/kg p.o.) produced significant ($p < 0.05$) prolongation of duration of pentobarbitone-induced sleep in mice (Table 5).

Conversely, rats treated cumulatively for six days with the aqueous methanolic extract had a slightly reduced onset of pentobarbitone (40 mg/kg i.p.)-induced sleep at 100 mg/kg dose while the doses of 200 and 400 mg/kg p.o. slightly increased the sleep onset time. These effects were non-significantly different from the control. However, the duration of pentobarbitone sleep was prolonged by all the doses of the leaf base extract (100 - 400 mg/kg p.o.). These effects were not dose-dependent and was only significant at dose of 400 mg/kg p.o. Phenobarbitone (1 mg/kg p.o.) produced some reduction in onset and duration of pentobarbitone-induced sleep while cimetidine (100 mg/kg p.o.) produced a significant ($p < 0.05$) prolongation of the sleep (Table 6).

Effect on motor co-ordination (Rota-rod Performance)

The aqueous methanolic extract of *S. bicolor* leaf base (100 - 400 mg/kg i.p.) did not produce significant effect on the rota-rod performance of the mice. Most of the mice were able to stay on the rotating rod through the 3 min (180 s) cut-off time point without falling (Table 7).

DISCUSSION

The spontaneous motor activity is a model that has been used in laboratory animals to evaluate the gross behavioural effects of drugs (Hsieh et al., 1991; Carpenedo et al., 1994; File and Fernandes, 1994). The model measures the level of excitability of the central nervous system (Mansur et al., 1971) which correlates well with drug effects in humans. Agents that suppress this behaviour usually do so through central inhibition (Adzu et al., 2002). The significant ($p < 0.05$) reduction in the spontaneous motor activity by the *S. bicolor* leaf base extract therefore suggests a reduction in the excitability of the central nervous system which could be suggestive of sedative activity. Ozturk et al. (1996) reported that the decrease in the activity may be closely related to sedation

Table 7. Effect of aqueous methanolic extract of *S. bicolor* leaf base. (100 - 400 mg/kg i.p.) on motor coordination (rota-rod performance) of mice.

Treatment (i.p.)	Time (second)					
	30	60	90	120	150	180
Normal saline (control; 20ml/kg) *S. bicolor*	180.0 ± 0.0	180.0 ± 0.0	180.0 ± 0.0	180.0 ± 0.0	180.0 ± 0.0	180.0 ± 0.0
100 mg/kg	180.0 ± 0.0	180.0 ± 0.0	180.0 ± 0.0	180.0 ± 0.0	180.0 ± 0.0	180.0 ± 0.0
200 mg/kg	180.0 ± 0.0	176.6 ± 3.4	180.0 ± 0.0	180.0 ± 0.0	180.0 ± 0.0	180.0 ± 0.0
400 mg/kg	180.0 ± 0.0	180.0 ± 0.0	180.0 ± 0.0	180.0 ± 0.0	180.0 ± 0.0	180.0 ± 0.0

Values are expressed as mean ± SEM (n = 5).

resulting from central nervous system (CNS) depression. Similar effect was seen in the significant (p < 0.05) reduction of the number of head dips in the hole board test by the leaf base extract. This test is a measure of exploratory behaviour (File and Wardill, 1975; Crawley, 1985) that reveals sedative activity of agents (File and Pellow 1985; Amos et al., 2001). The test has also been accepted as a parameter for the evaluation of anxiety conditions in animals (Crawley, 1985). The extract therefore possibly has I sedative property. Apomorphine acts directly on the post-synaptic dopamine D-2 receptors to induce hyperactivity and stereotypic behaviour. Inhibition of apomorphine-induced climbing behaviour in mice is suggestive of D2 receptor inhibition (Moore and Axton, 1988). The ability of a drug to antagonise apomorphine-induced climbing behaviour has been correlated to central depressant activity with potential neuroleptic effect (Protais et al., 1976; Costal et al., 1978). The inability of *S. bicolor* leaf base extract to inhibit apomorphine-induced stereotypic behaviour possibly suggests non-inhibition of the D-2 receptors and also indicates that the extract may not be a potential neuroleptic. Potentiation of pentobarbitone-induced hypnosis may be attributed to an action on the central mechanisms involved in the regulation of sleep (Chindo et al., 2003) or an inhibition of pentobarbitone metabolism (Kaul and Kulkarni, 1978). Endogenous neurotransmitters in the brain especially dopamine and gamma-aminobutyric acid (GABA) are implicated in the mechanism of sleep (Osuide and Wambebe, 1980). It is generally accepted that the sedative effects of drugs can be evaluated by measurement of pentobarbitone sleeping time in laboratory animals (Ming-Chin Lu, 1998; Carpenedo, 1994; Gamaniel et al., 1998). Prolongation of pentobarbitone-induced hypnosis is suggestive of centra depressant activity of a compound (Perez et al., 1998). The present study showed that the aqueous methanolic extract of *S. bicolor* leaf base administered once prolonged pentobarbitone-induced hypnosis. This indicates that the extract may not have acted via dopaminergic pathway as indicated by apomorphine-induced stereotypic behaviour test but possibly by enhancing the central inhibitory effect of GABA or by inhibiting pentobarbitone

metabolism or via other mechanisms that may be remotely involved in the mechanism of sleep. These effects were not seen in the aqueous and ethylacetate fractions of the leaf base extract indicating that the pharmacological constituents of the plant responsible for this effect may have been lost or distorted due to the fractionation.

This result was further buttressed by the microsomal enzyme test result that also showed prolongation of pentobarbitone-induced hypnosis after six (6) days treatment with the leaf base extract. This observation was similar to that of cimetidine (100 mg/kg p.o.), which is a known microsomal enzyme inhibitory drug. Microsomal enzymes are associated with a number of drug metabolisms. Administration of microsomal enzyme inhibitor reduces metabolic effect of the microsomal enzyme, producing effects of the drug with longer duration (Grant, 2001). The leaf base extract may have therefore inhibited the metabolic effect of microsomal enzymes on pentobarbitone thereby prolonging its hypnotic effects as did cimetidine.

The test for motor coordination (rota rod performance) was adopted to evaluate the effect of the extract on the physical performance, endurance and possible neuromuscular inhibition. The study revealed that the extract did not produce any effect on motor coordination. This therefore suggests that the extract has centrally-mediated actions (based on the inhibitory effects observed in the previous studies) and not through peripheral neuromuscular blockade (Perez et al., 1998).

In conclusion, the study has shown that the leaf base extract of *S. bicolor* has sedative activity which is central nervous system related effect. This sedative effect can be taken advantage of therapeutically. The knowledge of this sedative effect is also useful in listing the precautionary measures to be taken when *S. bicolor* extract is being indicated for use as medicine.

ACKNOWLEDGEMENTS

The authors are grateful to U.S. Inyang, the Director General, National Institute for Pharmaceutical Research and Development (NIPRD) and his Management team for funding this investigation. They are also grateful to Ibrahim Muazzam, a plant Taxanomist with NIPRD's herbarium for the ethnobotanical information he provided on the study plant. The technical assistance offered by Sunday Dzarma is also appreciated.

REFERENCES

Adzu B, Amos S, Dzarma S, Wambebe C, Gamaniel K (2002). Effect of *Zizypus spinachristi* wild aqueous extract on the central nervous system in mice. J. Ethnopharmacol. 79: 13 – 16.

Amos S, Kolawole E., Akah P., Wambebe C., Gamaniel K. (2001): Behavioural effects of the aqueous extract of *Guiera senegalensis* in mice and rats. Phytomedicine 8 (5):356 - 361.

Carpenedo R, Chiarugi A, Russi P, Lombardi G, Carla V, Pellicciari R, Mattoli L, Maroni F (1994). Inhibitors of Kynurenine hydroxylate and kynureniase increase cerebral formation of kynureniase and have sedative and anti-convulsant activities. Neuroscience 61: 237 – 243.

Chiej R (1984). Encyclopedia of Medicinal Plants. MacDonald.

Chindo BA, Amos S, Odutola AA, Vongtau HO, Abbah J, Wambebe C, Gamaniel KS (2003). Central nervous system activity of the methanolic extract of *Ficus platyphylla* stem bark. J. Ethnopharmacol. 85: 131 – 137.

Costal B, Naylor RJ, Nohria V (1978). Climbing behaviour induced by apomorphine in mice. A potent model for the detection of neuroleptic activity. Eur. J. Pharmacol. 50: 39 – 50.

Crawley JN (1985). Exploratory behaviour models of anxiety in mice. Neurosci. Behav. Rev. 9: 37- 44.

Duke JA, Wain KK (1981). The Medicinal Plants of the World, Computer index with more than 85,000 enteries, Vol.3.

File SE, Wardill AG (1975). Validity of head dipping as a measure of exploration in a modified hole-board. Psychopharmacologia, 44: 53 – 59.

File S, Pellows S (1985). The effect of triazolobenzodiazepines in two animal tests of anxiety and on the hole-board. Br. J. Pharmacol. 86: 729 – 735.

File SE, Fernandes C (1994). Dizocilpine prevents the development of tolerance to the sedative effects of diazepam in rats. Pharmacol. Biochem. Behav, 47: 823 – 826.

Fujimori H, Cobb D (1965). Central nervous system depressant activity of Ma1337, 3-[3,4- M- chlorophenyl – 1-piperazyl propyl]-1-2-4 (1H, 3H) quinozotinedione hydrochloride. J. Pharmacol. Exp. Ther. 148: 151– 157.

Gamaniel K, Amos S, Akah PA, Samuel BB, Kapu S, Olusola A, Abayomi AO, Okogun JI, Wambebe C (1998). Pharmacological profile of NIPRD 94/002/1 – 0. A novel herbal antisickling agent. J. Pharmaceut .Res. Dev. 3(2): 89 – 94.

Grant R, Wilkinson (2001). Pharmacokinetics - The Dynamics of Drug: Asorption, Distribution and Elimination. *In:* Goodman and Gilman, Joel Hardman and Lee Limbird (10th ed.). The Pharmacological Basis of Therapeutics. McGraw Hill, New York, Toronto pp. 3 - 29

Grieve M (1931). A Modern Herbal. Reprint (1974). Hafner Press, New York.

Grieve M (1984). A Modern Herbal. Penguin. ISBN 0 – 14-046-440-9.

Hsieh MT., Peng WH., Tsai HY., Chang TS. (1991). Studies on anti-convulsive, sedative and hypothermic effects of *Periostracum cicadae* extracts. J. Ethnopharmacol. 35: 83 – 90.

Kaul PN, Kulkarni SK. (1978). New drug metabolism inhibitor of marine origin. J. Pharm. Sci. 67: 1293 – 1296.

Kenneth SK, Kenneth ID (1984). Genetic control of apomorphine-induced climbing behaviour in two inbred mouse strains. Brain Res. 293: 343 – 351.

Lorke D (1983). A new approach to acute toxicity testing. Archives of Toxicol. 54: 275 – 287.

Marin-Bettolo GB (1980). Present aspects of the use of medicinal plants in traditional medicine. J. Ethnopharmacol. 2: 5 - 7

Mansur J, Martz RMW, Carlini EA (1971). Effects of acute and chronic administration of *Cannabis sativa* and (-) 9- traus-tetrahydro cannabinol on the behaviour of rats in an open field arena. Psychopharmacology 19: 338 – 397.

Ming-Chin Lu (1998). Studies on the sedative effects of *Cistanche deserticola*. J. Ethnopharmacol. 59: 161 – 165.

Miya TS, Holck HGO, Yui GKW, Spratto GR (1973). Laboratory guide in pharmacology. Burgess Publishing Company. Minneapolis MN pp. 44 – 46.

Moore NA, Axton MS (1988). Production of climbing behaviour in mice requires both D1 and D2 receptor activation. Psychopharmacology, 94: 263 – 266.

Morton JF (1981). Atlas of Medicinal Plants of middle America. Bahamas to Yucatan. CC. Thomas, Springfield, II.

Okokoh L. (1999). Quick guide to Natural Health Care. Capstone Herbal Health Centre, Lagos. Pp 29

Osuide G, Wambebe C. (1980). Antagonism of pentobarbitone sleep by dopamine, levodopa and apomorphine in chicks. Clin. Exp. Pharmacol. Physiol. 7: 237 – 248.

Ozturk Y, Aydine S, Ben R, Baser KHC, Berberoglu (1996). Effects of *Hypericum perforatum* L. and *Hypericum calycinum* L. extracts on the central nervous system in mice. Phytomedicine 3 (29): 139 – 146.

Perez RMG, Perez JAL, Garcia LMD, Sossa HM (1998). Neuropharmacological activity of *Solanum nigrum* fruit, J. Ethnopharmacol. 62: 43 – 48.

Perry LM (1980). Medicinal Plants of East and Southeast Asia. MIT Press, Cambridge.

Protais P, Costertin J, Schwartz JC (1976). Climbing Behaviour induced by apomorphine in mice. A simple test for the study of dopamine receptors in the striatum. Psychopharmacology 50: 1 – 6.

Ramirez TED, Ruiz NN, Arellano JDQ, Maldrigal BR, Michel MTV, Garzon P (1998). Anticonvulsant effect of *Mogolia grandiflora* L. in rats. J. Ethnopharmacol. 61: 143 – 152.

UNDP/World Bank/WHO (2001). Introduction of the OECD principles of GLP. Special Programme for Research and Training in Tropical Diseases (TDR) – Good Laboratory Practice Training Manual for the Traiee pp. 3 – 19.

Wambebe C (1985). Influence of some agents that affect 5HT meta-bolism and receptors and nitrazepam-induced sleep time in mice. Br. J. Pharmacol. 84: 185 – 191.

Watt JM, Breyer-Brandwijk MG (1962). The medicinal and poisnous plants of southern and eastern Africa. (2nd ed.) E & S. Livingstone, Ltd., Edinburgh and London.

Wolfan C, Viola H, Paladini AC, Dajas D, Medina JH (1994): Possible anxiolytic effects of Chrysin, a central benzodiazepine receptor ligand isolated from *Passiflora coeruiea* Pharmacol. Biochem. Behav. 47: 1 – 4.

17

Comparative effects of smoke and ethanolic extract of *Nicotiana tabacum* on hippocampus and neurobehaviour of mice

Adeniyi P. A. O.* and Musa A. A.

Department of Anatomy, P. M. B 1515, College of Health Sciences, University of Ilorin, Ilorin, Nigeria.

The effects of tobacco use on health are well known, and are documented in reliable scientific reports. The aim of this study is to investigate some of the effects of both ethanolic and smoke tobacco on the hippocampus and behaviour of mice. The presumably healthy 32 mice were used for this study, the animals were randomly divided into four groups, A, B, C and D, of eight animals each. Group A were given 10.72 mg /kg body weight of the extract in 0.2 ml of normal saline, group B 10.72 mg /kg body weight of the tobacco smoke exposure for 3 min, group C were given 0.2 ml of normal saline and group D were exposed to the smoke of equal weight (0.02 g) of cotton wool for 3 min for 21 experimental days. The mice were sacrificed by cervical dislocation and the brains excised, blotted, weighed and fixed in formol calcium for neurohistological analysis, using Haematoxylin and Eosin and Cresyl Fast Violet. There were significant decreases in the body weight, brain weight and relative brain weight, pyramidal and granular cell layers and neurological scores between nicotine administered groups compared to the control group (p<0.05). The results suggested that consumption of *Nicotiana tabacum* leaves, either through smoking or chewing may lead to some level of neurohistoarchitectural alterations, brain weight changes and neurobehavioural disruption or also help in reduction in weight.

Key words: *Nicotiana tabacum*, hippocampus, nicotine, neurohistoarchitecture, neurobehaviour.

INTRODUCTION

Smokeless tobacco products have been in existence for thousands of years among different populations. Over time, these products have gained popularity throughout the world (such as Tombak in Sudan, Snus in Sweden and Khaini in India) with mass marketing of new forms sold under different brand names (Kumar et al., 2006; Foulds et al., 2003; Idris et al., 1995). The term chewing tobacco is often associated with dipping tobacco (split tobacco, moist snuff) where users place a dip of tobacco between the lower or upper lip and the gum by resting the dip on the inside lining of the mouth. 'Maras powder' (MP), which is a kind of powder obtained from the shields of tobacco, is widely used in the south-east region of Turkey as smokeless tobacco and it is taken through

buccal mucosa or together with cigarette (Erenmemısoglu et al., 1999). The same research group has also found that Turkish smokeless tobacco MP prepared from *Nicotiana tabacum* L. leaves contain low amounts of nicotine (1.17%), nornicotine (0.04%), and 0.06% anabasine. International Agency for Research on Cancer (IARC) reported that moist snuff contains aliphatic and aromatic hydrocarbons, formaldehyde, ketones, alcohols, phenols, amines, amides, alkaloids, metals, radio elements such as polonium-210, uranium-235, 238. Carcinogens in tobacco, the most abundant and strongest being tobacco-specific N-nitrosamines (TSNA), such as N-nitrosonornicotine (NNN) and 4-(methylnitrosamino)-1-(3-pyridyl)-1-butanone (NNK) are formed by N-nitrosation of nicotine (Kurucu et al., 1998). Tobacco consumption continues to grow all over the world. Inhalation of tobacco smoke, with its numerous toxic and mutagenic substances (for example, carbon monoxide, nicotine, polynuclear aromatic hydrocarbons,

---

*Corresponding author. E-mail: adephiladex.ng@gmail.com

N-nitrosamines), may have toxic effects on brain function. Hippocampus is the structure that lies on the fringes of the medial aspect of each cerebral hemisphere (the limbic system) of the brain and it is involved in memory and learning. Exposure to tobacco nicotine either from cigarettes and other forms of tobacco including cigars, pipe tobacco, snuff, and chewing tobacco, has been reported to be associated with alteration in the normal functions of the brain and the whole nervous system (NIDA, 2009a; Charles, 2000; Katzung, 2005; and NIDA, 2009b). Nicotine has been reported to be the highest and most toxic compound of aqueous extract of tobacco leaves (Carla et al., 1997; Penton and lester, 2009; Grunberg, 1982). Nicotine is used to aid smoking cessation and other nicotine addictions (Charles, 2000; Katzung, 2005). Using a controlled amount of nicotine helps to reduce nicotine withdrawal symptoms when one attempts to quit the use of tobacco products (NIDA, 2009b; Charles, 2000; Adeniyi, 2007). Annually, about 5 million deaths are attributed to tobacco smoking contributing the second leading cause of mortality among adults worldwide (Aghaji, 2008; Uwakwe and Modebe, 2008). This frightening data attests to the death of about three million people in the year 2007 alone (NIH, 1993; Wilson and Philpot, 2002), these findings and reports suggest the need for thorough experimental and clinical studies of the effects of tobacco intake on the body systems, most especially the brain. The aim of this study therefore, was to investigate some of the effects of both ethanolic and smoke tobacco on the hippocampus of mice.

MATERIALS AND METHODS

Animal care

All experimental investigations were done in compliance with humane animal care standard outlined in the "Guide to the care and use of Animals in research and teaching", as approved by the Institute of Laboratory Animal Resource, National Research Council, DHHS, Pub. No NIH 86 – 23 (Anne, 2004). The study was carried out using presumably healthy 32 mice of both sexes (18 to 25 g) of three (3) months old. The animals were kept under standard and good laboratory conditions (12 h light and 12 h darkness, temperature (30°C ± 4.5°C), humidity and ventilation). They were given standard rat diet, purchased from the same company, Bethel Feeds, Ilorin, Nigeria.

Extract preparation

The N. tabacum leaves were collected from Igboho, the northern part of Oyo State, Nigeria. Plant samples were authenticated at the Department of Plant Science, University of Ilorin, Nigeria. The leaves were air-dried at room temperature. Grinded leaves (50 g) were dissolved in 500 ml of 70% alcohol for 24 h at room temperature. The filtrate was thereafter obtained from the solution using Whatman's No 1 filter paper and evaporated to dryness in an air - dry oven at 40°C, the residue of the extract obtained in form of paste was stored in a capped bottle and kept in a desiccators (Obembe et al., 2010). The pH of the extract was determined before and after concentrating it, to be 4.19 and 5.72 respectively,

using pH meter (pH – 25 Model, Germany). The yield of the tobacco extract was determined to be 41.35% (Adeniyi, 2010).

Animal treatment

The animals were given the N. tabacum are shown as follows:

Tobacco extract: This was given orally with the aid of an orogastric tube.

Tobacco smoke: It was administered by exposing each animal to dried N. tabacum leaves wrapped with 0.02 g of cotton wool in a burning chamber for 3 min (Burning time (BT); this was determined by allowing three of the N. tabacum leaves of known weight (equivalent of 10.72 mg/kg body weight) to burn and the average burning time was determined).
Administration was done for 21 days and 4 h after which mice from each group were sacrificed for analysis, while the rest were sacrificed by 7 days (a week) after the last administration, to study the withdrawal effects of the N. tabacum exposure on the animals.

Experimental design

A total of 32 mice (16 males and females each), were used for this study. The animals were randomly divided into four (4) groups, A, B, C and D, of eight (8) animals each. Group A was given 10.72 mg /kg body weight of the extract in 0.2 ml of normal saline, group B 10.72 mg /kg body weight of the tobacco smoke exposure for 3 min, group C 0.2 ml of normal saline and D was exposed to smoke of equal weight (0.02 g) of cotton wool for 3 min for 21 experimental days.

Neurobehavioural observations

The neurobehavioural analysis was done at 08:00 h of the day using elevated plus maze (EPM) to study the locomotion, exploration, and motor coordination in both the treated and control animals. The results are shown in Figure 3.

Animal sacrifice

After administration, the mice four (4) from each group were sacrificed by cervical dislocation on day 21 and 28 of the treatment and their brains were excised, blotted with filter paper and the wet weights were taken and recorded and brains were quickly transferred to a specimen bottle containing 10% formol calcium and fixed for 2 days (Adeniyi et al., 2010a; Baron, 1986). Thereafter, the hippocampus was excised to process for histological analysis and the wet weights of the brain and volumes were recorded for analysis. The brain volume was determined by liquid (water) displacement method and recorded in millimeter (Ofusori et al., 2008).
Relative brain weight (RBW) changes: The RBW for each animal was calculated using the formula:

$$RBW = \frac{Brain\ weight}{Body\ weight} \times 100\%$$

Brain volume (BRV) changes: The RBV change for each group was calculated using the formula:

$$Percentage\ BRV\ change = \frac{BRV\ at\ day\ 21 - BRV\ at\ day\ 28}{BRV\ at\ day\ 21} \times 100\%$$

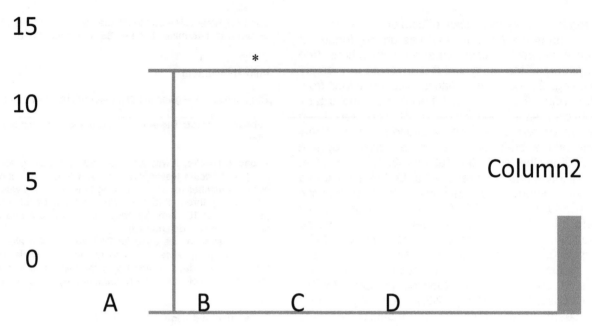

Figure 1. Showing the head dipping (HD) of mice after 21 days of *N. tabacum* exposure. * Statistical significant difference (p< 0.05).

Neurohistology

The brains are fixed in 10% formol calcium, hippocampus was excised and processed for Haematoxylin and Eosin (H & E) and Cresyl Fast Violet (CFV) staining techniques (Adeniyi et al., 2010a; Baron, 1986). The tissues were excised, imbedded in paraffin and processed for routine histologic studies. The slices of 5 μ were sectioned with the Letiz rotary microtome. The sections were mounted and examined with the light microscope and the photomicrography of each slide was recorded.

Neurohistometry

The pyramidal (PCL) and granular (GCL) cell layers thickness was measured using the method of W.H.O and Ofusori et al. (2008) in which an occulometer was inserted into the microscope and focused through stained slides.

Statistical analysis

The data were expressed as means ± Standard Error of Mean (SEM). Significance was determined using the student's t-test. A p-value of less than 0.05 was considered statistically significant, using SPSS software version 16.0.

RESULTS

Gross observations

There were no significant changes in the skin colour and arrangement, the colour of their eyes was normal compared to the control groups. Also, the gross anatomy of the brain of the nicotine administered groups appeared normal compared to the control groups.

The animal weight changes

The average weight gain recorded for the treatmen group during the experimental period was reduced during the first 14 days in group A and B compared to C and D However, they all gained weight during the 7 withdrawa days.

Animal behavior

The general behaviour of the animals was comparatively normal. However, the rate of head deeding (HD) stretching (S), quadrate duration (QD) and transition (T were significantly (p<0.05) different between nicotine administered groups and the control groups (Figures 1 t 4).

Brain weight (BWT) changes

The average brain weight recorded for treatment grou during the experimental period reduced during the 7 days of withdrawal (Table 1).

Relative brain weight (RBW) changes

The RBW (Table 1) changed between the nicotine administered groups, group A had the highest RBW compared to C and as in group B compared to D after 21

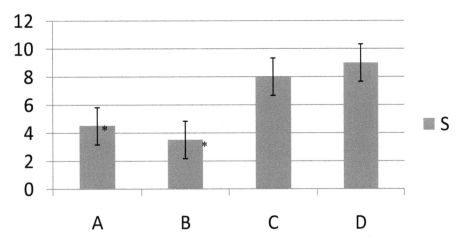

Figure 2. Showing the stretching attempt (s) of mice after 21 days of *N. tabacum* exposure. * Statistical significant difference (p < 0.05).

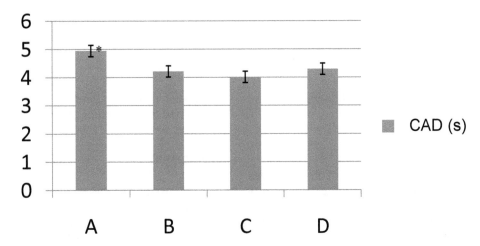

Figure 3. Showing the close arm duration (CAD) in second of mice after 21 days of *N. tabacum* exposure. * Statistical significant difference (p<0.05).

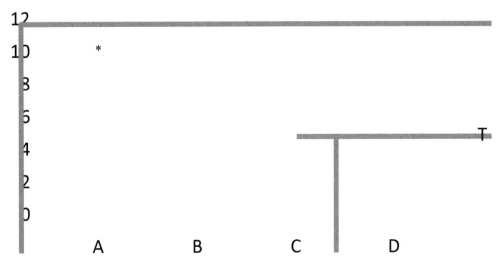

Figure 4. Showing the transition (T) of mice after 21 days of *N. tabacum* exposure. * Statistical significant difference (p<0.05).

Table 1. Brain weight (BWT) (g) and relative brain weight (RBW) changes in control animals and those exposed to tobacco smoke and extract for the experimental period (mean ± SEM).

Groups	Day 21		Day 28	
	BWT	RBW (%)	BWT	RBW (%)
A	0.5172*±0.0112	2.57	0.3786*±0.0209	1.89
B	0.4121±0.0121	1.93	0.3667±0.0072	1.66
C	0.3434±0.0122	1.61	0.3080±0.0066	1.28
D	0.03623±0.0212	1.52	0.3480 ±0.0370	1.42

*Significantly different from control mice (P<0.05).

Table 2. Brain volume (ml) changes in animals exposed to tobacco smoke and extract for the experimental period (mean ± SEM).

Groups	Day 21	Day 28	Percentage brain volume changes (%)
A	4.0±0.00	3.5±0.50*	(12.50)
B	4.0±0.00	4.0±0.00	0.00
C	4.0±0.00	4.0±0.00	0.00
D	4.0±0.00	4.0±0.00	0.00

*Significantly different from control mice (P<0.05).

days of treatment and this was dose dependent.

Brain volume (BRV) changes

The volume of brain of the animals (Table 2) was relatively the same in nicotine administered and control groups. Although, there was slight (12.5%) increase in the brain volume in group A, the brain volume changes were relatively the same across the groups.

Hippocampal neurohistology

Cell body stain intensity: The cell bodies were more densely stained in the nicotine administered groups in a dose dependent manner compared to the control groups but the architectural arrangement appeared normal Table 3.

Vaculations: There were more vaculations in the nicotine administered groups compared to the control group C.

Cell population: The population of the neural cells (pyramidal cells) appeared to be more in the nicotine administered groups compared to the control groups in a dose dependent pattern.

Pyramidal cell layer: This appeared uniformly normal with cell bodies of nicotine administered groups densely stained compared to the control group.

Granule cell layer: Appeared uniformly normal with cell

bodies of nicotine administered groups densely stained compared to the control group (Figure 5).

DISCUSSION

The observed reduction in weight of the animals in the experiment may implicate nicotine in the tobacco plant use as reported by Adeniyi et al. (2010a) and Chen et al., (2005) and this may be associated with reduction in food intake by the tobacco users. Also the brain weights after administration and withdrawal were significantly different from the mice in group A compared to those in groups C and D (p<0.05), but relative brain weight (RBW) of those in group A have the highest RBW compared to C (p<0.05) and as in group B compared to D (p<0.05) after 21 days of treatment and it was dose dependent. These results are related to our findings on the leaf extract of aqueous of *N. tabacum* in Wistar rats (Adeniyi et al., 2010b). The observed increase in locomotory activities of mice (Figures 1 to 4) in the treated groups compared to the control groups is in agreement with our earlier report (Adeniyi et al., 2010b), reflecting the possibility of tobaccoto increasing anxietic characteristics in the treated groups. This may probably explain the reason for increased cell density observed in the treated groups compared with the control groups (Adeniyi et al., 2010a, b). The stretch – attempt (S) of the control was higher than the rest of the groups. S postures are 'risk - assessment' behaviour which indicates that the animal is resistant to move from its present location to the new position (Ekong et al., 2008; Blanchard et al., 2001), and thus high frequency of these activities indicates high level

Table 3. Hippocampal histometry analytic changes in animals on day 21 of tobacco exposure (mean ± SEM).

Groups	PCL (× 10^{-3}mm)	GCL (× 10^{-3}mm)
A	5.2000±0.6633	7.3333*±1.4530
B	6.8000±0.9695	10.5000*±1.3229
C	6.0000±0.4083	9.2500±1.1087
D	5.4000±0.4000	9.8000±1.2806

*Significantly different from control mice (P<0.05), PCL: Pyramidal cell layer, GCL: Granular cell layer.

NEUROPHOTOGRAPHS

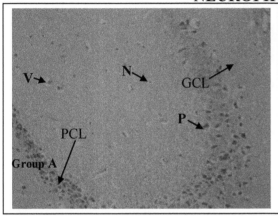

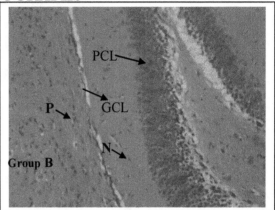

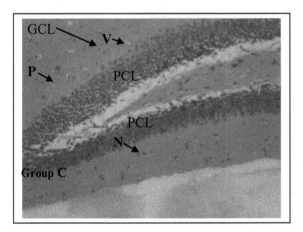

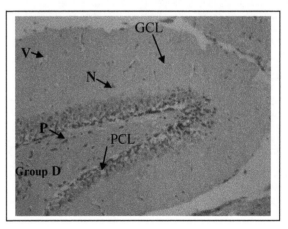

Figure 5. Hippocampus (H & E) day 21 *N. tabacum* exposures: Mg X 480: PCL: Pyramidal cell layer; GCL: Granular cell layer; P – pyramidal cell, N – neuroglia cell, and V – vacuole.
Note: The population of the neural cells (pyramidal and neuroplia cells) appeared to be more in the nicotine administered groups compared to the control groups in a dose dependent pattern and there were more vaculations in the nicotine administered groups compared to the control group C.

of anxiety (Ekong et al., 2008).

Conclusion

Tobacco has been reported to cause different neurological effects in both human and experimental animal, from all the changes observed between the treated and control groups, it is worthy to conclude that the administration of tobacco leaves smoke and extract, as revealed from this study, can result in brain weight loss, distorted neurohistoarchitecture and alterations in locomotory activities.

REFERENCES

Adeniyi PA (2007). Tobacco use and your health. Christ Focused. News letter of Atunbi Baptist Church, 39(3): 4.

Adeniyi PAO (2010). Comparative effects of smoke and ethanolic extract of Tobacco (Nicotiana tabacum) leaves exposure on the frontal cortex and hippocampus of adult mice – Rhabdomys pumpilio M. Sc. Research Thesis, Department of Anatomy, University of Ilorin, Ilorin, Nigeria.

Adeniyi PAO, Ghazal OK, Musa AA, Caxton – Martins EA (2010a). The neurobehavioural effects of smoke and ethanolic extract of Nicotiana tabacum leaves exposure in Mice. Res. J. Anim. Sci., 4(4): 99-102.

Adeniyi PAO, Ghazal OK, Enaibe BU, Adefolaju GA, Oyewopo AO, Caxton-Martins, E A (2010b). The Cytoarchitectural alterations in the neocortex of Wistar rats: Effects of aqueous tobacco (Nicotiana tabacum) leaves   extract exposure. Afr. J. Biotechnol., 9(44): 7539-7543.

Aghaji MN (2008). Cigarette Smoking and Quitting among young Adults in Enugun, Nigeria. Niger. Med. J., 49(2): 27–30.

Anne C (2004). Medicinal uses of tobacco in history. J. R. Soc. Med., 97(6): 292-296.

Baron JA (1986). Cigarette smoking and Parkinson's disease. Neurol., 36: 1490-1496.

Blanchard DC, Griebel G, Blanchard RJ (2001). Mouse defensive behaviours: pharmacological and behavioural assays for anxiety and panic. Neurosci. Behav. Rev., 25: 205-218.

Carla C, Hank F, Iain N, Tomoko M, Donna G, Sonya V (1997). Tobacco smoke is a source of toxic reaction glycation roducts, Proceedings of the National Academy of Sciences of the United States of America, Manhasset, NY 11030, pp. 1-32.

Charles RC (2000). Drugs in Modern Society; 5th ed. McGraw Hill Publication, pp. 161-186.

Chen H, Ross V, Steve B, Jessica J, Gary PA, Margaret JM (2005). Effect of Short- Term Cigarette Smoke Exposure on Body Weight, Appetite and Brain Neuropeptide Y in Mice. Neuropsychopharmacol., 30: 713-719.

Ekong MB, Igidi AO, Mesembe OE (2008). The effects of administration of Amodiaquine on some parameters of neurobehaviour of Wistar rats. Niger. J. Physiol. Sci., 23(1-2): 51-54.

Erenmemısoglu A (1999). Turkish smokeless tobacco"Maras powder". Prev. Med., 28: 616-617.

Foulds J, Ramstrom L, Burke M, Fagerström K (2003). Effect of smokeless tobacco (snus) on smoking and public health in Sweden. Tobacco Control, 12: 349-359.

Grunberg NE (1982). The effects of nicotine and cigarette smoking on food consumption and taste preferences. Addictive Behaviors. 7(4): 317-331.

Idris AM, Ahmed HM, Malik MO (1995). Toombak dipping and cancer of the oral cavity in the Sudan: a case control study. Cancer, 63: 477-480.

Katzung BG (2005). Basic and Clinical Pharmacology, the McGraw-Hill companies, 9th ed, pp. 100-106.

Kumar S, Pandey U, Bala N, Tewar V, Oanh KT (2006). Tobacco habit in northern India. J. Indian Med. Assoc., 104: 19-24.

Kurucu S, Kartal M, Erenmemisoglu A (1998). HPLC analysis of Nicotianarustica L. and chewing tobacco (Maras Powder) alkaloids. FABAD J. Pharm. Sci., 23: 61-64.

NIDA Research Report Series (2009A). Tobacco Addiction. U. S.Department of health and human services, pp. 1-11.

NIDA Research Report Series (2009B). Infofacts. U. S. Department of health and human services, pp. 1-5 (www.drugabsue.gov)

NIH Publication No. 93-3605 (1993). US Department of Health and Human Services.

Obembe OO, Ukwenya OV, Ige AO, Oyeyipo IP, Fasanmade AA (2010). Effects of prenatal exposure to passive cigrate smoke and nicotine on nitric oxide and blood glucose levels of rats. Int. J. Biomed. Health Sci., 6(4): 235-240.

Ofusori OA, Enaibe BU, Falana BA, Adeeyo OA, Yusuf UA, Ajayi SA (2008). A comparative morphometric analysis of stomach in rat (Rattus norvegicus), bat (Eidolon helvum) and pangolin (Manis tricuspis). J. Cell. Anim. Biol., 2(3): 079-083.

Penton RE, Lester RAJ (2009). Cellular events in nicotine addiction. Seminars cell Dev. Biol., 20: 418-431.

Uwakwe R, Modebe I (2008). The Prevalence of cigarette Smoking in a Nigerian Community. Trop. J. Health Sci., 5(2) 13-34.

Wilson MMG, Philpot C (2002). Cigarette Smoking and Weight Loss in Nursing Home Residents. Medicine on-line. http://priory.com/med/cigsmoking.htm.

18

Privatisation of the Central Medical Supplies (CMS) public corporation: Why not?

Gamal K. M. Ali[1] and Abdeen M. Omer[2]*

[1]Former Department of Pharmaceutical Services and Planning Manager, Federal Ministry of Health, Khartoum, Sudan.
[2]Occupational Health Administration, Ministry of Health, Khartoum, Sudan.

To improve the effectiveness of the public pharmacy, resources should be switched towards areas of need, reducing inequalities and promoting better health conditions. Medicines are financed either through cost sharing or full private. The role of the private services is significant. A review of reform of financing medicines in Sudan is given in this article. Also, it highlights the current drug supply system in the public sector, which is currently a responsibility of the Central Medical Supplies Public Corporation (CMS). In Sudan, the researchers did not identify any rigorous evaluations or quantitative studies about the impact of drug regulations on the quality of medicines and how to protect the public against counterfeit or low quality medicines, although it is practically possible. There is need to continually evaluate regulations put in place to ensure that the public is protected by promoting the marketing of high quality medicines rather than commercial interests, and that the drug companies are held accountable for their conducts.

Key words: Sudan, healthcare, medicines, essential drugs, pharmacy management.

INTRODUCTION

The present policy of the national health-care system in Sudan is based on ensuring the welfare of the Sudanese people through increasing national production and upgrading of the productivity of individuals. A health development strategy has been formulated in a way that realises the relevancy of health objectives to the main goals of the national development plans. The strategy of Sudan at the national level aims at developing the Primary Health Care (PHC) services in the rural areas as well as urban areas. In Sudan, 2567 physicians provide the public health services (554 specialists, 107 medical registrars, 1544 medical officers, 156 dentists, and 206 pharmacists) (Gamal and Omer, 2008). The proposed methods of preventing and controlling health problems are: (a) Promotion of food supply and proper nutrition (b) An adequate supply of safe water and basic sanitation; (c) Maternal and child health-care; (d) Immunisation against major infectious diseases; (e) Preventing and

control of locally endemic diseases, and (f) Provision of essential drugs. This will be achieved through a health system consisting of three levels (state, provincial and localities), including the referral system, and secondary and tertiary levels. In such a system, Pharmacy management should be coordinated and integrated with other various aspects of health in which the aspects considered subsequently have to be put into consideration

First, the community must be the focus of benefits accruing from the restructuring, and legislature to protect community interest on the basis of equity and distribution should be put in place. Handing of the assets to the community should be examined and the communities should be encouraged to transfer the management of health schemes to a professional entity. Secondly, the private sector should be used to mobilise and strengthen the technical and financial resources, from within and without the country, to implement the services with particular emphasis on utilisation of local resources. Thirdly, the government should provide the necessary financial resources to guide the process of community

---

*Corresponding author. E-mail: abdeenomer2@yahoo.co.uk

management of pharmacy supplies. The government should move from being a provider of services to being a facilitator through setting standards, specifications and rules to help harmonise the private sector. A legally independent body should be established by an act of parliament to monitor and control the service providers. The government should assist the poor communities, who cannot afford service cost, and alleviate social-economic negative aspects of privatisation. The fourth aspect is that the sector actors should create awareness to the community about the roles of the private sector and government in the provision of health and pharmacy services. These should be crowned with support agencies providing the financial and technical support, training facilities, coordination, development and dissemination of health projects, as well as evaluation of the projects.

The health system in Sudan is characterised by heavy reliance on charging users at the point of access (private expenditure on health is 79.1% (WHO, 2004)), with less use of prepayment system such as health insurance. The way the health system is funded, organised, managed and regulated affects health workers' supply, retention, and the performance. Primary Health Care was adopted and introduced during the last decade as a main strategy for health-care provision in Sudan with the following new strategies: (a) Polio eradication by 1988; (b) Integrated management of children illness (IMCI) initiative; (c) Rollback malaria strategy; (d) Basic developmental need approach by 1997, and (e) Safe motherhood involving an initiative of making pregnancy safer, eradication of harmful traditional practices and emergency obstetrics' care programmes.

The strategy of price liberalisation and privatisation has been implemented in Sudan over the last decade, and has had a positive result on government deficit. The investment law approved recently has good rules and regulations on the above strategy particularly pertaining to health and pharmacy areas. The privatisation and price liberalisation in the health fields has undergone re-structuring but it is not complete yet. There is still need to provide adequate pharmacy supplies to the major sectors if pharmacy services are to be perfected.

Basing on the fact that the government of Sudan has great experience in privatisation of public institutions as exemplified by Sudanese free zones and markets, Sudan telecommunications (Sudatel) and Sudan airlines, it should be in position to implement the privatisation process in the health privatisation policy with efficiency and effectiveness. Through privatisation, government is not evading its responsibility of providing health-care to the inhabitants, but merely shifting its role from being a provider to a regulator and standard setter. Drug financing was privatised early in 1992 and currently; the Federal Ministry of Health (FMOH) has privatised certain non-medical services in hospitals such as catering services, security and cleanings. Therefore, implementing

this policy cannot come as a surprise. The overall goal of the CMS ownership privatisation is to improve access to essential medicines and other medical supplies in order to improve health status of the inhabitants particularly in far states (e.g., western and southern states).

If alternative ownership of the CMS is established by selling the majority of shares to the private sector, the following objectives will be achieved: (a) Easy access to essential medicines of good quality and affordable prices to the states' population and governments; (b) Efficiency and effectiveness in drug distribution system to avoid the serious pitfalls and incidences that have been reported during the last ten years of the CMS; (c) Equity by reaching all remote areas currently deprived of the formal drug distribution channels, and (d) Improvement of the quality and quantity of delivery of medicines to the public health facilities.

Achievement of the aforementioned objectives is expected to: (a) Increase geographical and economic access to essential medicines in all states (that is, in both rural and urban areas) to reach at least 80% of the population (currently less than 50% of population has access to essential medicines); (b) improve the tax collection from the new business by becoming more efficient (the tax revenues could be used to finance other health-care activities), and (c) Enable the government to reserve some shares (not more than 50%) in the new business and then use its shares' profit to finance a free medicines project in hospital outpatients' clinics, and other exempted medicines, e.g., renal dialysis and haemophilic patients treatment.

PRIVATISATION OF PUBLIC PHARMACEUTICAL SUPPLIES

The term privatisation has generally been defined as any process that aims to shift functions and responsibilities (totally or partially) from the government to the private sector. In broader meaning, it refers to restricting government's role and to putting forward some methods or policies in order to strengthen free market economy (Aktan, 1995). Privatisation can be an ideology (for those who oppose government and seek to reduce its size, role, and costs, or for those who wish to encourage diversity, decentralisation, and choice) or a tool of government (for those who see the private sector as more efficient, flexible, and innovative than the public sector) (Kamerman et al., 2009; Gormley, 1991). Scarpaci (1991) contends that "the invisible hand of the market is more efficient and responsive to the consumer needs while the public administrative budgets consume a large portion of tax monies that could otherwise be used for service delivery". The emphasis is on improving the efficiency of all public enterprises, whether retained or divested. Privatisation may take many forms first among which are the elimination of the public function of government and its assignment to the private sector for financial support as well as delivery of services (police, and fire departments, schools, etc.). Opponents characterise this as "load-shedding" (Bendick, 2009). The second form is deregulation, which involves transfer of responsibility of setting standards and rules concerning goods or services from government to the private sector (Gormley, 1996; 1997). Privatisation also includes the selling of public assets (city buildings, sports stadiums) to private firms in which the government issues vouchers, financed cards or slips of paper that permit private individuals to purchase goods or services from a private provider (food stamps) or circumscribed list of providers (Kettl, 1995). There is also franchising which is the establishment of models by the public sector that are funded by government agencies, but implemented by approved private providers. The process also involves contracting through which the government finances services, service providers have been chosen and the specifications of the various aspects of the services have been laid out in contracts with the private-sector organisations that produce or deliver the services. Another aspect of privatisation is the introduction of user fees in public facilities such as hospitals enables these institutions to generate income or finance some goods from private sources, either through drug sales or other services. This kind of privatisation has been applied in Sudan since early 1990s, as the health financing mechanism (especially for medicines).

In Sudan, the government decided to distance itself from direct involvement in business, and thus to divest most of its interests whether in loss or profit making public enterprises. The public reform programme was implemented in the context of the broader reforms, which were introduced in 1992. The reforms started with the liberalisation of local currency, foreign exchange transactions, internal and external trade, prices and health services (e.g., user fee as a mechanism of drug financing and other services). They were based on the transfer of activities vested in the government institutions to the private sector. It signalled the government intention to reduce its presence in the economy, and to reduce the level and scope of public spending and to allow market forces to govern economic activities. Privatisation also forms part of the government strategy of strengthening the role of the private in the development to achieve the vision of the 25 years strategy in which the private sector would be the engine for economic growth. Although it has become clear that the previous policies delivered very disappointing results, this reform has led to greater reliance on individual initiative and corporate accountability rather than on government as a decision-maker in business matters.

Since the privatisation policy goal is to improve the performance of the public sector companies, it can contribute to the growth and the development of the economy by broadened ownerships, participation in

management, and stimulation of domestic and foreign private investment.

The following are the primary objectives, which have been defined in the government's policy statement on public sector reform: (a) Improving the operational efficiency of enterprises that are currently in the public sector by exposing business and services to the greatest competition for the benefit of the consumer and the national economy (b) reducing the burden of public enterprises on the government's budget by spreading the shares' ownership as widely as possible among the population. (c) Expanding the role of the private sector in the economy (permitting the government to concentrate on the public resources abandoning its role as provider of basic public services, including health, education, social infrastructure, and to compact the side effects of the privatisation) and (d) encouraging wider participation of the people in the ownership and management of business.

In pursuing the primary objectives, the privatisation policy aims at transforming the performance of most significant enterprises in the public sector and ensuring liquidation of all viable and non-viable public enterprises as soon as possible through commercialisation, restructuring and divesture.

Public sector reform efforts are thus aimed at reducing government dominance and promoting a larger role for the private sector, while improving government's use of resources. Movement towards those goals in some countries is supported by components of a structural adjustment loan, which help to initiate the programme and establish the legislative and institutional base.

Contrary to the ideas advanced previously, however, opponents of the privatisation policy argue that the original objectives of state ownership ensured that the corporate sector of the economy was in national hands rather than being controlled by either foreign investors or the minorities that enjoyed business dominance upon independence. With privatisation, they further argue that the use of investment in state firms to accelerate development in situations where the private sector could be reluctant to take risks is lost.

PUBLIC SECTOR MEDICINES SUPPLY SYSTEM

In Sub-Saharan African countries (Sudan inclusive), discussions about the medicine distribution system reform have concentrated on ways of improving sustainability and quality of access to essential medicines. These discussions also have include debate on the impact of privatisation of public drug supply organisations on effectiveness, efficiency, quality and cost of medicines in the public health facilities, as well as on the respective role of the public and private sectors (Leighton, 1996). Until the mid 1980s, governments in Africa assumed responsibility for providing drugs to the inhabitants in some countries such as Mali and Guinea. The private distribution of all drugs including aspirin was illegal (Vogel et al., 1989). In many countries, including Sudan, there were two parallel government distribution systems. The public health network of hospitals and health centres were gratuitously supplied with drugs while in the public sector pharmacies, the drugs were sold to the public at subsidised prices.

During the 1990s, Sudan introduced a number of initiatives to establish drug-financing mechanisms as part of the health reform process and decentralised decision-making at a state level. In 1992, when a law was passed, medicines in public health system were not free-of-charge anymore. The aim of the government was to increase equitable access to essential medicines, especially at states' level. As a result, the central medical stores, which were responsible for the medicines supply system of the public health facilities, became an autonomous drug supply agency, and was renamed the Central Medical Supplies Public Corporation (CMS) and operated on cash-and-carry basis. It was capitalised and an executive board was installed. Since that time, it implied that the states and federal hospitals have to buy their own medicines and other medical supplies. They have to organise their own transport means for distribution of medicines to their primary health-care facilities and hospitals. In addition, all hospitals became financially autonomous entities and had to organise their own medicine procurement systems.

Before the introduction of the public drug supply system in Sub-Saharan Africa, Sudan inclusive, there were serious shortages or no medicines at all, particularly in rural areas. A study in Cameroon found the rural health centres received only 65% of the stock designated for them, and 30% of the medicines that arrived at the centres did not reach the clients. The loss rate after arrival in hospitals was estimated at 40% (Stephens, 1982). In Sudan, Graff and Evarard (2003) who visited the country on a WHO mission reported that, despite the cash-and-carry system taking off well, the lack of sufficient foreign exchange hampered the CMS procurement activities and that this resulted in low stock levels of all medicines including failure to stock life-saving products. Hospitals had to purchase the medicines from elsewhere and often had to buy from private sector. Despite large budget allocations to hospital, the allocations were not sufficient to cover the purchase of needed medicine supplies. This resulted in the medicines not being available most of the times. The in- or outpatients with their prescriptions were directed to the private pharmacies. In 2003, Khartoum Teaching Hospital, the biggest hospital in Sudan (not farther than 5 km away from the CMS), had medicine stock of only LS 83,000 (US$ 31). This would not fill one prescription for an anaemic patient with renal failure. It was a common practice for patients or their relatives to be given prescriptions to buy any pharmaceutical supplies that were needed including drugs and other disposables, from private sector pharmacies.

Many ministries of health, service providers and researchers have identified many characteristics that lead to poor performance in Africa's public drug supply systems. The systems are characterised by (1) absence of competition (2) insufficient funding (3) inefficient use of available resources and (4) poor management.

Competition is the best way to ensure that the goods and services desired by the consumer are provided at the lowest cost. Given the customers (that is, public health facilities) freedom of choice enables market forces to provide sustained pressures on companies to increase efficiency. Privatised companies generally operate in a competitive market environment.

With regard to inability to provide sufficient funding, Sudan provides a good example. In Sudan, with exception of Khartoum, Gezira and Gedaref states, all the states do not have enough funds to establish efficient drug supply system. In spite of being profit-making organisation, the CMS has failed to avail such funds during the past 14 years.

Public control promotes inefficient use of available resources. The CMS has worked as a profit-making organisation since its establishment in early 1990s. Due to the absence of privatisation, the CMS engaged in the establishment of a repackaging joint venture pharmaceutical factory in 1999 and recently announced its commitment to build a pharmaceutical city with not less than US$ 20 million, regardless of the fact that there is lack of life-saving medicines in the public health facilities. Had it not been lack of prioritisation, a typical symptom and sign of most public organisations, such an amount could be sufficient to establish a reliable supply system for all states of Sudan.

There are a number of constraints inherent in operating government drug supply service, which leads to poor management. These constraints comprise:

1. Hiring civil servants rather than persons with business experience and skills. Managers confront different challenges in public setting. They are not easily hired or fired. The lack of accountability results from the lack of shareholders, who would be free to remove incompetent administrators.
2. Too low wages. Even if the services were able to recruit outside of civil service, the wages paid are often too low to attract experienced managers. In addition, the managers do not share in dividends or other monetary activities as do private managers and incentives for doing well are often attenuated in a bureaucracy.
3. Cultural and structural conditions that promote corruption. These, include enormous pressure of wage earners to support an extended family and a strong incentive to more than their fixed government wage traditional gift giving practice as well as having a proprietary view of public offices (Van der Geest, 1982).

PRIVATISATION OF THE CMS'S OWNERSHIP

The public sector drug supply institutions, CMS inclusive, have not succeeded in as far as organising reliable and regular essential drug supply for the public health facilities is concerned (Huss, 1996). One of the many criticisms levelled on the public drug supply system, generally in Africa and particularly in Sudan, is how badly they are internally managed. There are those who agree that, despite the experience of autonomy and the stabilised role of the private sector organisations, a greater amount of real pharmaceutical resources could still be made available to the public health-care system. They argue that the access to essential medicines could be significantly increased, if managerial efficiency of the system were improved and were able to overcome the constraints inherent in operating a government drug supply organisation (Akin, 1987).

ADVANTAGES OF PRIVATE AGENCIES

There are many arguments in favour of privatisation of public institutions. Advocates of this method claim that privatisation has a large number of advantages (Savas, 1987; Hartley, 1986; De Hoog, 1984; Moore, 1987; Ascher, 1987). First, it is argued that privatisation is efficient and effective because it fosters and initiates competition. The competition among firms drives the cost down. Empirical studies have clearly proved that the cost of the services provided by the government is much higher than when the services are provided by private contractors. For example CMS's declared mark-up on cost (35%) amounted to 2.3 times the private mark-up (15%). In addition, private sector pays taxes, customs and other governmental fees (CMS exempted).

Furthermore, it has also been shown that privatisation provides better management than the public management since decision making under privatisation is directly related to the costs and benefits. In other words, privatisation fosters good management because the cost of the service is usually obscured.

Another important aspect advanced is that privatisation would help to limit the size of government at least in terms of the number of employees; it is an established fact that overstaffing is common in publicly owned enterprises. With competition established privatisation can help to reduce dependence on a government monopoly, which causes inefficiencies and ineffectiveness in services.

It is also argued that the Private sector is more flexible in terms of responding to the needs of citizens. Greater flexibility in the use of personnel and equipment can be achieved for short-term projects, part-time work, among others. Bureaucratic formalities are very common when government delivers the service. Less tolerance and strict hierarchy in bureaucracy are the reasons of the inflexibility in publicly provided services.

RATIONAL OF THE CMS PRIVATISATION

Even in the absence of broader adjustment context, however, it has long been clear that the CMS reform is needed and that it is actually unavoidable. Patients, administrators (at both hospitals and ministries of health), doctors and other health-care professionals, the regulatory authority and others are fully aware that the performance of the CMS is poor and that patients still suffer even after the privatisation of medicine financing in 1992. Although it is a profit-making organisation, neither the Ministry of Finance nor FMOH is getting any returns from the CMS. The Ministry of Finance, after more than 14 years, still has to inject annual money to cover the cost of certain budget lines such as free medicine projects. The following are the main three justifications, which summarise the inefficiency of the CMS as a public organisation:

1. The existence of widespread dissatisfaction with the situation of pharmaceuticals in public facilities: For instance, 79% of the population pay for their medicines out of pockets (WHO, 2004). The access to essential medicines in Sudan is still less than 50% (Quick, 1997).
2. The ever increasing cost of health care. There is no satisfactory estimate of the total capital invested in the CMS. Rather than receiving a sustained flow of dividends from its investments, the Ministry of Finance still finances the free medicines and drugs for certain diseases. For example, in Khartoum State, the CMS employs large capital, which is more than 10 times that of the Revolving Drug Funds (RDF) but the RDF, with a small capital of US$ 2 million supports the Ministry of Health activities with two billion every year. In contrast, the CMS has never contributed anything to health services since it was established in 1992. Instead, the strong stream of dividends and tax revenues, which should support public spending on other health activities, is lost. Hence, it is the poor who suffer as a result (Gamal and Omer, 2008).
3. Violation of pharmaceutical regulation at the expense of the public health by creating a big loophole in the pharmaceutical legal framework, which inevitably, leads to marketing of counterfeit medicines. This practice also suppresses the private sector (the government encourages it heavily to grow) by making inappropriate barriers to the private sector provision of drugs.

This is not to say the CMS has no future; there are substantial investment opportunities. Many can be turned around under new ownership and may succeed. It has been the experience of state enterprises worldwide that, in both socialist and in mixed economies, it is exceedingly difficult to remain competitive if enterprises are run by boards of public servants with multiple objectives and without real accountability to shareholders. The constraints on investment, from government and other business decisions also contribute to stifling competition especially if the enterprises are cut off by virtue of ownership from the latest technologies, and marketing and management trends.

This mainly stems from the fact that public sector boards and civil servants are not in touch with markets and commercial trends and those government-run companies have conflicting objectives that do not stress commercial accountability and thus jeopardise survival and commercial success (Gamal and Omer, 2008).

Reform is a matter of practical necessity rather than ideology. For example, the government of Cuba is still committed to socialist policies, and has recently chosen for pragmatic reasons, to privatise its telephone company. The final pragmatic reason compelling the government towards swift public sector reform is that the resources are being misused.

STRATEGIES TO OVERCOME THE CMS PRIVATISATION OBSTACLES

It is not surprising some obstacles and resistance from some CMS members of staff will confront this reform. The following strategies may help to overcome such resistance and obstacles: (a) Consensus should be built by negotiation with relevant ministries, public and private sectors, and interest groups so that all "buy into" the process and participate in formulating the goals (b) Promotion of research and development and dissemination of research information for community use. The WHO Mission Report of 2003 will be of great value and expected outcomes with being more focused on the patients after adoption of user fee policy.

THE ROLE OF THE FMOH

Private enterprise functions most efficiently if market forces are allowed to operate independently and completely unfettered. Nonetheless, some FMOH involvement is necessary to ensure the availability of proper use of good quality and affordable pharmaceuticals. Therefore, FMOH will continue its current responsibility of importing, licensing, inspecting and regulating the distribution system without any discrimination between different organisations, including the new established businesses. This has to be done by facilitating the development of adherence to the national drug list in the public health facilities, encouraging cheap purchase of registered medicines from reliable sources, quality control of medicines and maintenance of quality through out the system, as well as enforcement of the price control system. The FMOH could also be involved in informing private distributors and the public about the appropriate use of medicines.

At the public health facilities, however, freedom-of-choice arguments that would justify a laissez-fair

approach to private sector importing do not apply. There is the overriding merit aspects required in the management of medicines, the related requisites of availability, cost-efficiency, and quality control. Some pharmaceuticals are more cost-effective than others. And therefore, the enforcement of a government-mandated essential drug list lowers the real resource cost of a given quantity of pharmaceuticals necessary for alleviation of common diseases. Standard treatment guidelines alleviate unsuitable medicating practices particularly over-medication, and reduce costs to consumers (Gamal and Omer, 2008).

RECOMMENDATIONS

By resurrecting competition, which could be achieved mainly through privatisation of the CMS ownership, many of the mentioned pitfalls can be avoided. The new business should be responsible (of course without any kind of monopoly) for drug supply and distribution to the public health facilities on competition basis. The initial capital of the drug stocks for the different health facilities should be given to this new business by signing a clear agreement with interested states' ministries of health.

The government may retain a special (or "golden") share ranging from 30 to 50% to protect a newly privatised business from unwelcome take-over on national security grounds, or as temporary measure, to provide an opportunity for management to adjust to the private sector. The special share requires certain provisions in the articles of incorporation of a company, which may not be changed without the specific consent of special shareholder. The presence of a special share is a useful tool but is not intended to be a government straitjacket on the management. The management and not the government are generally responsible for ensuring that the special share's provisions are observed (Omer, 1994; Gibbon, 1996). In order to develop a free market in shares, special shares should be time limited as far as possible. The purpose of privatisation is to remove the government from ownership of the CMS. In some cases, especially where there are major uncertainties about the probable market of the business, for example, United Kingdom and other governments have sold their ownership interest gradually over a period of years (Gibbon, 1996; Bryman, 2004; MOH, 2003; WHO, 2007; Andalo, 2004).

CONCLUSIONS

The CMS reform is stronger today than it was in the early 1990s, when the reforms were started. There are many highly committed and able individuals throughout the public sector in the absence of the single-minded pursuit of commercial success. Also, in the long-term interest of employment growth and the public at large, narrower concerns have prevailed. Managements and boards are less able and less willing to impose accountability for results on themselves and their employees. Stock-out of life saving items is common, and sanctions for non-performance are often absent altogether. To overcome those common symptoms of all public owned enterprise, and achieve the strategic objectives of the FMOH by increasing the access of population to the essential medicines, the privatisation of the CMS's ownership is the best solution of choice.

REFERENCES

Akin JS, Birdsall N, De Ferranti DH (1987). *Financing health services in developing countries: an agenda for reform.* World Bank, Washington, D.C: USA.

Aktan CC (1995). An introduction to the theory of privatisation. J. Soc. Pol. Econ. Stud., 20(2): 187-217.

Andalo D (2004). Counterfeit drugs set alarm bells ringing. Pharm. J., pp. 273- 341.

Ascher K (1987). The politics of privatisation contracting out public services. New York: St Martin's Press. P. 23-28.

Bendick MJ (2009). Privatising the Delivery of Social Welfare Services. Privatisation and Welfare State, Eds. Princeton, N.J: Princeton University Press. pp. 15-23.

Bryman A (2004). Social Research Method. (2nd Edition). Oxford University Press.

De Hoog RH (1984). Contracting out for human services-economic, political and organisational perspectives. New York: State University of Albania. Pp. 34-42.

Gamal KMA, Abdeen MO (2008). The Impact of the Pharmaceutical Regulations on the Quality of Medicines on the Sudanese Market: Importers' Perspective. Sudan Knowledge. Pp. 1-16.

Gibbon H (1996). A guide for divesting government-owned enterprises. How to Guide. July 15. Geneva, Switzerland. Pp. 4-19.

Gormley WT (1996). Regulatory privatisation: a case study. J. Pub. Adm. Res. Theor., 6(2): 243-260.

Gormley WT (1997). Regulatory Enforcement: Accommodation and conflict in four states. Pub. Adm. Rev., 37(4): 285-293.

Graff PJ, Evarard MM (2003). *WHO mission to Sudan: travel report. WHO/HO: EXD/HTP.* World Health Organisation: Geneva. Pp. 23-28.

Hartley K (1986). Contracting-out: A step towards competition. Econ. Affairs, 6: 5.

Huss R (1996). Pharmaceutical consumer co-operative - the third path? CRAME: a case study of from Central African Republic. World Hospitals. 31(3): 13-15.

Kamerman SB, Khan AJ (2009). Privatisation and Welfare State. Princeton, N.J: Princeton University Press. pp. 25-30.

Kettl DF (1995). Privatisation as a tool of reform. The Lafollette Policy Report. 7.

Leighton C (1996). Strategies for achieving health-financing reform in Africa. World Development. 24(9): 1511-1525.

Ministry of Health (MOH). (2003). 25 years Pharmacy Strategy (2002-2027). Khartoum: Sudan. Unpublished Report. Pp. 3-17.

Moore S (1987). Contracting-out: A painless alternative to the budget cutter's knife. Steve H. Hankie (Ed.). Prospect for privatisation. New York: The Academy of political science. Pp. 16-27.

Omer AM (1994). Socio-cultural aspects of water supply and sanitation in Sudan. *NETWAS*, Nairobi: Kenya. 2: 4.

Quick JD (1997). *Managing Drug Supply: The Selection, Procurement, Distribution and Use of Pharmaceuticals.* 2nd ed. West Hardford, CT: Kumarian Press. Pp. 5-15.

Savas, E.S. (1987). Privatisation: The key to better government. Chatham House Publishers Inc., New Jersey. Pp. 18-26.

Scarpaci JL (1991). Health Services Privatisation in Industrial Societies. London: Jessica Kingsley Publishers.

Stephens B (1982). *Cameroon health centre study. Prepared for Population, Health Nutrition Department: World Bank.* International Science & Technology Institute, Inc., Washington, D.C. Pp. 7-25.

Van der Geest S (1982). The efficiency of inefficiency: medicine distribution in South Cameroon. Soc. Sci. Med., 16: 2145-2153.

Vogel RJ, Stephen B (1989). Availability of pharmaceutical in Sub-Saharan Africa: roles of the public, private and church mission sectors. Soc. Sci. Med., 29(4): 479-86.

WHO (2004). *The World Medicines Situation.* World Health Organisation (WHO): Geneva, Switzerland. WHO/EDM/PAR/2004.5

WHO (2007). *The World Medicines Situation.* World Health Organisation (WHO): Geneva, Switzerland. WHO/EDM/PAR/2004.5

19

The effect of oral administration of honey and glucophage alone or their combination on the serum biochemical parameters of induced diabetic rats

M. Sheriff[1], M. A. Tukur[2], M.M. Bilkisu[3], S. Sera[1] and A.S. Falmata[1]

[1]Department of Biochemistry, Faculty of Science, University of Maiduguri, Borno State, Nigeria.
[2]Department of Human Physiology, College of Medical Sciences University of Maiduguri, Borno State, Nigeria.
[3]Department of Medicine, College of Medical Sciences University of Maiduguri, Borno State, Nigeria.

Accepted 24 December, 2010

The effects of feeding honey on normal and alloxan induced diabetes rats treated and untreated were studied. In the experimental design, 25 rats were divided into five groups of five rats each, with Groups I and II serving as the normal and diabetic control, while Groups III, IV and V were the diabetic test groups administered with glucophage 500 mg/kg, glucophage in combination with honey (500 and 10 mg) and only honey (10 mg wet wt) per kilogram body weight respectively. All groups, (I - V) were fed with growers mash and water *ad libitum* for six weeks. The following parameters were assayed using standard methods; serum blood glucose, lipid profile, urea and creatinine. The differences observed in the serum level of HDL, triglycerides and total cholesterol in the test groups and diabetic control were statistically significantly ($p \geq 0.05$) compared to the normal control. The same was the case for low-density lipoprotein (LDL) serum level in the test groups which was statistically insignificant to the normal control while LDL serum level in diabetic control was significantly ($p \geq 0.05$) higher than the normal control. The difference in the LDL and total cholesterol level in the test groups were statistically significant to the diabetic control except cholesterol level of the Test III that was statistically insignificant to the diabetic control. High-density lipoprotein (HDL) and triglycerides in the test groups were statistically insignificant to the diabetic control. The blood glucose level in the combined therapy group (Test II) gave an acceptable range in both the fasting and 2 h postprandial compared to the diabetic and honey control group respectively. In conclusion, honey should be administered along with hypoglycemic agent in diabetic condition for use as alternative sweetener.

Key words: Diabetes, honey, glucophage.

INTRODUCTION

Sweeteners are ingredients that add sweetness to foods. There are two categories of sweeteners: nutritive and non-nutritive sweeteners. Example of nutritive sweetener is honey (Lynn, 2001).

Honey is sweet and viscous fluid produce by honey bees (genus Apis) and other insects from the nectar of flowers. Honey is also a popular sweetener and groups as a common house hold product used through out the world. Popularity comes not only of its being a natural sweetener but also many benefits proven or unproven associated with it. It has many medicinal uses described in traditional medicine. Modern system of medicine is also finding the honey efficacious in various medicinal and surgical conditions (Frankel et al., 1998; Lubsy et al. 2003). Antimicrobial, antioxidant and wound healing properties of honey are being evaluated with successful outcome. Prevention and treatment of various infections due to wide variety of organisms and promoting surgical wound healing are some of the areas where honey is making its mark (Bansal et al., 2005). Obi et al. (1994) reported 5% v/v concentration of honey decreases the duration of diarrhoe in cases of bacterial gastroenteritis. Honey lowers glycaemic index in patients with diabetes (Chen et al., 2000; Ahmed et al., 2008).

In one of the clinical trials of Type I and II diabetes, the use of honey was associated with significantly lower

---

*Corresponding author. E-mail: shemodu@yahoo.com.

glycaemic index than with glucose or sucrose in normal as well as Type I diabetes (Al-Walli, 2004). Type II diabetes had values similar to honey. Honey compared with dextrose caused a significantly lower rise in plasma glucose levels in diabetes subjects. It also cause reduction of blood lipids, homocystein levels and protein levels in normal and hyperlipidaemic subjects (Al-Walli, 2004). The active ingredient is honey is fructose. Fructose generates a small hyperglycaemic effect as it is absorbed slowly by our body as opposed to either sucrose or glucose (Brand, 2003).

Diabetes is a metabolic disorder which is due to insulin resistance or deficiency (Shulaman, 2000). It is a complex disease characterized by grossly abnormal fuel usage where by glucose is over produce by the liver and underutilized by organs. It is the most common serious metabolic disease in the world. Type I is caused by auto immune destruction of the insulin-secreting beta cells in the pancreas, Type II diabetes, by contrast, has a different cause and it is the most prevalent while gestational diabetes occurs during pregnancy. Diabetes and its associated complication have affected about 200 million people world wide representing 6% of the population. In diabetes condition, the blood sugar level is high, a condition referred to as hyperglycaemia. In this condition, the renal tubular glucose re absorption threshold is exceeded and glucose is excreted in urine, a process called glucosuria. The metabolic derangement is frequently associated with permanent and irreversible function and structural changes in the cell of the body, those of the vascular system being particularly susceptible. The changes lead to the development of well-defined clinical entities, when glucose concentration in the blood exceeds the capacity of the renal tubules to reabsorb, its forms a glomerular filtrate, glucosuria occurs. Glucose increases the osmolality of the glomerular filtrate and thus prevents the reabsorption of the water as its passes down the renal tubular system. This way, the volumes of urine is markedly increase and polyuria occurs. This in turns lead to lost of water and electrolyte which result in thirst and polydipsia (Stanley and Passmore, 1973; Allan et al., 2004). A stricking feature of diabetes is the shift in fuel usage from carbohydrate to fats. Triacylglycerols are mobilized and ketone bodies are formed to an abnormal extent. Since ketones are acids, this high concentration put a strain on the buffering capacity of the blood and on the kidney which controls the PH by excreting excess H into the urine. H excretion is accompanied by Na, K, PO_4 and H_2O excretion causing severe dehydration leading to a decreased blood volume.

Diabetes complication may lead kidney failure thereby causing changes in urea and creatinine levels. Urea level become elevated in the blood principally due to increase in the breakdown of amino acids for energy since insulin uptake of glucose by cell is impaired (http://www.cufpallief.com/test.htm). Accelerated ketone body formation can lead to acidosis, comma and death in untreated insulin-dependent diabetes.

Hyperlipidemias are common with patients with diabetes and further increase the risk of ischemic heart disease, especially in Type II diabetes. Detection and control of hyperlipidemia can reduce myocardial infraction, coronary deaths and overall mortality. In deed, even when low density lipoprotein (LDL) cholesterol concentration is normal or slightly raised in Type II diabetes (the major abnormalities being low HDL cholesterol and high triglycerides concentrations) the LDL particles may be qualitatively different and more atherogenic than those in non diabetic patients (Watkins, 2003).

AIMS AND OBJECTIVES

The research is aimed at evaluating the effect of administration of honey alone, glucophage alone or their combination for use as an alternative sweetener in the management of diabetes mellitus.

MATERIALS AND METHODS

Experimental design

Twenty five rats used in this investigation were albino rats (adult male)that were in-bred in the animal colony of the Department of Biochemistry, University of Maiduguri.

The weight of the rats ranges from 120 - 250 g. They were stabilized on standard laboratory feed (Grower's mash EGWA feed Jos, Nigeria) which contains 54% of carbohydrate, 13% fat, 10% protein, 20% fiber, 2% normal supplement and 1% vitamin and water.

They were kept in a well ventilated animal house and weighed weekly for four weeks. After which they were grouped into five groups of five (Making a total of 25 rats) as follows:

Group A: Normal control: Rats were not induced and untreated. They were given normal feed and parameters from this group serve as a base live data (control).

Group B: Rats were induced with Alloxan monohydrated (0.2 ml/200 g body weight) and untreated, this serves as the diabetic control group and in addition were given normal feed/water *ad libitum.*

Group C: Rats were induced with Alloxan monohydrate (0.2 ml/200 g body weight) thereafter they were treated with Glucophage hydrochloride tablet B.P 500 mg/100 g body weight twice a day with urine sugar monitored, this group served as the test Group (I).

Group D: Rats were induced with Alloxan monohydrate (0.2 ml/200 g body weight and then treated with glucophage (as described in group B) for one week then treated with 1 ml of honey which was administered for 1 week this represents test Group II.

Group E: Rats were induced with Alloxan monohydrate as described above and then treated with honey (1 ml/200 g body weight) for 1 week. (Honey control).

Table 1. Shows the effect of feeding honey on lipid profile in normal rats.

Parameters/Groups	Total cholesterol	HDL	LDL	Triglycerides
Normal control	2.06 ± 0.15^a	1.86 ± 0.21^a	0.36 ± 0.1^a	0.96 ± 0.5^a
Diabetic control	2.86 ± 0.38^a	1.26 ± 0.64^a	0.96 ± 0.11^b	1.9 ± 0.63^a
Test I	2.06 ± 0.17^a	1.62 ± 0.19^a	0.52 ± 0.13^a	1.06 ± 0.21^a
Test II	2.22 ± 0.3^a	1.82 ± 0.4^a	0.48 ± 0.13^a	1.18 ± 0.61^a
Test III	2.3 ± 0.4^a	1.4 ± 0.12^a	0.54 ± 0.11^a	1.44 ± 0.79^a

Values are mean ± SD, n = 5, Values with different superscript along a column vertically are statistically significant ($p\leq0.05$).

Table 2. Serum glucose level in normal, diabetic controls and test groups.

Parameters/Groups	Fasting blood glucose (Mmol/l)	2 h Posporangial
Normal control	3.86 ± 0.38^a	4.26 ± 0.64^a
Diabetic control	11.57 ± 2.22^b	16.45 ± 3.11^b
Test I	5.28 ± 1.33^b	6.26 ± 1.00^b
Test II	6.22 ± 1.03^b	7.82 ± 1.04^b
Test III	8.44 ± 1.66^b	11.05 ± 2.11^b

Values are mean ± SD, n = 5, Values with different superscript along a column vertically are statistically significant ($p\leq0.05$).

Method of intubation

The intubations were done using stomach tube. The rats were maintained on a daily administration of glucophage 500 mg/100 g body weight b.d. (twice a day) 1 ml of honey /100 g body weight was administered to the test group treated with honey.

Method of blood collection (Serum)

At the end of the experiment, the rats were sacrificed and the blood was collected in a plain container. The blood was allowed to clot and centrifuged in an ultra centrifuge at 3500 r pm to obtain the serum. The serum was used for analyzing cholesterol, HDL, LDL, Triglycerides and Blood glucose level.

Determination of serum cholestorol

Free and esterified cholesterol in the sample originates by means of the coupled reactions with a colored complex formation that was measured spectrophotometrically as described by the (National Cholesterol Program Expert Panel, 2001; Fossati and Prencipe, 1982).

Determination of high density of lipoprotein (HDL)

VLDL and LDL in the sample precipitate with phosphotungstate and magnesium ions. The supernatant contains HDL. The HDL cholesterol is then spectrophotometrically measured by means of the coupled reactions described by Bustein et al. (1980), Bucole et al. (1973) and National Cholesterol Program Expert Panel (2001).

Determination of blood glucose

The enzymatic method of glucose oxidase was used as described

by Trinder (1965) and urine sugar was estimated using the clinistex test strips (Burgett, 1974).

RESULTS AND DISCUSSION

Table 1 shows the result of total cholesterol HDL, LDL, and total triglycerides level before and after the administration of honey. A test of significant was carried out between the normal control against the diabetic control and within test groups. The serum level of total cholesterol was significantly higher ($p\geq0.05$) than the normal control; the same pattern was also observed in the test groups. HDL serum level in diabetic control was insignificantly lower than normal control and the same was observed down the groups. Triglycerides and LDL in the diabetic control were significantly higher than the normal control, except the serum level of LDL in the diabetic control that was significantly ($p\leq0.05$) higher than normal control. The level of total cholesterol in the Test I was significantly lower than the diabetic control, the same was observed in Test II expect Test III that was statistically insignificant to the diabetic control.

HDL serum level in the test groups was significantly ($p\geq0.05$) higher than the diabetic control. LDL serum level in the test groups was statistically significantly ($p\leq0.05$) to the diabetic control while triglycerides serum level in the test groups was statistically insignificant to the diabetic control.

In Table 2 the diabetic control which is the groups that have not received any treatment after diabetic induction, they have a high cholesterol level than those that

Table 3. The effect of administration of honey on ASAT, ALAT and total protein in treated and untreated diabetic rats.

Group	Parameter		
	ASAT	ALAT	Total protein
Normal control	437.7±5.8	132.7±25.0	97.2±1.0
Diabetic control	486.3±108.5	167.3±44.5	95.2±18.0
Test I	426.8±29.8	143.0±41.9	90.5±2.7
Test II	377.6±41.3	117.2±30.5	82.6±64
Test III	422.7±143.1	94.7±41.9	80.3±7.6

Table 4. Electrolytes, urea and creatinine in normal, treated and untreated alloxan induced diabetic rats.

Group	Parameter					
	Na^+	K^+	Cl^-	HCO_3^-	Urea	Creatinine
Normal control	147.2±1.3	4.7±0.4	92.8±1.3	23.0±2.1	5.5±0.7	60.4±4.7
Diabetic control	136.0±3.8	8.1±0.7	120.6±4.2	14.6±0.6	15.6±3.1	78.4±4.2
Test I	141.2±1.9	5.9±0.6	93.2±2.6	20.4±1.1	7.7±0.9	58.4±3.5
Test II	146.6±7.1	8.5±1.3	102.0±7.5	22.0±4.3	8.8±3.4	57.8±2.4
Test III	141.2±0,8	6.4±0.8	92.0±2.8	18.8±1.8	8.0±3.3	58.2±4.9

received treatment. In the test groups, the group that have received treatment only glucophage have lower cholesterol level compared to those that have received both glucophage and honey or those that received only honey. The HDL also shows that it is higher in the group that received honey alone or honey with glucophage. LDL is higher in the diabetic control than in the group that received treatment. While those that received only honey have the lowest LDL level. Triglycerides are higher in the diabetic group when compared to the test groups. Wile in the test groups, the group that received combination therapy with honey and glucophage have a higher value of triglycrides compared to those that received only honey or glucophage.

Table 2 shows the serum blood glucose level of in the test groups in comparism with the normal and diabetic control. The blood glucose of the diabetic control is significantly higher when compared to both the normal control and the all the test groups, both at fasting and 2 h postprandial. This is consistent with earlier reports by Modu et al. (2008). The group that was given administered only glucophage, had a near normal blood glucose level both at fasting and 2 h postprandial compared to diabetic and honey control (Test III). This effect might be attributed to the increased peripheral absorption of glucose by glucophage (Sfikakis, 1988). But the group that was administered glucocphage in combination with honey recorded a slightly higher glucose level both at the fasting and 2 h postprandial. Even though the increase is within the normal range. This shows that honey when used in combination with a hypoglyceamic drugs, can serve as an alternative sweetener (Daisy and Ezira, 2007). While the group that served as the honey control, recorded much higher blood glucose concentration both at fasting as well as 2 h postprandial compared to the normal control and Test I and II respectively. This result revealed that, the use honey singly in diabetic condition will result into hyperglyceamia and its continuous use under such conditions might result into complications associated with diabetes mellitus.

In Table 3, ALAT level is found to be higher in the normal control than in the test groups, while the diabetic controls have the highest level of ASAT. The ALAT is higher in the normal than the test group. The diabetic controls also have higher value of ALAT than the test group. The diabetic controls have higher ALAT value than the other test groups but the group that received only honey have the lowest ALAT concentration, followed by the group that received both glucophage and honey.

The normal controls have higher concentration of total serum protein than the other groups. The diabetic control also has higher concentration of total protein compared to the other test groups. The group that received only honey has the lowest total protein level.

From Table 4, the normal control have higher Na and HCO₃ concentration than all the other groups, while creatinine level is higher in the normal control than the test group, but the creatinine on the other hand is higher in the diabetic control than in the test groups as well as the normal control.

The K level is higher in the diabetic control and those taking only honey, while it is lower in the normal control group.

The normal control have lowest urea level, while diabetic control have the highest urea level which is followed by the group treated with only honey.

REFERENCES

Al-Walli NS (2004). Natural honey lowers plasma glucose, C-reactive protein, homocysteine and blood lipids in healthy diabetic and hyperlipidemic subjects: Comparism with dextrose and sucrose. J.Med. Food, 7: 100-107.

Bansal V, Medhi B, Pandhi P (2005). Honey-A remedy rediscovered and its therapeutic utility. Kathmandu University Med. J., 3(11): 305-309.

Burgett DW (1974). Glucose oxidase: A food protective mechanism in social hymenoptera. An Entomon. Soc. Am. Adv. Food Res. (C.O.Chichester Eds). Academic press New York. 24: 54-60.

Bustein M, Schnolnick HR, Morfin R (1980). Rapid method for the isolation of lipoproteins from human serum by precipitation with polyanions. Scand J. Clin. Lab. Investig., 40: 583-595.

Chen L, Melita A, Berenbaum M, Zangeri AR, Engeseth NJ (2000). Honeys from different flora sources as inhibitors of enzymatic browning. In fruits and vegetable homogenates. Afri. Food Chem., 48: 4997-5000.

Daisy P, Ezira J (2007). Hypoglycemic property of polyherbal formulation in sreptozocin induced diabetic rats. Biochem. cell. Arch., 7: 135-140.

Fossati P, Prencipe L (1982). Serum triglycerides determine colorimetrically with an enzyme that produces hydrogen peroxide. Clin. Chem., 28: 2077-2080.

Frankel S, Robinson GE, Berenbaum MR (1998). Antioxidant capacity and correlated characteristics of the unifloral honeys. J. Agric., pp. 27-37.

Lubsy PE, Combes A, Wilkinson JM (2003). Honey: A potent agent for wound healing? Wound Oslo my continence. Nursing, 29: 295-300.

Lynn MO (2001). Honey as a nutritive sweetener. J. Food Adv. Food Res., (C.O.Chichester Eds). Academic press New York, 32(2): 212-216.

Modu S, Ibrahim S, Muas A, Mshelia DS, Arjinoma Z (2008). Effect of combined feeding of various doses of honey and caraway oil on some biochemical and heamatological parameters in normal health rats. Kanem J. Med. Sci., 2(1): 22-27.

National Cholesterol Education Program Expert Panel (2001). Third report of the National Cholesterol Education Program (NCEP). Expert on detection, evaluation and treatment of high blood cholesterol in adult. NIH Publication Bethesda, National Heart, Lung and Blood Institute. pp. 451-476.

Obi CL, Ugoji EO, Edun SA, Lawal SF, Anyiwo CE (1994). Anti bacterial agents isolated in Lagos, Nigeria. Afr. J. Med. 23: 257-260.

Sfikakis P (1988). Metabolic effects of honey (alone or combined with other foods) in type II diabetes. Entrez Pub.Med. Abs.

Shulaman GI (2000). Cellular mechanism of insulin resistance. The J. Clin. Investig. 26(2): 250-254.

Watkins PJ (2003). ABC of Diabetes: Cardiovascular disease, hypertension and lipids. 5th edition. BMJ-PG Books Nigeria. 376: 874-876.

20

Phytochemical and biological study of *Striga hermonthica* (Del.) Benth callus and intact plant

Faisal Hammad Mekky Koua[1]*, Hind Ahmed Babiker[1], Asim Halfawi[2], Rabie Osman Ibrahim[1], Fatima Misbah Abbas[3], Eisa Ibrahim Elgaali[3] and Mutasim Mohamed Khlafallah[3]

[1]Department of Biochemistry, Faculty of Science and Technology, Al Neelain University, P. O. Box 12702, Al Baladya St. Khartoum, Sudan.
[2]Deparment of Pharmacognosy, Faculty of Pharmacy, University of Medical Sciences and Technology, P. O. Box: 12810, Khartoum, Sudan.
[3]Commission for Biotechnology and Genetic Engineering, National Center for Research P. O. Box 2404 Khartoum, Sudan.

Preliminary phytochemical screening of *Striga hermonthica* was carried out to assess the chemical contents and biological activity of callus comparing to that of intact plant (upper and underground parts). The results show the presence of terpenes, tannins, coumarins, cardiac glycosides, flavonoids, saponins, anthracenosides and alkaloids. Further, ethanol extracts analysis-using thin layer chromatography (TLC) revealed differences in chemical constituents between calli, and different parts of the plant with five fractions in callus, three fractions in upper-parts and two fractions in underground-parts based on solvent systems. Antimicrobial assay of S. *hermonthica* extracts revealed various activities against *Staphylococcus aureus*, *Pseudomonas aeruginosa*, *Escherichia coli* and *Candida albicans* using agar well-diffusion method. The richest extract with phytochemical constituents and most effective one was the ethanol extracts of the different parts.

Key words: *Striga hermonthica*, phytochemical screening, thin layer chromatography, callus, flavonoids, antimicrobial assay.

INTRODUCTION

Striga hermonthica (Del.) Benth (Scrophulariaceae) is an ubiquitous hemi-parasitic plant growing in wide spectrum of food crops, e.g., rice (*Oryza sativa* L.), millet (*Pennisetum glaucum* L. Leeke), maize (*Zea mays* L.) and sorghum (*Sorghum bicolor* L. Moench) roots (Tarr, 1962; Hutchinson and Dalziel, 1963; Carson, 1988; Press et al., 2001). It is widespread in West and East Africa (Mohamed, 1994; Mohamed et al., 2001; Musselman et al., 1991). *S. hermonthica* is a well-known medicinal plant that has been used widely in folkloric medicine in some parts of Africa (Choudhury et al., 1998; Kokwaro, 1976; Atawodi et al., 2003). It has a wide range of medicinal uses; the pharmacological abortificient effect, dermatosis, leprosy ulcer, pneumonia and jaundice remedy, trypanocidal effects, antibacterial and anti-plasmoidal

activities have been reported (Choudhury et al., 1998; Hussain and Deeni, 1991; Kokwaro, 1976; Nacoulma, 1996; Okpako and Ajaiyeoba, 2004). The plant has also revealed antioxidant property due to its diverse content of phenolic compounds, e.g., luteolin, apigenin, anthocyanins and tannins (Chouldhury et al., 2000; Khan et al., 1998; Kiendrebeogo et al., 2005). *In vitro* propagation of plants holds tremendous potential for the production of high-quality plant based on medicines (Murch et al., 2000). However, the medicinal effectivity of this plant has been studied extensively; nevertheless, none of these reviews has attempted to harness the advantages of *in vitro* propagation and subsequent phytochemical screening for medicinal purposes. In the current study, we successfully induced the callus of S. *hermonthica* using an entire *in vitro* system. The preliminary phytochemical screening of this plant indicated the presence of saponins, tannins, flavonoids, volatile oils and cardiac glycosides (Okpako and

*Corresponding author. E-mail: faisalkoua@gmail.com

Ajaiyeoba, 2004). In this contribution, we have initially screened the *in vitro* produced calli of this plant for its phytochemical constituents in compare to phytochemicals of different parts of the intact plant. We have also studied very initially the antimicrobial activity of various extracts of *S. hermonthica* against several standard microorganisms.

MATERIALS AND METHODS

Plant Materials and Microbial Growth Condition

The intact plant was collected from Shambat Forages Field, Khartoum, Sudan. The samples were divided into upper (shoot) and underground (haustoria) part and air-dried at room temperature (25°C). *S. hermonthica* callus was produced using a standard method (Zhou et al., 2004). The calli of different ages of weeks four, six and eight were collected, freeze-dried and stored at - 80°C till used. Petroleum ether, ethanol and water extract were used for phytochemical screening following the standard method (Vaghasiya and Chanda, 2007). *Escherichia coli* ATCC25922, *Pseudomonas aeruginosa* ATCC27853, *Staphylococcus aureus* ATCC25923 and a fungal strain *Candida albicans* ATCC7596 were obtained from the Department of Microbiology, Institute of Medicinal and Aromatic Plants, National Centre for Research, Ministry of Science and Technology, Khartoum, Sudan.

Phytochemical screening

The presence of triterpenes, sterols, tannins, coumarins, cardiac gylcosides, flavonoids, saponins, anthrocenosides, carotenoids, glycosides and alkaloids were appraised was conducted following the standard protocols (Culei, 1989; Harborne, 1973; Trease and Evans, 1989).

Thin layer chromatography technique

Frozen dry callus of different ages, upper and underground parts of *S. hermonthica* were defrosted and 250 mg extracted with 2.50 ml of 75% ethanol in water bath for 2 h with intermittent cooling every 30 min to avoid decomposition of components. The extracts were transferred to micro-tubes and centrifuge (6000 rpm) for 3 min. Aliquots (5 µl) of the respective solution was applied into Silica gel 60_{254} aluminum plates (Merck, Germany) in four different solvent systems with different polarity (well known for flavonoids separation), Ethyl acetate/Formic acid/Acetic acid/Water (100:11:11:27), Ethyl acetate/Methanol/Water (100:13.5:10), Ethyl acetate/Formic acid/Water (68:8:8) and Butanol/Acetic acid/Water (100:25:125) (Males et al., 2006; Wagner and Bladt, 1996). The experiments were conducted in pre-saturated thin layer chromatography (TLC) chamber. The TLC plates were air-dried at room temperature for 30 min and visualized under 365 nm UV-lamp (UVP, Upland, CA 91786, U.S.A) before and after treating with the detecting reagent (iodine vapor) (Jork et al., 1994). The retention factor (R_f) for the separated spots was calculated using the following equation:

$$R_f = [\text{Distance traveled by the sample} / \text{Distance traveled by the solvent}]$$

Antimicrobial activity

The well diffusion method (Bauer et al., 1966; Schillinger and Lucke, 1989) was used to test antimicrobial activity of *S. hermonthica* extracts. Mueller-Hinton Agar medium was pre-swabbed with tested microorganisms and four wells in each plate were made using cork-borer of 0.6 mm diameter. The extracts at final concentration 2 mg/ml and positive control Kanamycin were used at concentration of 50 µg/ml, with 50 µl per well for each. For the native control solvents alone were applied following the same protocol. The cultures were incubated at 35°C for 24 h and the zones of inhibition were measured. The experiment was done in triplicates and the means of inhibition zones were calculated manually.

RESULTS AND DISSCUSION

Preliminary phytochemical screening

Medicinal plants constitute an effective source of both traditional and modern medicines, herbal medicine has been shown to have genuine utility and about 80% of rural population depends on it as primary health care (WHO, 1978). *S. hermonthica* is one of these plants, which plays a vital role in the folk medicine in some parts of Africa (Keindrebeogo et al., 2005). Phytochemical screening of *S. hermonthica* callus and intact plant was carried out to appraise the scientific aspects of the traditional uses of this plant. The preliminary screening revealed the presence of various active principle metabolites; these are alkaloids, flavonoids, coumarins, cardiac glycosides, anthracenosides, saponins, tannins, reducing compounds, terpenes and steroids (Table 1). To some extent these results are consistent with Okpako and Ajaiyeoba (2004), who reported the presence of saponins, tannins, flavonoids, volatile oils and cardiac glycosides of the intact plants. In contrast, this is the first reports for coumarins and anthracenosides. The data obtained during this study revealed that *S. hermonthica* callus and intact plant shown the presence of flavonoids, terpenes, sterols and glycosides in approximately high amounts. Kiendrebeogo et al. (2005) estimated the flavonoids content of the *S. hermonthica* acetone aqueous extract to be about 4% mainly as luteolin flavonoid. However, tannins, coumarins, cardiac glycosides, reducing sugar and alkaloids were found in various levels among the tested parts (Table 1). Anthracenosides and emodols were not detected among all tested parts, except in underground (haustoria) parts, which revealed the presence of anthracenosides in trace amount. Thus, the preliminary screening tests may be useful in the detection of the bioactive principles and subsequently may lead to exploring novel compounds. Furthermore, these preliminary investigations facilitate the subsequent quantitative estimation and qualitative separation of pharmacologically active chemical compounds. The curative properties of medicinal plants are perhaps due to the presence of various secondary metabolites such as alkaloids, flavonoids, glycosides, phenols, saponins, sterols, etc (Hassan et al., 2004). *S. hermonthica* has been used extensively in folkloric remedies of many diseases, such as malaria,

Table 1. Phytochemical constituents of *S. hermonthica* different parts of intact plant and callus.

Phytochemical constituents	Screened plant parts		
	Aerial part	Underground parts	Callus
Triterpenes / sterols	++	+	+
Tannins	+	±	±
Coumarins	−	+	+
Cardiac glycosides	+	+	±
Flavonoids	++	+	++
Saponins	++	+	+
Anthracenosides	−	±	−
Emodols	−	−	−
Carotenoids	±	−	−
Glycosides	+	+	+
Reducing compounds	+	+	+
Alkaloids			
-Wagner's test	−	+	+
-Mayer's test	±	+	±

++ = reasonable amount, + = moderate amount, ± = trace amount, − = not detected. These amount remarks estimated by observing the test color intensity which was used as indicative for the phytochemical quantity.

trypanosomasis, and some bacterial infections (Okpako and Ajaiyeoba, 2004). The wide spectrum curative ability of this plant may be due to the diverse phytochemicals that have been reported in this plant (Keindrebeogo et al., 2005; Okpako and Ajaiyeoba, 2004). Nonetheless, still there is shortage in the scientific information about the phytochemical composition of *S. hermonthica* and its active ingredients. Claims in this respect to the therapeutic success of the plant still need more research to prove the scientific usage of this plant in remedies. No attempt has been made by any worker to purify the compounds contained in the plant extract; however, the plant crude extract proved its effectiveness against many diseases (Kokwaro, 1976; Atawodi et al., 2003).

Thin layer chromatography

For further investigation on the chemical constituents of *S. hermonthica* callus and intact plant, a thin layer chromatography screening of richest extracts (alcohol extracts) was carried out using different solvent systems. Since phenolic compounds, e.g., flavonoids were observed in all of the *S. hermonthica* analyzed materials (Table 1). Flavonoids were selected for further analysis using TLC technique for more comparative study between *S. hermonthica* calli and the different parts of the intact plants. TLC plates showed different results illustrated in the figures of TLC chromatograms (Figures 1A to C). Solvent system I (system I hereafter) revealed the best results, followed by solvent system II. System I separated five clear spots from all callus extracts of different ages and three and two spots from the haustoria

and shoot respectively (Tables 2 to 5). The spot with Rf ~0.54 showed similarity between all parts of *S. hermonthica*, these similar spots suspected to be chemically identical compounds. In addition, there was a high similarity between chemical constituents of upper parts (shoot) and callus tissues of different ages except in one fraction with Rf ~ 0.24, which appear in the calli extracts and it is not in shoot extract. We observed that the calli tissues of different ages revealed no differences on the TLC chromatograms, which contained five spots with R_f values ~0.24, 0.38, 0.47, 0.57 and 0.94 and thus we found no indication of age impact on the chemical constituents of the calli. Lack of comparative studies made it difficult to assign these separated spots to any of the well-known reference phenolic compounds; however, one of these separated compounds is likely to be luteolin, apigenin, flavone and/or anthocyanins, which was found in high amount (Choudhury et al., 2000; Khan et al., 1998; Kiendrebeogo et al., 2005). The same results of TLC chromatogram were obtained in solvent system II with few differences in number of separated spots in each plant parts. Solvent systems III and IV seem to be not suitable, which separated unclear, less and diffusing-like spots (Figure 1A). Generally, the spots were unclear in most of the preparations and appeared pale yellow, yellowish green and green in some when visualized by eye, however, under UV-lamp in long wave length 365 nm the spots colors were fluorescent blue with exception of the spots of calli and shoot with R_f values ~0.94, 0.95, 0.91 and 0.97 gave orange to red fluorescent color under 365 nm UV-lamp (Figure 1C). The similarity of shoot and calli of *S. hermonthica* in most of their flavonoids components suggests that the callus is a possible

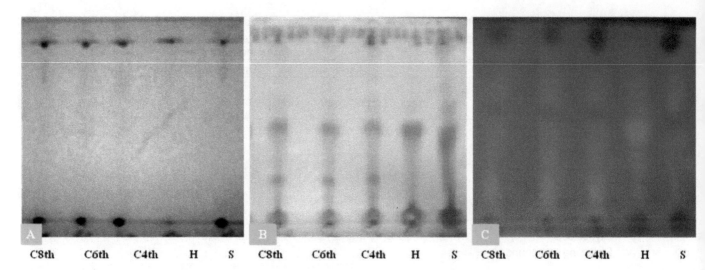

Figure 1. TLC chromatograms of alcoholic extracts of *S. hermonthica* (C4th, C6th and C8th represent calli of week 4, 6 and 8, respectively. H = haustorium part, S = shoot); (A) TLC chromatogram developed on system IV before treating with iodine vapor; (B) TLC chromatogram developed on system I, spots color after treating with iodine vapor; (C) TLC chromatogram of system I under UV-lamp of long wavelength 365 nm.

Table 2. TLC remarks of alcoholic extract components of *S. hermonthica* developed on system I (Ethyl acetate/formic acid/Acetic acid/Water, 100:11:11:27).

Plant parts	No. of spots	R_f (values)*	Separated spots remark	Spots under UV-lamp at (365nm)
	1	0.26	Pale yellow green/-	Blue fluorescent
Shoot	2	0.39	Pale yellow green/-	Blue fluorescent
	3	0.97	Green	Orange/Red fluorescent
Haustoria	1	0.57	Pale yellow/-	Blue fluorescent
	2	0.91	Pale yellow/-	Blue Fluorescent
	1	0.24	Pale yellow green/-	Blue fluorescent
	2	0.38	Pale yellow green/-	Blue fluorescent
Callus of week (4)	3	0.47	Pale yellow/-	Blue fluorescent
	4	0.57	Pale yellow/-	Blue fluorescent
	5	0.94	Green	Orange/Red fluorescent
	1	0.26	Pale yellow green/-	Blue fluorescent
	2	0.38	Pale yellow green/-	Blue fluorescent
Callus of week (6)	3	0.48	Pale yellow/-	Blue fluorescent
	4	0.57	Pale yellow/-	Blue fluorescent
	5	0.95	Green	Orange/Red fluorescent
	1	0.26	Pale yellow green/-	Blue fluorescent
	2	0.39	Pale yellow green/-	Blue fluorescent
Callus of week (8)	3	0.47	Pale yellow green/-	Blue fluorescent
	4	0.57	Pale yellow green/-	Blue fluorescent
	5	0.95	Green	Orange/Red fluorescent

*Values represent Means calculated from triplicates experiments. (-) means these sports are almost invisible in some.

alternative source for the production of the phytochemical constituents. The results suggest further studies in this field.

Antimicrobial activity of *Striga* extracts

The antimicrobial effects of medicinal plants are well

Table 3. TLC remarks of alcoholic extract components of *S. hermonthica* developed on system II (Ethyl acetate/Methanol/Water; 100:13.5:10).

Plant parts	No. of spots	R$_f$ (values)*	Separated spots remark	Spots under UV-lamp at (365nm)
Shoot	1	0.49	Pale yellow green/-	Blue fluorescent
	2	0.56	Pale yellow green/-	Blue fluorescent
	3	0.94	Green	Orange/Red fluorescent
Haustoria	1	0.54	Pale yellow/-	Blue fluorescent
	2	0.93	Pale yellow/-	Blue fluorescent
Callus of week (4)	1	0.24	Pale yellow green/-	Blue fluorescent
	2	0.54	Pale yellow/-	Blue fluorescent
	3	0.61	Pale yellow green/-	Blue fluorescent
	4	0.95	Green	Orange/Red fluorescent
Callus of week (6)	1	0.24	Pale yellow green/-	Blue fluorescent
	2	0.54	Pale yellow green/-	Blue fluorescent
	3	0.63	Pale yellow/-	Blue fluorescent
	4	0.94	Green	Orange/Red fluorescent
Callus of week (8)	1	0.26	Pale yellow green/-	Blue fluorescent
	2	0.56	Pale yellow green/-	Blue fluorescent
	3	0.61	Pale yellow/-	Blue fluorescent
	4	0.95	Green	Orange/Red fluorescent

*Values represent MEANS calculated from triplicates experiments. (-) means these sports are almost invisible in some.

Table 4. TLC remarks of alcoholic extract components of *S. hermonthica* developed on system III (Ethyl acetate/Formic acid/Water; 68:08:08).

Plant parts	No. of spots	R$_f$ (values)*	Separated spots remark	Spots under UV-lamp at (365nm)
Shoot	1	0.74	Pale yellow/-	Blue Fluorescent
	2	0.88	Pale yellow/-	Blue Fluorescent
Haustoria	1	0.83	Pale yellow	Blue Fluorescent
Callus of week (4)	1	0.75	Pale yellow green/-	Blue Fluorescent
	2	0.88	Pale yellow/-	Blue Fluorescent
Callus of week (6)	1	0.74	Pale yellow/-	Blue Fluorescent
	2	0.88	Pale yellow/-	Blue Fluorescent
Callus of week (8)	1	0.74	Pale yellow/-	Blue Fluorescent
	2	0.86	Pale yellow/-	Blue Fluorescent

* Values represent means calculated from triplicates experiments. (-) means these sports are almost invisible in some.

documented (Valero and Salmeron, 2003). The increasing failure of chemotherapeutic and antibiotic resistance exhibited by pathogenic microbial infectious agents has led to the screening of several medicinal plants for their potential antimicrobial activity (Colombo et al., 1996; Iwu et al., 1999). The antimicrobial activities of the different extracts of the different parts of *S. hermonthica* were assayed *in vitro* using agar well diffusion method. Three bacterial strains, *S. aureus* ATCC 25923, *E. coli* ATCC25922, *Ps. aeruginosa* ATCC 27853, and one fungal species *C. albicans* ATCC7596 were used. The results represent the microbial growth inhibition by petroleum ether, ethanol and aqueous extracts of *S. hermonthica* at a concentration 5 mg/ml (Tables 6).

Table 5. TLC remarks of alcoholic extract components of *S. hermonthica* developed on system IV (Butanol/Acetic acid/Water; 100:25:125).

Plant parts	No. of spots	R$_f$ (values)*	Separated spots remark	Spots under UV-lamp at (365nm)
Shoot	1	0.47	Pale yellow green/-	Blue Fluorescent
	2	0.90	Pale yellow green/-	Blue Fluorescent
	3	0.96	Pale green	Orange/red fluorescent
Haustoria	1	0.10	Pale yellow/-	Blue Fluorescent
	2	0.91	Pale yellow/-	Blue Fluorescent
Callus of week (4)	1	0.10	Pale yellow green/-	Blue Fluorescent
	2	0.55	Pale yellow/-	Blue Fluorescent
	3	0.93	Pale green	Orange/Red fluorescent
Callus of week (6)	1	0.12	Pale yellow green/-	Blue Fluorescent
	2	0.55	Pale yellow green/-	Blue Fluorescent
	3	0.91	Pale green	Orange/Red fluorescent
Callus of week (8)	1	0.10	Pale yellow green/-	Blue Fluorescent
	2	0.55	Pale yellow green/-	Blue Fluorescent
	3	0.91	Pale green	Orange/Red fluorescent

*Values represent Means calculated from triplicates experiments. (-) means these sports are almost invisible in some.

Table 6. Antimicrobial activities of *S. hermonthica* extracts agains tested standard microorganisms.

Plant parts	Standard microorganisms	Zones of inhibition (mm)*			
		Ether extract	Ethanol extract	Water extract	Kanamycin antibiotic
Upper parts (intact plant)	*S. aureus*	0.00	5.70	0.00	21.00
	P. aeruginosa	0.00	3.30	0.00	20.00
	E. coli	0.00	3.00	0.00	12.00
	C. albicans	1.00	2.70	0.00	n.t
Haustorium (intact plant)	*S. aureus*	0.00	2.70	0.00	21.00
	P. aeruginosa	0.00	3.70	1.30	20.00
	E. coli	0.00	2.00	0.00	12.00
	C. albicans	1.00	3.00	0.00	n.t
Callus	*S. aureus*	0.00	3.00	0.00	21.00
	P. aeruginosa	0.00	2.00	3.70	20.00
	E. coli	0.00	4.00	0.00	12.00
	C. albicans	1.00	2.00	0.00	n.t

*Values represent means of triplicates; n.t = not tested.

Controls were maintained where pure solvents were used instead of the extracts. Moreover, Kanamycin antibiotic at a concentration of 5 mg/L was used against bacterial strains as positive control (Figure 2). The petroleum ether extracts of different parts of *S. hermonthica* showed no antibacterial properties against all bacterial strains and weak antifungal activity against *C. albicans* with 1.00 mm inhibition zone. In different *Striga* spp. Hirematch et al. (1996), found that the petroleum ether extract of both *Striga densiflora* Benth and *Striga orobanchioiedes* Benth has an antibacterial activity against pathogenic and non-pathogenic bacteria. The inactivity of ether extract of *S. hermonthica* may be due to the absence or insufficient and effective concentration of the antimicrobial agents in the petroleum ether extract of *S. hermonthica*. On the other hand, the ethanol extracts

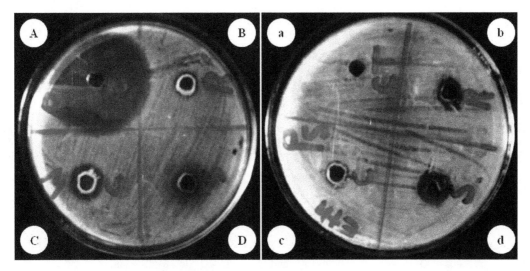

Figure 2. Antimicrobial activity of *S. hermonthica* extracts on *P. aeroginosa*, Left: the effects of water extracts (A) Kanamycin, (B) Intact plant (haustoria), (C) Callus and (D) Intact plant (shoot); Right: the effects of ethanol extracts (a) negative control, (b) Intact plant (haustoria), (c) callus and (d) Intact plant (shoot).

of almost all parts of *S. hermonthica* were used in this study (callus, upper-parts or under-ground parts) exhibited antimicrobial activity with various actions against the tested microorganisms. The maximum antimicrobial activity was achieved by ethanol extracts of the upper-parts of *S. hermonthica* against Gram-positive *S. aureus* ATCC25923 with inhibition zone of 5.7 mm as highest inhibition zone among all extracts, followed by ethanol extract of callus which showed activity against *E. coli* ATCC25922 with 4.00 mm inhibition zone. The lowest activity was obtained from ethanol extracts of both callus and under-ground parts with 2.00 mm zone inhibition against *C. albicans* ATCC7596 and *P. aeruginosa* ATCC27853 in callus and *E. coli* ATCC25922 in under-ground parts. Previous work done by Hirematch et al. (1997) on *Striga sulphurea* revealed that the ethanol (95%) extract exhibited high activity against *S. aureus*, *E. coli*, *P. aeruginsoa* and *Aspergillus niger*. These findings support our results obtained with the ethanol extracts, which may be due to the richness of the ethanol extract with active principle compounds, such as flavonoids, cardiac glycosides, alkaloids. The aqueous extracts of different parts of *S. hermonthica* showed no effect against all tested microorganisms, except the water extracts of callus and under-ground parts, which exhibited activity against *P. aeruginosa* ATCC27853. Kanamycin antibiotic was used at concentration 5 mg/ml against tested bacterial strains, the results obtained revealed high differences between Kanamycin and *S. hermonthica* extracts. The variations in the results obtained from different extracts of the different parts of *S. hermonthica* may reflect the influence of the tested microbial strains, plant parts and solvents used in the extraction, which play important roles as restriction factors affecting the antimicrobial activity. The differences in the antimicrobial

effects of the different parts of *S. hermonthica* may strongly be attributed to the phytochemical properties and differences among the various parts of the plant. More comprehensive studies regarding the phytochemistry and the pharmaceutical properties of this plant will eventually enrich the knowledge about the scientific aspect of its medicinal uses.

REFERENCES

Atawodi SE, Bulus T, Ibrahim S, Ameh DA, Nok AJ, Mamman M, Galadima M (2003). *In vitro* trypanocidal effect of methanolic extract of some Nigerian savannah plants. Afr. J. Biotechnol., 2: 317-321.

Bauer AW, Kirby WM, Sherris JC, Turk M (1966). Antibiotic susceptibility testing by a standardized single disk method. Am. J. Clin. Pathol., 45: 493-496.

Carson AG (1988). *Striga*: Improved management in Africa. In: Robson T O and Broad HR (Eds) Proceeding of FAO/OAU All-Africa Government Consultation on *Striga* Control. Cameroon, p. 250.

Choudhury MK, Marting ZG, Agbaji AS, Nok AJ, Mukhopadyay S (2000). Chemical investigation of the flowers of *S. sensegalensis*. Indian J. Pharm. Sci., 62: 396-397.

Choudhury MK, Phillips AL, Mustapha A (1998). Pharmacological Studies of *Striga senegalesis* Benth (Schrophulariaceae) as an Abortifacient. Phytother. Res., 12: 141-143.

Colombo D, Scala A, Taino IM, Toma L, Ronchetti F, Tokuda H, Nishino H, Nagatsu A, Sakakibara J (1996). 1-*O*-, 2-*O*- and 3-*O*-ß-glycosyl-*sn*-glycerols: structure − anti-tumor-promoting activity relationship. Bioorg. Med. Chem. Lett., 6: 1187-1190.

Culei I (1989). Methodology for Analysis of Vegetable Drugs. Practical Manuals of the Industrial Utilization of Medical and Aromatic Plants. Bucharest Office of Joint UNIDO, Bucharest.

Harborne JB (1973). Phytochemical Methods: A Guide to Modern Techniques of Plant Analysis. Chapman A & Hall, London.

Hassan MM, Ayewale AO, Amupitan JO, Abduallahi MS, Okonkwo EM (2004). Preliminary phytochemical and antibacterial investigation of crude extracts of the root bark of *Detarium microcarpum*. J. Chem. Soc. Niger., 29: 26-29.

Hirematch SP, Rudresh K, Bandami, S (1997). Antimicrobial activity of various extracts of *Striga sulphurea* and Heridesmus indicus. Indian J. Pharm. Sci., 59: 145-147.

Hirematch SP, Swamy HKS, Badami S, Meena S (1996). Antimicrobial and antifungal activity of *Striga densiflora* and *Striga orobanchioiedes*. Indian J. Pharm. Sci., 58: 174-176.

Hussain HS, Deeni YY (1991). Plants in Kano ethnomedicine; screening for antimicrobial activity and alkaloids. Int. J. Pharmacognosy, 29: 51-56.

Hutchinson J, Dalziel JM (1963). Flora of West Tropical Africa. In: Hepper FN (Ed.) Crown Agents for Overseas Governments and Administrations, Milbank, London SW1, pp. 370-373.

Iwu MW, Duncan AR, Okunji CO (1999). New antimicrobials of plant origin. In: J Janick (ed.), Perspectives on new crops and new uses. ASHS Press, Alexandria, VA, pp. 457-462.

Jork H, Funk W, Fishcer W, Wimmer H (1994).TLC Reagents and Detection Methods – Physical and Chemical Detection Methods: Activation Reactions, Reagent Sequences, Reagents, II, Vol 1b. Wiley, NY.

Khan IZ, Aqil M, Kolo B (1998). 5-Hydroxy-6,8–dimethoxyflavone 7,4'-*O*- diglucoside from *Striga hermonthica* (DEL) Benth. Ultra Sci. Phys. Sci., 10: 278-280.

Kiendrebeogo M, Dijoux-Franca M-G, Lamien CE, Meda A, Wouessidjewe D, Nacoulma OG (2005). Acute toxicity and antioxidant property of *Striga hermonthica* (Del.) Benth (Schrophulariaceae). Afr. J. Biotechnol., 4: 919-922.

Kokwaro JO (1976). Medicinal Plants in East Africa. In: Van Puyvelde L and Geysen D (Eds.) Flowering Plant families of East Africa. East African Literature Bureau, Nairobi, Kenya, pp. 92-93, 203.

Males Z, Plazibat M, Vundac VB, Zuntar I (2006). Qualitative and quantitative analysis of flavonoids of the Strawberry tree- *Arbutus unedo* L. (Ericaceae). Acta Pharm., 56: 245-250.

Mohamed KI (1994). Biosystematics and diversification in the genus *Striga* Lour. (Scrophulariaceae) in Africa. Ph.D thesis, Old Dominion University, Norfolk, p. 170.

Mohamed KI, Musselman LJ, Riches CR (2001). The Genus *Striga* (Scrophulariaceae) in Africa. Ann. Missouri. Bot. Gard., 88: 60-103.

Murch SJ, Krishna Raj S, Saxena PK (2002). Tryptophan is a precursor for melatonin and serotonin biosynthesis in *in-vitro* regenerated St. John's wort (*Hypericum perforatum* L. cv. Anthos) plants. Plant Cell Rep., 19: 698-704.

Musselman LJ, Bharathalasksmi SB, Knepper DA, Mohamed KI, White CI (1991). Recent research on the biology of *Striga asiatica*, *S. gesnerioides* and *S. hermonthica*. In: Kim SK (Ed.) Combating Striga in Africa. Proceedings International Workshop, Ibadan, Nigeria, 1988. IITA, Ibadan, pp. 31-41.

Nacoulma OG (1996). Plantes Medicinales et pratiques medicales traditionnelles au Burkhina-Faso: cas du plateau central. These da'etat Universite de Ouagadougou, Ouagadougou, Burkina-Faso. p. 261.

Okpako LC, Ajaiyeoba EO (2004). *In vitro* and *in vivo* antimalarial studies of *Striga hermonthica* and *Tapinanthus sessilifolius* extracts. Afr. J. Med. Med., Sci. 33: 73-75.

Press MC, Scholes JD, Riches CR (2001). Current status and future prospects for management of parasitic weeds (*Striga* and *Orobanche*). In: Riches CR (Ed.) The World's Worst Weeds. British Crop Protection Council, Brighton, UK, pp. 71-90.

Schillinger U, Lucke F (1989). Antimicrobial activity of Lactobacillus sake isolated from meat. J. Appl. Environ. Microbiol., 55: 1901-1906.

Tarr SAJ (1962). Disease of Sorghum, Sudan Grass and Broom Corn. Commonwealth Agriculture Bureaux. (CAB), the Commonwealth Mycological Institute, Kew, Surry, U.K., pp. 229-302.

Trease GE, Evan WC (1989). Pharmacognosy. 13th edn. Bailliere Tindall, London, pp. 176-180.

Vaghasiya Y, Chanda SV (2007). Screening of methanol and acetone extracts of fourteen Indian medicinal plants for antimicrobial activity. Turk. J. Biol., 31: 243-248.

Valero M, Salmeron MC (2003). Antibacterial activity of 11 essential oils against *Bacillus cereus* in tyndallized carrot broth. Int. J. Food Microbiol., 85: 73-81.

Wagner H, Bladt S (1966). Plant Drug Analysis. Springer, Berlin, pp. 195-197.

World Health Organization (WHO) (1978). The promotion and development of traditional medicine. Technical report series, p. 622.

Zhou WJ, Yoneyama K, Takeuchi Y, Iso S, Rungmekarat S, Chae SH, Sato D, Joel DM (2004). *In vitro* infection of host roots by differentiated calli of the parasitic plant *Orobanche*. J. Exp. Bot., 55: 899-907.

21

Evaluation of *Sesamum indicum* gum as a binder in the formulation of paracetamol granules and tablets

Clement Jackson[1]*, Ekaette Akpabio[1], Romanus Umoh[2], Musiliu Adedokun[1], [1]Peace Ubulom and Godwin Ekpe[3]

[1]Department of Pharmaceutics and Pharmaceutical Technology, Faculty of Pharmacy, University of Uyo, Akwa Ibom State, Nigeria.
[2]Department of Pharmacognosy and Natural Medicine, Faculty of Pharmacy, University of Uyo, Akwa Ibom State, Nigeria.
[3]Department of Clinical Pharmacy and Biopharmacy, Faculty of Pharmacy, University of Uyo, Akwa Ibom State, Nigeria.

Comparative evaluation of *Sesamum indicum* gum as a binder in the formulation of paracetamol (PCM) granules and tablets was performed using acacia, gelatin, and Sodium carboxyl methylcellulose (SCMC) as standard binders for comparison. The properties of granules and tablets such as; flow rate, angle of repose, density, weight uniformity, crushing strength, friability, disintegration rate and release profiles, were evaluated. The compact granules had good flow properties. However, binder concentration influenced flow characteristics. SIG gave the highest hardness/friability ratios. It also prolonged disintegration and dissolution time and dissolution rate. Hence, SIG may not be useful as a binder in conventional tablet formulation but may serve as a binder or hydrophilic polymer in sustained release tablet formulation.

Key words: *Sesamum indicum* gum, binder, paracetamol tablets.

INTRODUCTION

Excipients of plant origin are of particular interest to Formulation scientists because they are reliable, sustainable and will minimize reliance upon fossil fuels derived products (Liu et al., 2007). Vegetable products are therefore suitable alternatives to synthetic products because of their minimal toxicity, cost effectiveness and affordability compared to synthetic products. Additives from plant sources are also generally non toxic renewable means for the sustainable supply of less expensive pharmaceuticals (Patel et al., 2007; Liu et al., 2007). Gums from plant sources have various applications in drug delivery as disintegrating agents (Alfa et al., 1999), emulsifier (Nasipuri et al., 1999a), and suspending agents (Nasipuri et al., 1999b) and as binding agents (Sinha et al., 2002). They have also been utilized in formulating immediate and controlled release products (Ibrahim et al., 2002).

Sesame (*Sesamum indicum* L.) is an essential oilseed crop worldwide. it has been cultivated in Korea from time immemorial for use as a traditional health food. Sesame seeds are used in the manufacture of tahin (sesame butter) and *halva*, and for the preparation of crackers, cakes and pastry products in commercial bakeries. There are many varieties of sesame adapted to various ecological conditions (Nzikou et al., 2009). The plant also grows in China, Ethiopia, Mexico, United States and Nigeria.

As a medicinal plant, traditional uses of sesame include limited application as demulcent and emollient. The oil is also used as a laxative and tonic. Etukudo (2003) reported the use of sesame oil as a pharmaceutical solvent, and a constituent of the oil (sesamolin) as synergist for pyrethrum insecticide.

The aim of this research is to assess the suitability of *Sesamum indicum* gum (SIG) as a binder for pharmaceutical tablet formulations. A comparative evaluation of *Sesamum indicum* gum as a binder in the formulation of paracetamol (PCM) granules and tablets

---

*Corresponding author. E-mail: clementjackson1@yahoo.com.

Table 1. Composition of tablets batches.

Materials	(1%W/W Binder	(2% W/W) Binder	(3% W/W) Binder	(4% W/W) Binder	(5% W/W) Binder
Paracetamol(mg)	500	500	500	500	500
Lactose (mg)	45	40	35	30	25
Binder(mg)	5	10	15	20	25

was performed. Acacia, gelatin and Sodium carboxyl methylcellulose (SCMC) was employed as standard binders for comparison.

MATERIALS AND METHODS

Paracetamol powder was a gift from SKG Pharma, Lagos, Nigeria, Lactose and maize starch were purchased from BDH, England. Magnesium stearate was purchased from Sigma Aldrich, USA. All other chemicals and reagents used were of laboratory grade.

Isolation of gum

The bark and other extraneous materials of the gum was removed manually and dried in an oven at 50°C for 8 h. The dried gum was separated into light colored and dark colored grades. The light colored grade was selected for further processing by milling in a domestic blender into fine powder and designated as crude *S. indicum* gum (CSIG). The gum mucilage was prepared by dissolving 100 g of SCIG in 200 ml of distilled water and kept for 24 h with intermittent stirring. Insoluble debris was removed by the use of calico while 96% ethanol was used to effect precipitation. The precipitate was re-filtered and washed with ether and dried in an oven at 50°C for 8 h. The dried purified gum was milled and screened through 180 μm sieve. The powdered gum was used in subsequent tests and analysis as purified *S. indicum* gum (PSIG).

Production of paracetamol tablets

Tablets of paracetamol were prepared by a wet granulation technique. Lactose was used as diluents while magnesium stearate was used as lubricant. SIG gum was incorporated in the formulations in different proportions as binder. The composition of different formulations used in the research containing 500 mg of paracetamol (PCM) in each case (Table 1). In all the formulation batches, PSIG and the binders were sieved (<500 μm) separately before use and mixed with Paracetamol powder and lactose (<150μm) in a blender. The blend were mixed for 10 min in a tumbler mixer (Karl Kolb, D 6072 Dreieich, Germany) and granulated with water for 5 min. After passage through the screen, granules were dried at 50°C for 2 h in a hot air oven (Salvis, Switzerland). The dried granules were re-screened through a 1.7 mm sieve and lubricated with 1.0% magnesium stearate for 5 min. The final blend was compressed using a single station tablet press (THP Shanghai, Tianxiang ad Chentai Pharmaceutical Machinery Co. Ltd, China) fitted with 12.5 mm punch. The tablet weight was approximately 550 mg.

Evaluation of granules

The granules were evaluated for bulk density and tapped density (Shah et al., 1977), angle of repose (Carr, 1965; Cooper and Gunn, 1986), hausner ratio and compressibility index (USP, 2007).

Evaluation of tablets

Hardness test

The hardness of 10 tablets chosen at random from each of the batches after storing at ambient temperature for 24 h was determined in a hardness tester (Erweka, Model TBH - 28). The mean hardness was calculated.

Friability

The weight of 20 tablets chosen from each batch was determined collectively as initial weight, WA. The tablets were placed in a friabilator (Erweka); set to rotate at 25 rpm for 4 min, after which the tablets were de-dusted and weighed (WB). Friability was calculated from the equation:

$$F = (WA - WB)/W_A \times 100$$

The mean value was determined.

Disintegration time determination

Five tablets from each batch were used for the test. Erweka disintegration test apparatus (Model DT4) was used (British Pharmacopoeia, 2003). The disintegration medium was 0.1 N HCl, maintained at 37 ± 0.5°C. The disintegration time was taken as the mean time required for the tablets to break into small particles that can pass through the screen into the disintegration medium.

Dissolution rate determination

British Pharmacopoeia 2003 method was also used. One tablet was placed in the apparatus and rotated at 100 rpm. The dissolution medium was 1000 ml 0.1 N HCL, maintained at 37 ± 0.5°C. 5 ml portions of the dissolution medium were withdrawn using at predetermined time intervals. Each 5 ml sample withdrawn was replaced by an equivalent fresh dissolution medium to maintain sink conditions. The solution was analyzed after colour development using a Sp6-450 UV/VIS spectrophotometer at 240 nm.

RESULTS AND DISCUSSION

Granule properties

The flow properties of paracetamol granules were expressed as hausner's ratio and angle of repose (Table 2). Results show good to excellent flow.

Granules with Hausner ratio less than 1.25 have good flow properties (Panda et al., 2008) and granules with angle of repose less than 30° show good flow (Reddy et

Table 2. Physical properties of paracetamol granules.

Binder conc.(%w/w) Acacia	Bulk Density	Tapped density	Hausner's ratio	Angle of repose($\emptyset$)
1	0.4520	0.5125	1.13	34.75
2	0.4051	0.4680	1.16	33.60
3	0.4000	0.4605	1.15	33.82
4	0.3890	0.4518	1.16	33.45
5	0.3795	0.4390	1.16	32.95
Gelatin				
1	0.4325	0.4850	1.12	34.45
2	0.3970	0.4560	1.15	34.16
3	0.3895	0.4485	1.15	33.79
4	0.3856	0.4390	1.14	33.21
5	0.3796	0.4370	1.15	32.90
SCMC				
1	0.4225	0.4720	1.13	33.75
2	0.3986	0.4575	1.15	33.40
3	0.3907	0.4410	1.13	32.90
4	0.3875	0.4360	1.13	32.55
5	0.3820	0.4305	1.13	31.96
PSIG				
1	0.3675	0.4150	1.13	30.50
2	0.3655	0.4110	1.12	29.85
3	0.3630	0.4082	1.12	29.76
4	0.3588	0.4050	1.13	29.32
5	0.3545	0.3986	1.12	29.00

al., 2003). Therefore, granules prepared by using different binders - acacia, gelatin, SCMC and PSIG - exhibited good flow properties. Hausner ratio was below 1.25 for the different concentrations of the binders

Hardness and friability

The effect of binder concentration on tablet hardness and friability are shown in Table 3. An increase in binder concentration increased the hardness of the tablets. On the other hand, friability decreased as binder concentration increased. An increase in binder concentration will enhance the formation of stronger interparticulate bonds between the granules during compression in a tabulating machine (Esezobo and Pilpel, 1976). This means that the tablets would offer greater resistance to shock and abrasion since there is a stronger adhesive bonding of the granules at high binder concentrations. In general, the tablets showed good friability profiles, since most had friability values of less than 1.0% (Harwood and Pilpel, 1968).

Disintegration time

The effect of binder concentration on tablet disintegration time is shown in Table 3. The tablets formulated with PSIG failed the British Pharmacopoeia 2003 disintegration time test. However, tablets containing SCMC, acacia, and gelatin as binders disintegrated in less than 15 min. The binders follow this order of increasing tablet disintegration time: SCMC < acacia < gelatin < PSIG.

Dissolution profile

Tablets made with SCMC gave the highest drug release while PSIG had the lowest (Table 3). As the binder concentration increased, the rate of release of paracetamol from the tablets decreased.

In other words, there was an inverse relationship between binder concentration and release rate of drug.

PSIG displayed a very remarkable delay in the release rate at higher binder concentrations

Table 3. Physical properties of paracetamol tablets.

Binder conc.(%w/w) Acacia	Hardness(N)	Friability (%)	Disintegration time (min)	Dissolution at 30 min (cumulative% drug released)
1	3.13	0.90	5.40	100.80
2	3.24	0.89	6.92	95.45
3	4.85	0.85	10.00	86.75
4	6.35	0.81	12.50	75.00
5	6.70	0.76	14.15	72.50
Gelatin				
1	3.50	0.90	6.00	100.00
2	3.85	0.85	7.50	93.75
3	4.96	0.81	11.00	73.60
4	6.75	0.80	12.85	73.00
5	7.00	0.74	14.28	62.70
SCMC				
1	2.31	1.02	4.50	101.36
2	3.52	0.89	6.45	100.00
3	3.88	0.85	8.00	98.53
4	4.75	0.85	9.50	90.50
5	5.49	0.81	11.90	85.00
PSIG				
1	4.75	0.86	21.60	65.35
2	4.91	0.81	31.20	58.00
3	5.66	0.80	51.20	48.54
4	6.25	0.73	66.60	40.40
5	7.48	0.60	85.80	32.38

since none of the tablet batches formulated with PSIG released up to 75% of drug in 30 min (Esezobo and Pilpel, 1976).

Conclusion

The results of this study established, for the first time, some basic characteristics of tablets formulated with gum obtained from the *S. indicum*. The gum performs as a smart polymer, and may be utilized in sustained drug delivery. The gum produced powder granules with good flow properties and tablets with good physicotechnical characteristics.

PSIG could not be suitably utilized as a binder in formulation of immediate released tablets since it prolongs tablet disintegration time and also delays drug dissolution rate. It may be useful as a binder or hydrophilic polymer in sustained release tablet formulation.

REFERENCES

Alfa J, Chukwu A, Udeala OK (1999). Cissus stem gum as potential dispersant in Pharmaceutical liquid systems: rheological characterization. Boll. Chim. Farm., 140: 20-

27.

British Pharmacopoeia (2003). Her Majesty's Stationery Office, London, A246.

Carr RL (1965) Evaluating flow properties of solids. Chem. Eng., 72: 163 –168.

Cooper J, Gunn C (1986). Powder flow and compaction. In: Carter S.J, Tutorial Pharmacy, CBS publishers, New Delhi, pp: 211–233.

Esezobo S, Pilpel N (1976). Some formulation factors affecting tensile strength, disintegration and dissolution of uncoated oxytetracycline tablets. J. Pharm. Pharmacol., 28: 6–15.

Etukudo, I. Ethnobotany; Conventional and rational use of plants. The Verdiet press Ltd, Uyo, pp. 106-107.

Harwood CF, Pilpel N (1968). Granulation of griseofulvin. J. Pharm. Sci., 57: 478-481.

Ibrahim MA, Dawes VH, Bangudu AB (2002). Evaluation of cissus pupulnea polymer as a matrix Former for controlled drug release. J. Phytomed. Ther, 5: 23-32.

Liu M, Fan J, Wang K, He Z (2007). Synthesis, characterization and evaluation of phosphated cross linked konjac glucomannan hydrogels for colon targeted drug delivery. Drug. Deliv., 14: 397-402.

Nasipuri RN, Igwilo CI, Brown SA, kunle OO (1999). Mucilage from Abelmoschus esculentus (okra) Fruit: a potential pharmaceutical raw material part II-Emulsifying properties. J. Phytomed. Ther. 2: 27-34.

Nasipuri RN, Igwilo CI, Brown SA, Kunle OO (1999). Mucilage from Abelmoschus esculentus (okra) Fruit: A potential pharmaceutical raw material; part II-suspending properties. J. Phytomed. Ther., 1: 22-88.

Nzikou JM, Matos 1L, Bouanga-Kalou G, Ndangui CB, Pambou-Tobi NPG, Kimbonguila A et al (2009).Chemical Composition on the Seeds and Oil of Sesame (Sesamum indicum L.) Grown in Congo-Brazzaville. Advance J. Food. Sci. Technol., 1(1): 6-11

Panda D, Choudhury NSK, Yedukondalu M, Si S, Gupta R (2008). Evaluation of gum of Moringa oleifera as a binder and release retardant in tablet formulation. Indian J. Pharmac. Sci., 70(5): 614-618.

Patel DM, Prajapat DG, Patel NM (2007). Indian. J. Pharm. Sci., 69: 431-435.

Reddy K, Mutalik S, Reddy S (2003). Once-daily sustained-release matrix tablets of nicorandil: Formulation and in vitro evaluation. AAPS Pharm. Sci. Tech., 4(4): 480-488.

Shah D, Shah Y, Rampradhan M (1977). Development and evaluation of controlled release diltiazem hydrochloride microparticles using cross – linked polyvinyl alcohol. Drug. Dev. Ind. Pharm; 23: 567–574

Sinha VR, kumrie R (2002) binders for colon specific drug delivery: an in vitro evaluation. Int. J. Pharm., 249: 23-31.

United States of Pharmacopeia-National Formulary (2007). USP 30 – NF 25. The Unit States Pharmacopeial Convention, Rockville, MD. 1: 226.

22

Ketamine hydrochloride induces anxiety behaviour activities in adult male mice

Musa A. A.* and Adeniyi, P. A. O.

Department of Anatomy, PMB 1515, College of Health Sciences, University of Ilorin, Ilorin, Nigeria.

The trafficking and abuse of Ketamine are a concern to law enforcement and drug treatment providers because of the drug's increasing availability and its use in facilitating sexual assaults globally. The aim of this study is to investigate some of the effects of administration of ketamine intramuscularly (IM) on bebaviour in mice. The presumably 16 healthy male mice were used for this study; the animals were randomly divided in to two (2) groups, A and B, of eight (8) animals each. Group A were given 8 mg/ kg of the Ketamine (IM) and B were serve as control for 7 days. The exploratory and non – exploratory behaviours of the animals were assessed for 5 minutes using the elevated plus maze (EPM). The results suggested possible anxiolytic and schizophrenic symptoms after the administration.

Key words: Ketamine, behaviour, schizophrenic symptoms, intramuscular, elevated plus maze.

INTRODUCTION

Ketamine hydrochloride, a Schedule III drug under the Controlled Substances Act, is a dissociative anaesthetic that has a combination of stimulant, depressant, hallucinogenic, and analgesic properties. Ketamine produces dissociative anesthesia, which is characterized by catatonia, amnesia, and analgesia, with or without actual loss of consciousness (Katzung, 2004). The drug is an arylcyclohexylamine chemically related to phencyclidine (PCP), a drug frequently abused because of its psychoactive properties. The mechanism of action of ketamine may involve blockade of the membrane effects of the excitatory neurotransmitter glutamic acid at the N-metheyl-D-aspartate (NMDA) receptor (Katzung, 2004; Trevor et al., 2002). Legally used as a preoperative veterinary anesthetic, ketamine is abused for these properties and used to facilitate sexual assault. Common street names for ketamine are K, special K, ket, kit kat, vitamin K, purple, special la coke, cat valium, super acid, super C, lady K, super K, ketaject, and cat tranquilizers.

Distribution of liquid and powdered ketamine typically occurs among friends and acquaintances, most often at raves, nightclubs, and at private parties. Distribution of liquid and powdered ketamine typically occurs among friends and acquaintances, most often at raves, nightclubs, and at private parties; street sales of ketamine are rare (IB, 2004). Behrens (2009) reported that abusing ketamine, which inhibits the NMDA receptor, can result in symptoms indistinguishable from schizophrenia in the mouse prelimbic cortex. Ketamine produces its cardiovascular stimulation by excitation of the central sympathetic nervous system and possibly by inhibition of the uptake of norepinephrine at sympathetic nerve terminals. Increases in plasma epinephrine and norepinephrine levels occur as early as 2 min after intravenous ketamine and return to baseline levels 15 min later (Katzung, 2004; Trevor et al., 2002). The elevated plus maze test is used to asses anxiety in experimental animals; the basic measure is the animal's preference for dark, enclosed places over bright, exposed places. These findings and reports suggest the need for further experimental and clinical studies of the role of ketamine intake on the body systems, most especially the brain/ behaviour in particular. The aim of this study is to investigate some effects of ketamine on the explorative activities of mice using elevated plus maze (EPM).

---
*Corresponding author. E-mail:alwajud1423@yahoo.com, alwajud1423@gmail.com.

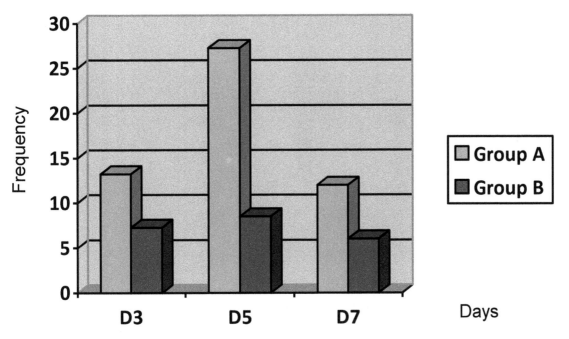

Figure 1. Showing head dipping (HD) of exploratory activity in mice.

MATERIALS AND METHODS

Animal care

All experimental investigations were done in compliance with human animal care standard outlined in the "Guide to the care and use of Animals in research and teaching", as approved by the Institute of Laboratory Animal Resource, National Research Council, DHHS, and Pub. No NIH 86 to 23. The animal right committee of the University of Ilorin, Nigeria gave the permission to carry out this work. The study was carried out using presumably healthy adult male mice with average body weight of 25.06 g. The animals were kept under standard and good laboratory conditions (12 hours light and 12 hours darkness, temperature, humidity and ventilation). They were given standard rat diet, purchased from Bethel Feeds, Ilorin, Nigeria.

Experimental design

Total of 16 adult male mice were used for this study. The animals were randomly divided in to two (2) groups, A and B of eight (8) animals each. Group A were given 8 mg/kg body weight of Ketamine (IM), produced by LABORATE Pharmaceutical, India, and B serve as control group for 7 experimental days.

Neurobehavioural observations

The neurobehavioural analysis was done at 0800 h of the day using elevated plus maze to study the locomotion, exploration, and motor coordination in both the treated and control animals (Brown, 2010; Iheanyi et al., 2010; Adeniyi et al., 2010). The results are shown in Figures 1 and 2.

Procedure

Both the treated and control animals were placed in the center of the apparatus to explore for 5 min. Measurements compared included total time spent in the closed arms (CAD) as well as, entries into the open and closed arms (T) and head dipping (HD) (Brown, 2010; Iheanyi et al., 2010; UCLA, 2011; Adeniyi et al., 2010).

Statistical analysis

The data were expressed as means ± Standard Error of Mean (SEM), and were statistically evaluated with SPSS software version 14.0 software. Data collected were analyzed using the student's t – test.

RESULTS

Gross observations

There were no significant changes in the skin colour and fur arrangement; the colour of their eyes was normal compared to the control groups.

The animal weight changes

The treated group lost shed weight drastically, especially between the 2nd and 4th days of treatment, when compared with the control group (Figure 3).

Animal behaviour

After administration of ketamine, the mice loss their gat within 1 to 2 min and become weak and sleep for about 5

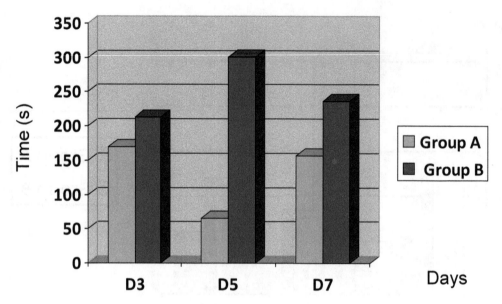

Figure 2. Showing closed arm duration (CAD) of exploratory activity in mice (in s).

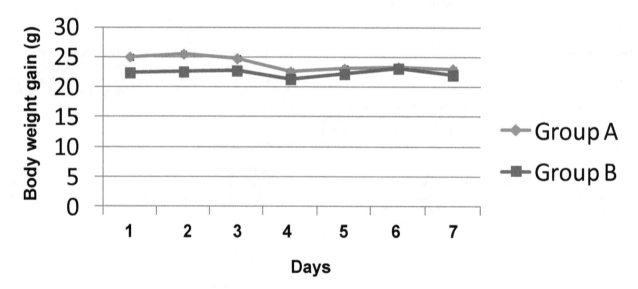

Figure 3. showing the average body weight changes (g) during experimental period.

minutes thereafter woke up. Rate of Head deeding (HD), Closed arm duration (CAD) and Transition (T) were significantly ($p < 0.05$) different between treated and the control group (Figures 1 to 2).

DISCUSSION

The intramuscular administration of 8 mg/kg body weight of Ketamine for 7 days resulted in reduction of closed arm duration (CAD) in mice that is, increase in activities of mice in the open arm of the maze; however there was a statistical increase ($p < 0.05$) in head dipping (HD) of

the mice. Ketamine and other drugs that block NMDA receptor channel have potent antiepileptic activity in animal models, though these drugs have yet to be tested clinically (Katzung, 2004; Trevor et al., 2002). Considerable evidence exists such that the release of glutamate during neuronal injury can, by activating the NMDA receptor, cause further cell injury and death (Katzung, 2004). Thus, a particularly exciting finding is that blocking the NMDA receptor can attenuate the neuronal damage caused by anoxia in treated animals. The mechanism of action of ketamine may involve blockade of the membrane effects of the excitatory neurotransmitter glutamic acid at the NMDA (N-methyl-

Daspartate) receptor subtype (Katzung, 2004). Ketamine is a highly lipophilic drug and is rapidly distributed into highly vascular organs, including the brain, and subsequently redistributed to less well perfused tissues with concurrent hepatic metabolism and both urinary and biliary excretion. Ketamine is the only intravenous anesthetic that possesses analgesic properties and produces cardiovascular stimulation. These characteristics may account for the anxiety behaviours, elevated HD and lowered CAD (Adeniyi et al., 2010) in mice treated with ketamine during 7 days of this study. Since Rodents, such as rats and mice, are most active in the dark (Benstaali et al., 2001; Kopp, 2001), they are expected to spend more time in the closed arm of the maze during the 5 min of their exposure (Schellinck et al., 2010) however, the opposite is the case in the treated animals; spending more time exploring open arm is an indication of hyperactivity/anxiety in these animals injected with Ketamine. The behavior of mice in the EPM represents anxiety-related behavior in humans has reported by Schellinck et al. (2010).

Conclusion

The intramuscular administration of 8 mg/kg body weight of Ketamine for 7 days resulted in reduction of closed arm duration (CAD) in mice that is, increase in activities of mice in the open arm of the maze; however there was a statistical increase ($p < 0.05$) in head dipping (HD) of the mice. The results suggested possible anxiolytic and schizophrenic symptoms after the drug administration.

From all the changes observed from comparism between the treated and control group, we thereby concluded that the administration of ketamine resulted in alterations in locomotory activities in treated animals.

REFERENCES

Adeniyi PAO, Ghazal OK, Musa AA, Caxton–Martins EA (2010). The neurobehavioural effects of smoke and ethanolic extract of Nicotiana tabacum leaves exposure in Mice. Res. J. Anim. Sci., 4(4): 99–102.

Behrens M (2009). In the Dana Alliance's Progress Report on Brain Research, p. 41.

Benstaali C, Mailloux A, Bogdan A, Auzeby A, Touitou Y (2001). Circadian rhythms of body temperature and motor activity in rodents: their relationships with the light–dark cycle. Life Sci., 68: 2645–2656.

Intelligence Bulletin (IB) (2004). Ketamine U.S Department of Justice. Product No. 2004 – L0424 – 007. pp.1-4.

Katzung BG (2004). Basic and Clinical Pharmacology, the McGraw-Hill companies, 9th ed., pp. 433-434.

Kopp C (2001). Locomotor activity rhythm in inbred strains of mice: implications for behavioural studies. Beh. Brain Res., 125: 93–96.

Brown RE (2010). Studying Neurobehaviour. Book of Abstracts of 3rd International Neuroscience congress of the institute of Neuroscience and Biomedical research (INBR). p. 17.

Schellinck HM, David PC, Richard EB (2010). Advances in the Study of Behavior. Burlington Academic Press. 41: 255-366.

Trevor AJ, Katzung BK, Masters (2002). Katzung and Trevor's Pharmacology, Examination and Board Review. Lange Medical Books/ McGraw – Hill, NY. pp. 233-234.

UCLA (2011). Elevated plus Maze. Behavioral Testing Core Facility

23

Technical report on laboratory outbreak investigation of sudden death syndrome in broiler chicken in Kathmandu valley Nepal 2009

Kedar Karki

Central Veterinary Laboratory Tripureswor, Kathmandu Nepal. E-mail: drkedar_karki@yahoo.com.

The incidence of death of broiler birds above 40 days suddenly increased in the month of July to October 2009 in Kathmandu valley. Birds that were presented for post-mortem examination at the Central Veterinary Laboratory Tripureswor Kathmandu were usually found dead on their backs with wings out-stretched. Gross abnormalities recorded on post mortem examinations were: muscle oedema, pulmonary, renal and liver congestion, dark black to pale yellow streaked liver bile filled gall bladder and congestive splenomegaly, blood clot in atrium haemorrhage in duodenal muscle, whitish yellow pasty fluid in proventriculus gland, greenish coloration marked intact feed particles in gizzard and excessive mucous filled swollen intestine. Incidence rate was recorded between 1.5 to 2.5% of the flock. The mean mortality rate due to sudden death syndrome was 1.3 to 9.6%. *Penicillium* spp. *Aspergillus* spp. with CFU ranging from 56×10^4 to 62×10^5, to uncountable mold count ' *Escherichia coli, Streptococcus* spp. and *Staphylococcus* spp. were the usual organisms isolated from culture samples of liver, lung, spleen and proventriculus. The condition seems to be related to mycotoxicosis. Reduction of mortality was achieved by feed restriction, with 8 to 10% reduction in nutrient density. Supplementation of glucose containing electrolyte, liquid toxin binder, immuno-modulator, acidifier and antibiotic therapy.

Key word: Sudden death syndrome, broiler birds, Kathmandu valley, *Penicillium*, CFU, ranging from 56×10^4 to 62×10^5 g, uncountable mold count.

INTRODUCTION

Sudden death syndrome (SDS) has been recognized for over 30 years, and is also referred to as acute death syndrome or "flip-overs". It is most common in males when their growth rate is maximized. Mortality may start as early as 3 to 4 days, but most often peaks at around 3 to 4 weeks of age, with affected birds being found dead on their back. Mortality may be found at 1.5 to 2.0% in mixed-sex flocks and as high as 4% in male flocks only (George, 2007). Sudden death syndrome has developed into a major problem to the broiler industry in many parts of the world. Broilers of all ages are affected starting as early as 2 days of age and continuing through to market age. Peak mortality usually occurs between 3 and 4 weeks of age (Gardiner et al., 1988). The syndrome has been reported to cause between 1.31 and 2.46% mortality with males more commonly affected than females (Riddell and Orr, 1980). However, Proudfoot et al. (1982) reported 0.90 to 3.61% mortality due to SDS in

broilers. From 0.71 to 4.07% as reported by Riddel and Springer (1985) whereas, Ononiwu et al. (1979) reported 1.0% mortality due to SDS in broilers. Brigden and Riddell (1975) reported that 70 to 80% of male mortality and 20 to 25% of female broilers chickens mortality could be attributed to acute death syndrome or "Flip-Over Disease". Thus, SDS is a leading contributor to mortality in broiler chicken production. Although, the precipitating event is yet to be ascertained," Cardiovascular failure" appears to be the immediate cause of death (Siddiqui et al., 2009).

OUTBREAK OF SUDDEN DEATH SYNDROME IN KATHMANDU VALLEY

From the first week of July to October 2009, there was a sudden increase in mortality of broilers above 6 weeks of

Table 1. Epidemiology of affected flock with sudden death syndrome in July to October, 2009.

Observation/duration	No.of farmers/flock	Population at risk	Morbidity (%)	Mortality (%)	No. of samples examined
July	63	16620	4250 (25.57)	369(2.22)	63
August	51	15450	1235 (7.99)	232 (1.50)	51
September	32	10260	848 (8.26)	157 (1.53)	32
October	30	15700	2380 (15.16)	149 (0.94)	30
Total	176	58030	8713 (15.01)	907 (1.56)	176

Table 2. Results of microbiological examination.

No. of samples	Bacterial isolated	Fungi isolated	Positive no.	Negative no.
176	Escherichia coli Streptococcus Staphylococcus		35	141
176		Aspergillus Penicillium	145	31

Table 3. Rapid test for AI, ND, IBD.

Variable	No. of samples	Positive	Negative
AI	20	0	20
ND	20	o	20
IBD	20	o	20

age (Table 1) in Kathmandu valley. There were no premonitory signs. Just before death, birds appear normal and it is common to observe the birds if they eat, drink or walk normally. Then birds use to exhibit clinical signs such as extending their neck, squawk and start wing beating as well as, leg extension before falling on their back.

POSTMORTEM FINDING OF SDS BIRDS

Gross abnormalities recorded on post mortem examinations were muscle oedema, pulmonary, renal and liver congestion, dark black to pale yellow streaked liver bile filled gall bladder and congestive splenomegaly, blood clot in atrium haemorrhage in duodenal muscle, whitish yellow pasty fluid in proventriculus gland, greenish coloration marked intact feed particles in gizzard and swollen intestine with excessive mucous filled. All these post mortem observations conform to the descriptions of the syndrome made by Ononiwu et al. (1979).

Laboratory finding of Mycobiota and Microbiota of postmortem tissue samples

A total 176 tissue samples of lung, liver, spleen, proventriculus and gizzard, were collected during postmortem examination and were subjected for both bacterial and mycological culture. Results of microbiological examination are given in Tables 2 and 3.

Treatment and preventive measure given to the rest of birds in flock

All birds remaining in flocks were subjected to restricted feed up to 8 to 10% these percentages differ from the ones in the abstract, and fed twice daily. Supplementation with glucose containing electrolyte, liquid toxin binders, immunomodulator, and simple broad-spectrum antibiotics and acidifiers were provided in water. Vitamin B complex supplementation was totally withdrawn. All birds remaining in all affected farms responded well to the management and there was a marked improvement in the overall condition of the flock.

RESULTS AND DISCUSSION

Sudden death syndrome (SDS) is an acute heart failure disease that affects mainly fast growing male chickens that seem to be in good condition. Although, a common feature in fast growing birds is that the pathogenesis remains unclear (Ononiwu et al., 1979). Cardiac arrhythmias are involved in the pathogenesis of SDS with ventricular arrhythmias (VA) being the most common observation representing premature ventricular contractions and fibrillation (Olkowski and Classen, 1997; 1998). It has been reported that broilers fed with high vitamin D3 diet above the recommended levels in an attempt to prevent commonly occurring leg problems were 2.5 fold more likely to succumb to acute heart failure and die of SDS (Nain et al., 2007). SDS was also experimentally induced by feeding diets containing the mycotoxin moniliformin that resulted into cardiac injury with subsequent alterations in cardiac electrical conductance (Reams et al., 1997) suggesting the possible role of chronic mycotoxicosis to the causation of SDS. Other implicated causes of SDS include continuous artificial lighting (Ononiwu et al., 1979b), deviations in dietary calcium and phosphorus (Scheideler et al., 1995), feeding crumble-pellet diets (Proudfoot et al., 1982), dietary fat content (Rotter et al., 1985) and feeding frequency (Bowes et al., 1988). The latter recommendation of restricted feeding supports well the previous observation that abdominal fat deposition increases the risk of SDS such that restriction on calorie: protein ratio decreases the incidence of SDS (Mollison et al., 1984).

CONCLUSION

The present investigation indicates that broilers in good body weight condition when not harvested timely and remaining in poultry shades for prolonged periods suffer stressful events and even die sudden. Also, it is possible that increased humidity and hot seasons favors the growth of mold and fungus in stored feeds increasing the risk of birds to mycotoxicosis. Detail Histopathological examination of affected organ need to be carried out for further verification of the involvement of mycotoxin for this syndrome.

REFERENCES

Bowes VA, Julian RJ, Julian LS, Stirtzinger L, Stirtzinger T (1988). Effect of feed restriction on feed efficiency and incidence of sudden death syndrome in broiler chickens. Poult. Sci., 67(7): 1102-1104.

George Q (2007). Reduction of Early Mortality in Broiler Chickens through Nutrition and Management: Champion Feed service limited: www.championfeeds.com, www.championfeeds.com., pp. 1-2.

Mollison B, Guenter W, Guenter BR, Boycott BR (1984). Abdominal fat deposition and sudden death syndrome in broilers: the effects of restricted intake, early life caloric (fat) restriction, and calorie: Protein ratio. Poult. Sci., 63(6): 1190-1200.

Nain SB, Laarveld BC, Wojnarowicz C, Olkowski AA (2007). Excessive dietary vitamin D supplementation as a risk factor for sudden death syndrome in fast growing commercial broilers. Comparative biochemistry and physiology. Part A, Mol. Integr. Physiol., 148(4): 828-833.

Olkowski AA, Classen HL (1997). Malignant ventricular dysrhythmia in broiler chickens dying of sudden death syndrome. Vet. Vet. Record. 15; 140(7): 177-179.

Olkowski AA, Classen HL (1998). High incidence of cardiac arrhythmias in broiler chickens. Zentralblatt für Veterinärmedizin. Reihe A., 45(2): 83-91.

Olkowski AA, Wojnarowicz C, Nain S, Ling B, Alcorn JM, Laarveld B (2008). A study on pathogenesis of sudden death syndrome in broiler chickens. Res. Vet. Sci., 85(1): 131-140.

Ononiwu JC, Thomson RG, Carlson HC, Julian RJ (1979). Pathological Studies of "Sudden Death Syndrome" in Broiler Chickens. Can. Vet. J., 20(3): 70–73.

Ononiwu JC, Thomson RG, Carlson HC, Julian RJ (1979b). Studies on effect of lighting on "Sudden death syndrome" in broiler chickens. Can. Vet. J., 20(3): 74-77.

Proudfoot FG, Hulan HW, McRae KB (1982). The effect of crumbled and pelleted feed on the incidence of sudden death syndrome among male chicken broilers. Poult. Sci., 61(8): 1766-1768.

Reams RY, Thacker HL, Harrington DD, Novilla MN, Rottinghaus GE, Bennett GA, Horn J (1997). A sudden death syndrome induced in poults and chicks fed diets containing *Fusarium fujikuroi* with known concentrations of *moniliformin*. Avian Dis., 41(1): 20-35.

Rotter B, Guenter W, Boycott BR (1985). Sudden death syndrome in broilers: dietary fat supplementation and its effect on tissue composition. Poult. Sci., 64(6): 1128-1136.

Scheideler SE, Rives DV, Garlich JD, Ferket PR (1995). Dietary calcium and phosphorus effects on broiler performance and the incidence of sudden death syndrome mortality. Poult. Sci., 74(12): 2011-2018.

Siddiqui MF, Patil MS, Khan KM, Khan LA (2009). Sudden Death Syndrome – An Overview: Vet. World, 2(11): 444-447.

24

Mechanisms of endothelial cell protection by quercetin in hypercholesterolemia

Sri Agus Sudjarwo

Department of Pharmacology, Faculty of Veterinary Medicine, Airlangga University, Surabaya 60115, Indonesia.
E-mail: ags158@yahoo.com.

Mechanism of quercetin for protection of endothelial cell was studied in cholesterol-fed rabbits. Thirty rabbits were randomly divided into five groups. The negative control group was fed with a standard diet; the positive control group was fed with the same diet with 2% cholesterol; the quercetin group was fed with the same diet with 2% cholesterol and quercetin 50, 100 or 150 mg/kg BW/day. The cholesterol-rich diet significantly increased Malondialdehyde (MDA) in the aortic blood vessels, as reflected by Thiobarbituric Acid-Reactive Substances (TBARS), inhibited endothelium-dependent vascular relaxations to acetylcholine, and decrease tissue content cyclic GMP with vessels from normal rabbits (negative control). In cholesterol-fed rabbits, quercetin treatment decreased MDA in plasma production, improved endothelium - dependent relaxations to acetylcholine, and increase cyclic GMP production. These results suggest that quercetin not only improves endothelium-dependent relaxations but also reduces lipid peroxidation (malondialdehyde) in the aorta and enhanced the tissue content cyclic GMP in hypercholesterolemic rabbits. These findings suggest that quercetin might play an important role in the protective effect on endothelial dysfunction in hypercholesterolemia.

Key words: Quercetin, malondialdehyde, endothelium-derived relaxing factor (EDRF), cyclic GMP.

INTRODUCTION

The vascular endothelium is important in a number of homeostatic functions including the regulation of blood flow, vascular tone and local platelet function (Shimokawa, 1999). Endothelium-dependent relaxant effects on vascular smooth muscle is thought to be mediated by releasing EDRF, NO or an NO related substance, followed by an increase in the cyclic GMP content in smooth muscle (Sausbier et al., 2000; Fujitani et al.,1993; Karaki et al.,1993). Endothelium dependent vascular relaxations are impaired in numerous disease states, including hypercholesterolemia, atherosclerosis, hypertension, and chronic heart failure (Shimokawa, 1999; Verbeuren et al., 1990).

Bioassay experiments have suggested that impaired synthesis or release of endothelium-derived relaxing factor might contribute to the abnormal endothelium-dependent relaxation in hypercholesterolemic animals (Stephanie et al., 2005). It has shown that short-term cholesterol feeding in rabbit increases endothelial O^{2-} production, seemingly from xanthine oxidase. Thus, there is substantial evidence that hypercholesterolemia can impair endothelium-dependent relaxation via oxidative inactivation of endothelium-derived relaxing factor (Ohara et al., 1992; Jiang et al., 2001). Administration of polyethylene glycolated superoxide dismutase (SOD) to increase vascular SOD levels improved endothelium-dependent relaxation in atherosclerotic rabbits (Siekmeier et al., 2007; Valko, 2007; Rui-Li et al., 2008). Also, administration of antioxidant such as Vitamin E, Vitamin C and probucol could improve endothelium-dependent relaxation, normalized endothelial O^{2-} production in hypercholesterolemic vessels and reduces lipid peroxidation in the plasmaa (Inoue et al., 1998; Mahfouz et al., 1997; Margurite et al., 2003). Quercetin is considered to be a strong antioxidant due to its ability to

Abbreviations: MDA, malondialdehyde; **EDRF,** endothelium-derived relaxing factor; **NO,** nitric oxide; **TBARS,** thiobarbituric acid reactive substances; and **SOD,** superoxide dismutase; **TCA,** trichloroacetic acid; **BW,** body weight.

scavenge free radicals and bind transition metal ions.

These properties of quercetin allow it to inhibit lipid peroxidation (Hollman and Katan, 1997; Sakanashi, 2008). Lipid peroxidation is the process by which unsaturated fatty acids are converted to free radicals via the abstraction of hydrogen (Young and McEneny, 2001). As a result, quercetin may aid in the prevention of certain diseases, such as cancer, atherosclerosis, and chronic inflammation (Hollman and Katan, 1997; Murota and Terao, 2003). The purpose of our studies was to investigate the molecular mechanisms by which quercetin protected endothelial cell in hypercholesterolemia.

METHODS

Animal preparation

New Zealand White rabbits 6 to 8 weeks old weighing between 1.8 and 2.0 kg, after 1 week of adaptation, were randomly divided into five groups. The negative control group was fed a standard diet; the positive control group was fed the same diet with 2% cholesterol; the quercetin group was fed the same diet with 2% cholesterol and quercetin 50 mg/kg BW/day, 100 mg/kg BW/day or 150 mg/kg BW/day. After 8 weeks of dietary treatment, the animals were euthanized by having their necks severed. Median thoracotomy was then performed, and the aorta was removed to obtain the rings for assessing endothelial function, MDA and c GMP content.

Preparations of solutions and measurement of muscle tension

The thoracic aorta was isolated from rabbits, cut into spiral strips (1-2 mm in width and 5-7 mm in length) and placed in normal physiological salt solution which contained (mM): NaCl 136.9, KCl 5.4, $CaCl_2$ 1.5, $MgCl_2$ 1.0, $NaHCO_3$ 23.8, ethylenediamine-tetraacetic acid 0.01 and glucose 5.5. A high K^+ solution was made by substituting 69.6 mM NaCl with equimolar KCl. These solutions were saturated with a mixture of 95% O_2 and 5 % CO_2 at 37°C and pH 7.4. Muscle tension was recorded isometrically with a force-displacement transducer. Each muscle strip was attached to a holder under a resting tension of 1 g and equilibrated for 60-90 min in a 10 ml muscle bath until the contractile response to the high K^+ solution had become stable.

The functional integrity of the vascular endothelium was assessed by measuring whether 1 μM Acetylcholine induced almost complete relaxation in aortas stimulated with 100 nM norepinephrine (Sudjarwo et al., 1992).

Measurement of TBARS levels in aorta

MDA levels measured by TBARS assay. The aortic samples were homogenized in cold TCA (1 mg of tissue per ml of 10% TCA). After centrifugation, a portion of the supernatant was added to an equal volume of thiobarbituric acid (0.6% v/v), and the mixture was heated at 100°C for 20 min. The MDA concentration was calculated by use of a spectrophotometer, with absorption of 532 nm and the results were expressed in n mol/mg of dry tissue.

Measurement of cyclic GMP

Aortic strips were incubated with krebs solution containing 100 nM norepinephrine for 5 min. Then the strips were incubated with concentration of 1 μM acetylcholine. After 20 s incubation, except where otherwise stated, the preparations were frozen quickly in liquid nitrogen. Aortic strips frozen in liquid nitrogen were transferred to 5% (W/V) trichloro acetic acid solution and homogenized in a Potter glass homogenizer on ice. The homogenates were centrifuged at 1700 × g for 15 min at 4°C. The supernatants were extracted 3 times with 3 volumes of water-saturated ether, and cyclic GMP contents were measured by ELISA kit from Cayman Chemical Co. (Ann Arbor, MI, U.S.A).

Statistics

Results were expressed as mean ± SEM. Statistical analysis was performed using one-way analysis of variance (ANOVA) followed by Dunnett's test, $p < 0.05$ was considered statistically significant.

RESULTS

Effect of quercetin on lipid peroxidation in aorta

The lipid peroxidation production was 0.12 ± 0.02; 0.67 ± 0.08; 0.71 ± 0.1; 0.41 ± 0.09, 0.26 ± 0.07 n mol/mg protein in negative control, positive control, treatment quercetin at dose 50, 100 and 150 mg/kg BW, respectively.

In the positive control (hypercholesterolemic) group, the level of TBARS was significantly increased compared to negative control group (p<0.05). Treatment with quercetin at dose 100 and 150 mg/kg BW but not at dose 50 mg/kg BW markedly reduced aorta TBARS in hypercholesterolemia which was significantly different from the positive control (p<0.05) (Figure 1).

Effect of quercetin on acetylcholine induced endothelium-dependent vasorelaxation

Table 1 shows the concentration response for the relaxant effect of acetylcholine in norepinephrine stimulated aorta. Endothelium-dependent relaxation evoked by acetylcholine was significantly impaired in aortic ring from the cholesterol-fed (positive control) group as compared to those in the negative control group (p<0.05). The aorta from hypercholesterolemic rabbits treated with quercetin at dose 100 and 150 mg/kg BW but not at dose 50 mg/kg BW showed marked improvement of the impaired endothelium-dependent relaxation which was significantly different from positive control group (p<0.05).

Effect of quercetin on acetylcholine induced c GMP increase

The cyclic GMP production was 29.4 ± 2.8, 16.7 ± 1.9, 17.4 ± 1.5, 21.5 ± 2.1 and 25.7 ± 1.6 f mol/μg in negative control, positive control, treatment quercetin at dose 50

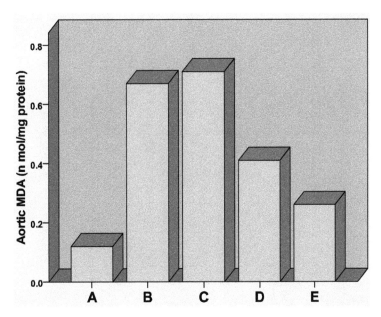

Figure 1. Bar graph showing plasma lipid peroxidation (Malondialdehyde) as determined by thiobarbituric reactive substances (TBARS). Negative control (A), Positive control (B), quercetin treatment at dose 50 mg/Kg BW (C), 100 mg/Kg BW (D) and quercetin treatment at dose 150 mg/Kg BW (E). Each point represents the mean of six experiments.

Table 1. Effect of quercetin on acetylcholine induced endothelium-dependent vasorelaxation.

Group	Vasorelaxation of acetylcholine (%)		
	10 nM	100 nM	1 μM
Negative control	18.9 ± 1.8	67.3 ± 4.4	84.1 ± 4.3
Positive control	4.1 ± 1.9	43.7 ± 3.1	57.6 ± 1.9
Quercetin 50 mg/kg BW	5.1 ± 1.2	45.1 ± 3.2	59.2 ± 4.1
Quercetin 200 mg/kg BW	7.3 ± 2.1	51.3 ± 3.7	64.3± 2.9
Quercetin 400 mg/kg BW	11.8 ± 2.2	59.4 ± 3.5	73.2 ± 4.1

Mean ± SEM, n = 6.

mg/kgBW, dose 100 mg/kg BW and dose 150 mg/kgBW, respectively.

In the positive control (hypercholesterolemic) group, the cyclic GMP production was significantly decreased compared to negative control group (p<0.05). The treatment with quercetin at dose 100 mg/kg BW and 150 mg/kgBW but not at dose 50 mg/kg BW markedly increase cyclic GMP production in hypercholesterolemia which was significantly different from the positive control (p<0.05) (Figure 2).

DISCUSSION

In the present study, we demonstrated that in the hypercholesterolemic, rabbit induced increase in lipid peroxidation. This was associated with the production of aortic TBARS. In the hypercholesterolemic, rabbit also induced decrease in cyclic GMP production and impaired endothelium-dependent relaxation. This is consistent with previous observations that in the hypercholesterolemic, rabbit and pig are associated with impairments of endothelium-dependent relaxation and is due, at least in part, to reduced production of EDRF and cyclic GMP by endothelial cells (Fujitani et al., 1993; Volker et al., 2004; Jiang et al., 2000). In addition, the blunted endothelium-dependent relaxation in hypercholesterolemic animals may also result from the destruction of EDRF by superoxide anion (Ohara et al., 1992; Inoue et al., 1998). The antioxidant such as beta carotene, alpha tocopherol and probucol have been reported to improve endothelium-dependent relaxation in hypercholesterolemic rabbits, suggesting that the free radical scavenging property of these antioxidants might

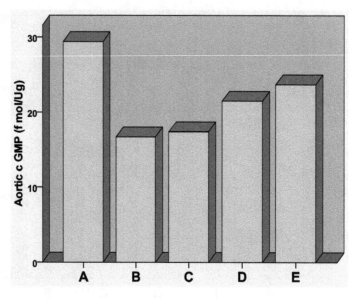

Figure 2. Effect of quercetin at dose 50 mg/kg BW, dose 100 mg/kgBW and 150 mg/kg BW on the increase in the cyclic GMP content in rabbits aortic strips after stimulation with 1 μM acetylcholine. Negative control (A), Positive control (B), quercetin treatment at dose 50 mg/kg BW (C), quercetin treatment at dose 100 mg/kg BW (D), and quercetin treatment at dose 150 mg/kg BW (E). Each columns represents the mean of six experiments and SEM, $p < 0.05$.

play an important role in the protective effect on endothelial dysfunction (Mahfouz et al.,1997; Marguerite et al., 2003). Recently, it has been reported that quercetin has potent antioxidant due to its ability to scavenge free radicals and bind transition metal ions. These properties of quercetin allow it to inhibit lipid peroxidation (Hollman and Katan, 1997; Sakanashi et al., 2008). Lipid peroxidation is the process by which unsaturated fatty acids are converted to free radicals via the abstraction of hydrogen (Young and McEneny, 2001). In our experiments, we also obtain several results indicating that this may be case: 1) in the hypercholesterolemic rabbits significantly inhibited acetylcholine induced endothelium-dependent relaxation, increase lipid peroxidation (malondialdehyde) and decrease cyclic GMP production, 2) the treatment with quercetin in hypercholesterolemic rabbits significantly reduced lipid peroxidation (malondialdehyde) production, augmented acetylcholine induced endothelium-dependent relaxation and increased cyclic GMP production. These results suggest that dietary treatment of rabbits with quercetin may prevent superoxide anion (O^{2-}), induced activation of EDRF, improve the endothelium-dependent relaxation to acetylcholine in the aortic blood vessels and increase cyclic GMP content in aortic of cholesterol-fed rabbits.

In conclusion, quercetin not only improves endothelium-dependent relaxations but also reduces lipid peroxidation (malondialdehyde) in the aorta and enhanced the tissue content cyclic GMP in hypercholesterolemic rabbits. These findings suggest that quercetin might play an important role in the protective effect on endothelial dysfunction in hypercholesterolemia.

REFERENCES

Fujitani Y, Ueda H, Okada T, Urade Y, Karaki H (1993). A selective agonist of endothelin type B receptors, IRL (1620). stimulates cyclic GMP increase via nitric oxide formation in rat aorta. J. Pharmacol. Exp. Ther., 267: 683-689.

Hollman PCH, Katan MB (1997). Absorption, metabolism and health effects of dietary flavonoids in man. Biomed. Pharmacother., 51: 305-310.

Inoue N, Ohara Y, Fukai T, Harrison DG,Nishida K (1998). Probucol improves endothelial-dependent relaxation and decreases vascular superoxide production in cholesterol-fed rabbits. Am. J. Med. Sci., pp. 242-247.

Jiang F, Gibson AP, Dusting GJ (2001). Endothelial dysfunction induced by oxidized low-density lipoproteins in isolated mouse aorta: a comparison with apolipoprotein-E deficient mice. Eur. J. Pharmacol., 424: 141-149.

Jiang JH, Valen G, Tokuno S, Thoren P, Pernow J (2000). Endothelial dysfunction in atherosclerotic mice: improved relaxation by combined supplementation with L-arginine-tetrahydrobiopterin and enhanced vasoconstriction by endothelin. Br. J. Pharmacol., 131: 1255-1261.

Karaki H, Sudjarwo SA, Hori M, Takai M, Urade Y, Okada T (1993). Induction of endothelium dependent relaxation in the rat aorta by IRL 1620, a novel and selective agonist at the endothelin ETB receptor. Br. J. Pharmacol., 109: 371-374.

Mahfouz MM, Kawano H, Kummerow FA (1997). Effect of cholesterol rich diets with and without added vitamin E and C on the severity of the atherosclerosis in rabbits. Am. J. Clin. Nutr., 6:1240-1249.

Marguerite ME, Mary BE, Mary J, Malloy MD, Elisa YC, Monique CS Steven MP, Markus S, Ken YL, John PC, Jason DM, Paul MR Nader R, Elizabeth M, Joseph LW, Michele MS (2003). Antioxidant vitamin C and E improve endothelial function in children with hyperlipidemia. Circulation, 108: 1059-1063.

Murota KJ, Terao (2003). Antioxidative flavonoid quercetin: implications of its intenstinal absorption and metabolism. Archiv. Biochem. Biophy., 417: 12-17.

Ohara Y, Peterson TH, Harrison DG (1992). Hypercholesterolemia increases superoxide anion production by the endothelium. Circulation. 86: 1-222.

Rui-Li Y, Yong H, Gang H, Wu Li, Guo-Wei L (2008). Increasing Oxidative Stress with Progressive Hyperlipidemia in Human: Relation between Malondialdehyde and Atherogenic Index. J. Clin. Biochem. Nutr., 43(3): 154–158.

Sakanashi Y (2008). Possible use of quercetin, an antioxidant, for protection of cells suffering from overload of intracellular Ca^{2+}: A model experiment. Life Sci. 83: 164-169.

Sausbier M, Schubert R, Voigt V, Hirneiss C, Pfeifer A, Korth M, Kleppisch T, Ruth P, Hofmann F (2000). Mechanisms of NO/cGMP-dependent vasorelaxation. Circ. Res., 87: 825-830.

Shimokawa H (1999). Primary endothelial dysfunction: atherosclerosis. J. Mol. Cell. Cardiol. 31: 23-37.

Stephanie ED, Cor de W (2005). Intact Endothelium-Dependent Dilation and Conducted Responses in Resistance Vessels of Hypercholesterolemic Mice in vivo. J. Vasc. Res., 42: 475-482.

Sudjarwo SA, Hori M, Karaki H (1992). Effect of endothelin-3 on cytosolic calcium level in vascular endothelium and on smooth muscle contraction. Eur. J. Pharmacol., 229: 137-142.

Siekmeier R, Steffen C, Marz W (2007). Role of Oxidants and Antioxidants in Atherosclerosis: Results of In Vitro and In Vivo Investigations. J. Cardiovasc. Pharmacol. Ther., 12(4): 265 - 282.

Valko M (2007). Free radicals and antioxidants in normal physiological functions and human disease. Int. J. Biochem. Cell Biol. 39: 44–84.

Verbeuren JJ, Van Hove VE, Herman AG (1990). Release and vascular activity of endothelium-derived relaxing factor in atherosclerotic rabbit aorta. Eur. J. Pharmac., 191: 173-184.

Volker OM, Delphine BR, Ulrike Z, Uttenthal LO, Jose R, Alain R, Tony JV, Arun Kumar HS, Harald HHWS (2004). Reduced c GMP signaling associated with neointimal proliferation and vascular dysfunction in late-stage atherosclerosis. PNAS, 101(47): 16671-16676.

Young IS, McEneny J (2001). Lipoprotein oxidation and atherosclerosis. Biochem. Soc. Trans., 29: 358-362.

25

Antioxidant activity of n-butanol extract of celery (*Apium graveolens*) seed in streptozotocin-induced diabetic male rats

Jabbar A. A. Al-Sa'aidi[1], Mohsen N. A. Alrodhan[2] and Ahmed K. Ismael[1]

[1]Physiology and Pharmacology Department, College of Veterinary Medicine, Al-Qadisiya University, Iraq.
[2]Deptartment of Internal and Preventive Medicine, College of Veterinary Medicine, Al-Qadisiya University, Iraq.

The potent of n-butanol extract of celery (*Apium graveolens*) seed in ameliorating the lipid peroxidation and antioxidant status were investigated in streptozotocin-induced diabetic rats. Thirty two mature male rats were assigned to four groups, non-diabetic control and three diabetic groups. Diabetes was induced by single injection with streptozotocin (60 mg/kg b.w., *i.p.*). Rats ≥ 200 mg/dl of blood glucose were used as diabetic. Diabetic groups (D, B, and I) were drenched with drinking water, n-butanol extract (60 mg/kg, b.w.), or injected with insulin (4 IU/animal), respectively for 21 days. On day 22, body weight gain was registered and male rats were sacrificed. Blood and liver subcellular fluid was obtained to assess blood glucose level and subcellular activity of Alanine aminotranferease (ALT), Aspartate aminotransferase (AST), catalase, Super oxide dismutase (SOD), Glutathione (GSH)-transferase and -reductase, and assessment of Malondialdehyde (MDA) and glutathione concentrations. Diabetic rats (D) showed marked increased blood glucose, decreased weight gain, increased activity of ALT, SOD, CAT, GSH-transferase, decreased GSH-reductase and normal AST. N-butanol extract of celery seed (B) or insulin (I) therapy moderated blood glucose within normal range, enhanced body weight gain and normalized the activities of all antioxidant enzymes. In conclusion, n-butanol extract of celery seed have potent role in ameliorating stressful complications accompanied by diabetes mellitus.

Key words: Celery, *Apium graveolens*, diabetes mellitus, antioxidants.

INTRODUCTION

Diabetes mellitus is the most important disease involving the endocrine pancreas. Its major manifestations include disordered metabolism and inappropriate hyperglycemia. Recent studies illustrated that uncontrolled hyperglycemia in rats was associated with oxidative stress (Koo et al., 2002, 2003). During diabetes, persistent hyperglycemia increases the production of reducing oxygen species (ROS) through glucose autoxidation (Hunt et al., 1990; Wolff et al., 1991). It is well known that in diabetes, oxidative stress has been found to be mainly due to an increased production of oxygen free radicals and a sharp reduction of antioxidant defense system. In addition, there is a relationship between diabetes and

between diabetes and impairment of lipid metabolism (Sharpe et al., 1998).

Although almost all organisms possess antioxidant defense and repair systems to protect them from oxidative damage, in some cases, these systems are insufficient to entirely prevent such damage. Currently, there is a trend towards replacement of the widely used synthetic antioxidants with antioxidants from natural sources to extend the shelf life of foods and to improve health conditions.

Flavonoids have attracted the interest of researchers because they show promise of being powerful antioxidants that can protect the body from free radicals and against oxidative stress (Bors et al., 1996). Flavonoids cannot be produced by the human body and are taken in through the daily diet. The evidence reported that flavornoids play a vital biological role, including the function of scavenging reactive oxygen species (Pietta and Simonetti, 1998). On the other hand, it has been shown

---

*Corresponding author. E-mail:jbr20042002@yahoo.com.

that phenolics from edible fruits and vegetables are also effective antioxidants (Karadeniz et al., 2005). The antioxidative properties of phenolics arose from their high reactivity as hydrogen or electron donors and from the ability of polyphenol-derived radicals to stabilize and delocalize the unpaired electron or from their ability to chelate transition metal ions (Rice-Evans et al., 1997). Hence, there is a strong interest to search for potential antioxidant agents derived from natural products.

A number of plants have shown a free radical scavenging activity in experimental animals, and one of it is the celery. Celery fruit (seed) extracts are extensively used as flavoring ingredients in many food products, including meat products, soups, frozen dairy desserts, candies, baked goods, gelatins, puddings, condiments and relishes, snack foods, alcoholic and non-alcoholic beverages and others (Momin and Nair, 2001). In the present study, we shall assess the activity of n-butanol extract of celery seed as antioxidant agent.

MATERIALS AND METHODS

Experimental animals

Mature male Sprague-Dawley rats have been used in the experiment. Male rats were allowed one week to acclimatize to the animal house environment before beginning of experiment. Animals were fed on the standard chow and drinking water *ad libitum* throughout the experiment. Room temperature was maintained at 22 ± 2°C, the light-dark cycle was on a 12:12 h with light on at 06:00 a.m and off at 06:00 p.m throughout the experimental period.

Preparation of n-butanol extract

Celery (*A. graveolens*) seed was purchased from the local market and classified by State Board for Seed Testing and Classification, Agriculture Ministry, Iraq (SBSTC). N-butanol extract of celery seed has been prepared from methanolic extract according to Harborne (1984) using Soxhlet apparatus. Using 1 kg of celery seed, methanolic extract was prepared, rotavaporated (40°C and 50 to 60 rpm), and lyophilized by dry freezer. Dried extract was weighted and stored in deep freeze. According to the polarity, three types of solvents have been used to separate different fractions of the crude extract; ethyl acetate, n-butanol, and distilled water, using a separating funnel in order to obtain the high, middle, and low polar fractions of the seed. N-butanol fraction of the celery seed has been evaporated, lyophilized, and kept at -4°C until use (Tsi and Benny, 1999).

Induction of diabetes in rats

Twenty four adult Sprague-Dawley rats weighting 240 to 251 g (56 days old) were used for inducing diabetes. Streptozotocin (STZ) was used to create animal models of type I diabetes (Mansford and Opie, 1968). The animals were injected by STZ (60 mg/kg b.w., i.p.) dissolved in 1 M of sodium citrate buffer (pH 4.5) STZ induces DM within 3 to 5 days by destroying the beta cells of Langerhans islets in the pancreas. The rats with plasma glucose ≥ 200 mg/dL were considered as diabetic rats and used for experiment (Cakatay and Kayali, 2006).

Experimental design

Eight non-diabetic and twenty four STZ-induced diabetic male rats were randomly assigned to 4 equal groups treated for three weeks as follows: non-diabetic control (C): daily drenched with 1 ml of drinking water and injected with 0.1 ml of normal saline; diabetic-control (D): daily drenched with 1 ml of drinking water and injected with 0.1 ml of normal saline; n-butanol treated (B): daily drenched with drinking water contains (60 mg/kg b.w) of n-butanol extract of celery seed and injected with 0.1 ml of normal saline and; insulin treated (I): daily drenched with drinking water and injected with single dose of insulin (4 IU/rat). Twenty four hours after the last treatment, rats were anaesthetized with pentobarbital (35 mg/kg b.w. ip), sacrificed, and liver subcellular fluid were obtained for evaluation of ALT, AST, GSH, SOD, Catalase, GSH-transferase and GSH-reductase.

Preparation of subcellular fluid

Liver tissues were perfused with distilled water until a pink color appeared. Tissues were homogenized by about 20 up and down strokes in a ground-glass tissue grinder. Sucrose (0.88 M) was used for homogenization, washing and re-suspension of the particulate fractions. Using cooled ultracentrifuge, homogenates were fractionated for obtaining subcellular fluid (Ayako and Fridovich, 2002).

Assessment of subcellular ALT and AST enzymes activity

Assessment has been performed by using the colorimetric method of Reitman and Frankel (1957).

Assessment of total GSH

The absorbance of the reduced chromagen was measured at 412 nm and was directly proportional to the GSH concentration (Burtis and Ashwood, 1999).

Assessment of superoxide dismutase (SOD) activity in liver subcellular fluid

By using the modified photochemical Nitroblue tetrazolium (NBT) method in utilizing sodium cyanide as peroxidase inhibitor, SOD levels were assessed (Winterbourn et al., 1975).

Determination of catalase (CAT) activity in liver subcellular fluid

According to Aebi (1974) and Kakkar et al. (1984), CAT activity was assessed by measuring the degradation rate of H_2O_2. The rate of disappearance of H_2O_2 was monitored spectrophotometrically at 230 nm.

Estimation of lipid peroxidation

The level of peroxidation product; Malondialdehyde (MDA) was measured according to Dillard and Kunnert (1982).

Glutathione reductase activity

This was measured by the method of Carlberg and Mannervik

(1975).

Glutathione-transferase activity

This was measured by the method of Habig et al. (1974). Protein was estimated by the method of Lowry et al. (1951).

Statistical analysis

All the values are expressed as mean ± SD. Data of the experiment were analyzed using one way analysis of variance (ANOVA 1), using F-test (Shiefler, 1980). Least significant difference (LSD) was carried out to estimate the significance of difference between individual groups. P value less than 0.05 was considered significant.

RESULTS

Body weight gain

The body weight of the rats at beginning of the study was similar in all groups. At the end of the treatment (after 21 days), all rats gained weight (Figure 1) but non-treated diabetic rats had a significantly ($p < 0.05$) lesser weight gain (20.5 ± 1.56 g) when compared with the rats in other three groups (control: 119.2 ± 4.63 g; B: 88.7 ± 3.55 g; and I: 92.9 ± 3.84 g).

Blood glucose

The blood glucose level of D group was significantly higher ($p < 0.05$) at the end of the experiment as compared with other groups (Figure 2). No significant differences were observed between B and I groups but control rats recorded the significant lesser level among the experimental groups.

Sub-cellular ALT and AST concentrations

As illustrated in Table 1, diabetic animals showed significant increased ($p < 0.05$) subcellular ALT concentration and normalized subcellular AST concentration in liver tissues, while n-butanol fraction of celery seed extract and insulin therapy normalized the two enzymes.

Sub-cellular anti-oxidant activity

Diabetic animals showed marked increased ($p < 0.05$) of MDA and GSH concentrations, and SOD CAT and GSH-transferase activity, and decreased ($p < 0.05$) GSH-reductase activity. N-butanol extract of celery seed and insulin therapy normalized the activities of all antioxidant enzymes (Table 2).

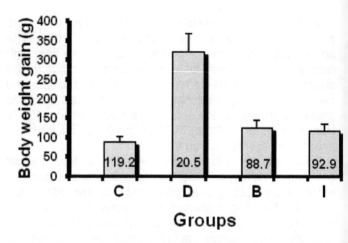

Figure 1. Effect of n-butanol extract of celery seed (*Apium graveolens*) on body weight gain (g) in STZ- induced diabetic mature male rats. C: non-diabetic control, D: diabetic control, B: diabetic treated with n-butanol extract, I: diabetic treated with insulin.

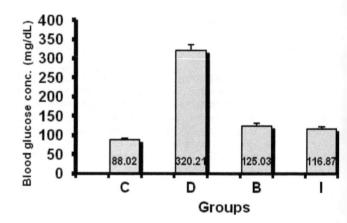

Figure 2. Role of n-butanol extract of celery seed (*Apium graveolens*) on blood glucose concentration in STZ- induced diabetic mature male rats. C: non-diabetic control, D: diabetic control, B: diabetic treated with n-butanol extract, I: diabetic treated with insulin.

DISCUSSION

The present experiment aimed to evaluate the antioxidant activity of n-butanol extract of celery (*A. graveolens*) seed in STZ-induced mature male rats. Since the finding that STZ possesses diabetogenic properties material by pancreatic beta cell destruction, this compound has been widely used to induce diabetes (Junod et al., 1969) and oxidative stress (Wright et al., 1999) in experimental animals. Recent studies evidenced that celery seed extract act as hypolipidemic and antioxidant as it has a scavenger to the free radicals (Cheng et al., 2008). Our results also registered hypoglycaemic effect of n-B extract of celery seed which may be attributed to the strong antioxidant of the phenolic compound in celery

Table 1. Effect of n-butanol extract of celery seed on subcellular concentration of ALT and AST in STZ-induced diabetic mature male rats.

Parameter	Group			
	C	D	B	I
ALT concentration (IU/L)	25.30±3.92[C]	40.62±4.77[A]	31.35±5.52[B]	25.61±4.34[C]
AST concentration (IU/L)	41.44±4.92[A]	41.55±5.38[A]	43.41±13.94[A]	18.93±5.04[B]

Numbers represent mean ± SD. Superscript letters represent the presence of significances between groups ($p < 0.05$). C: non-diabetic control, D: diabetic control, B: diabetic treated with n-butanol extract, I: diabetic treated with insulin.

Table 2. Effect of n-butanol extract of celery (*A. graveolens*) seed on serum antioxidants concentrations in STZ-induced diabetic mature male rats.

Parameter	Group			
	C	D	B	I
GSH concentration (nmol/mg protein)	842.2±90.500[A]	740.3±20.960[B]	847.6±70.330[A]	839.9±40.750[A]
SOD activity (U/L)	4.743±0.205[B]	6.003±0.313[A]	4.673±0.398[B]	5.968±0.425[A]
CAT activity (U/L)	0.039±0.002[B]	0.107±0.008[A]	0.052±0.006[B]	0.060±0.009[B]
MDA concentration (nmol/g tissue)	6.331±0.506[C]	55.898±6.001[A]	14.376±1.722[B]	18.187±1.709[B]
GSH-transferase activity (Unit/mg protein per min)	0.498±0.091[B]	0.776±0.098[A]	0.521±0.073[B]	0.593±0.088[A]
GSH-reductase activity (μmol of NADPH/mg protein)	49.328±3.779[A]	41.539±3.281[B]	43.632±4.718[B]	45.387±4.899[B]

Numbers represent mean ± SD. Superscript letters represent the presence of significances between groups ($p < 0.05$). C: non-diabetic control, D: diabetic control, B: diabetic treated with n-butanol extract, I: diabetic treated with insulin.

seed (Singh and Handa, 1995) or it can be suggested that the presence of alkaloids and flavonoids in high concentration in n-B extract of celery seed (Middeton et al., 2000) may be responsible for the oral hypoglycaemic effect registered in the present study.

It has been suggested that the lipid peroxidation may be a link between tissue injury and liver fibrosis by modulatory collagen gene expression (Parola et al., 1993). Our results show increased lipid peroxidation in non-treated diabetic group. The increase in oxygen free radicals in diabetes could be due to hyperglycemia, which upon auto-

oxidation generate free radicals. STZ has been shown to produce oxygen free radicals (Ivorra et al., 1989). Lipid peroxide mediated tissue damages have been observed in the development of type I and type 2 diabetes mellitus (Feillet-Coudary et al., 1999). Previous studies have reported that there was an increased lipid peroxidation in liver and kidney of diabetic rats (Pari and Latha, 2002; VenKateswaran and Pari, 2002).

STZ-treated rats registered increased liver subcellular concentration of ALT, whereas n-butanol and insulin-treated rats showed decreased concentrations of this enzymes. On the other

hand, the present study revealed that the n-BF of celery seed extract at the given dose has no harmful effect on liver function in normal rats. On the other hand, Tsi and Benny (1999) found that aqueous extract of celery did not produce any undesirable side effects such as weight loss or liver dysfunction as demonstrated by similar levels of subcellular ALT and AST in both the control and treated rats.

The antioxidant defense system, both enzymatic (SOD, CAT, GSH-transferase and GSH-reductase) and non enzymatic (GSH), has been studied here. The increased subcellular GSH content in liver of rats treated with n-BF and insulin may be one factor responsible for inhibition of lipid peroxidation. GSH, a major non protein thiol, involving many aspects of cellular metabolism and regulation, plays a crucial role in the cellular antioxidant defense system by scavenging free radicals and other reactive oxygen species (Wu et al., 2004). Under *in vivo* conditions, GSH acts as an antioxidant and its decrease was reported in diabetes mellitus (Baynes and Thorpe, 1999). We have observed significant decrease in GSH levels in liver during diabetes (D group). The decrease in GSH levels represent increased utilization due to oxidative stress (Anuradha and Selvam, 1993). The depletion of GSH content of liver may lower the antioxidant activity, as GSH is required as a substrate for this activity (Rathore et al., 2000).

Our results evidenced a parallel increase in both lipid peroxidation as determined by MDA concentration and antioxidant defense system represented by SOD, CAT and GSH-transferase in STZ-induced diabetic rats in response to oxidative stress. These results were reversed with n-BF and insulin treatment to a level comparable to that recorded with control rats. SOD and CAT are the two major scavenging enzymes that remove toxic free radicals. Previous studies have reported that the activity of SOD is low in diabetes mellitus (Vucic et al., 1997). Administration of n-BF increased the activity of these enzymes and may help to control free radical, as n-BF has been reported to be rich in flavonoids, a well known antioxidant (Middleton et al., 2000) which scavenges the free radical generated during diabetes.

CAT is a haem containing ubiquities enzyme, detoxify the hydrogen peroxide into water and oxygen. The elevated level of CAT in diabetic non-treated male rats was reduced and it was improved by the n-BF of celery seed treatment. However, improvement of SOD and CAT activities in the n-BF treatment rats could be due to the restoration of GSH. The result of antioxidant enzymes activity led to suggestions that n-BF of celery seed extract contains free radical scavenging activity which could exert a beneficial action against pathological alteration caused by the presence of free radicals. This action could involve mechanisms related to scavenging activity.

Some studies pointed to the relationship between the elevated xanthin oxidase (XOD) activity and production of oxygen radicals in diabetes (Swei et al., 1998; Desco et al., 2002). XOD inhibitor is known in clinical practice to reduce oxidative stress in diabetes. Thus, it can be said that active constituents of the n-BF of celery seed interact with the peroxy species Cl_3OO, thus reducing the activities of XOD, SOD and CAT enzymes. Our results demonstrated that n-BF of celery seed showed protective effect, probably to the presence of flavonoids. A hepatoprotective effect of celery has been observed in rats treated with paracetamol and thioacetamide (Singh and Handa, 1995). Flavonoids can act in the initiation stage of peroxidation interfering with the metabolism of oxidative agent either by scavenging the free radicals or by impairing the microsomal enzymatic system needed for this metabolism.

REFERENCES

Aebi H (1974). Catalase. In: Bergmeyer HU (ed.), Methods of Enzymatic Analysis. Verlag Chemie, Weinheim. pp. 673–8.

Anuradha CV, Selvam R (1993). Effect of oral methione on tissue lipid peroxidation and antioxidants in alloxan induced diabetes rats. J. Nutr. Biochem. 4:212-217.

Ayako OM, Fridovich I (2002). Subcellular distribution of superoxide dismutases (SOD) in rat liver. J. Biol. Chem. 276:38388-38393.

Baynes JW, Thorpe SR. (1999). Role of oxidative stress in diabetic complications. Diabetes 48:1-9.

Bors W, Heller W, Michel C, Stettmaier K (1996). Flavonoids and polyphenols: chemistry and biology. In: Cadenas E, Packer L (eds.), Handbook of Antioxidants. Dekker, New York. p 409.

Burtis C, Ashwood ER (1999). Tietz Fundamentals of Clinical Biochemistry, 4th Edition. WB Saunders Company. Chapter 22, p 414.

Cakatay U, Kayali R (2006). The evaluation of altered redox status in plasma and mitochondria of acute and chronic diabetic rats. Clin. Biochem. 39:907-12.

Carlberg I, Mannervik B (1975). Purification and characterization of the flavoenzyme glutathione reductase from rat liver. Biol. Chem. 250:5475-5480.

Cheng M C, Lin I Y,Tung H, Peng R (2008). Hypolipidemic and antioxidant activity of Mountain Celery essential oil. J. Agric. Food Chem. 56(11):3997-4003.

Desco MC, Asensi M, Marquez R, *Martinez*-Valls J (2002). Xanthine oxidase is involved in free radical production in type 1 diabetes: protection by allopurinol. Diabetes 51:1118–1124.

Dillard CJ, Kunnert KJ (1982). Effects of vitamin E, ascorbic acid and mannitol on alloxan induced lipid peroxidation in rats. Arch. Biochem. Biophys. 216(1):204-12.

Feillet-Coudray C, Rock E, Coudray C, Grzelkowska K, Azais-Braesco V, Dardevet D, Mazur A (1999). Lipid peroxidation and antioxidant status in experimental diabetes. Clin. Chem. Acta. 284:31-43.

Habig WH, Pabst MJ, Jakoby WB (1974). Glutathione-5-transferase, the first enzymatic step in mercapturic acid formation. J. Biol. Chem. 249:7130-7139.

Harborne JB (1984). Phytochemical Methods: A Guide to Modern Techniques of plant Analysis. Chapman and Hall, London, UK. pp. 1-34.

Hunt JV, Smith CC, Wolff SP (1990). Autoxidative glycosylation and possible involvement of peroxides and free radicals in LDL modification by glucose. Diabetes 39:1420-1424.

Ivorra MD, Paya M, Villar A (1989). A review of natural products and plants as potential antidiabetic drugs. J. Ethnopharmacol. 27:243-275.

Junod A, Lambert AE, Stauffacher W, Renold AE (1969). Diabetogenic action of streptozotocin: Relationship of dose to metabolic response. J. Clin. Investig. 48(11):2129–2139.

Kakkar P, Das B, Viswanathan PN (1984). A modified spectrophotometric assay of superoxide dismutase. Indian J. Biochem. Biophys. 21(2):130–132.

Karadeniz F, Burdurlu HS, Koca N, Soyer Y (2005). Antioxidant activity of selected fruits and vegetables grown in Turkey. Turk. J. Agric. 29:297-303.

Koo JR, Ni Z, Oviesi F, Vaziri ND (2002). Antioxidant therapy potentiates antihypertensive action of insulin in diabetic rats. Clin. Exp. Hypertens. 24:333–344.

Koo JR, Vaziri ND (2003). Effects of diabetes, insulin and antioxidants on NO synthase abundance and NO interaction with reactive oxygen species. Kidney Int. 63:195–201.

Lowry OH, Rosebrough NJ, Fair AL, Randall RJ (1951). Protein measurement with the folin phenol reagent. Biol. Chem. 193:265-275.

Mansford KR, Opie L (1968). Comparison of metabolic abnormalities in diabetes mellitus induced by streptozotocin or by alloxan. Lancet 1:670–671.

Middleton E, Kandaswami C, Theoharides TC (2000). The effects of plant flavonoids on mammalian cells: implications for inflammation, heart disease and cancer. Pharmacol. Rev. 52: 673–751.

Momin R, Nair MG (2001). Mosquitocidal, nematicidal and antifungal compounds from *Apium graveolens* L. seeds. J. Agric. Food Chem. 49:142–145.

Pari L, Latha M (2002). Effect of *Cassia auriculata* flowers on blood sugar levels, serum and tissue lipids in streptozotocin diabetic rats. Singapore Med. J. 43: 617-621.

Parola M, Pinzani M, Casini A, Albano E, Poli G, Gentilini A, Gentilini P, Dianzani MU (1993). Stimulation of lipid peroxidation or 4-hydroxynonenal treatment increases procollagen α1(I) gene expression in human liver fat-storing cells. Biochem Biophys. Res. Commun. 194:1044–1050.

Pietta PG, Simonetti P (1998). Dietary flavonoids and interaction with endogenous antioxidant. IUBMB Life 44:1069–1074.

Rathore N, Kale M, John S, Bhatnagar D (2000). Lipid peroxidation and antioxidant enzymes in isoproterenol induced oxidative stress in rat erythrocytes. Indian J. Physiol. Pharmacol. 44:161-166.

Reitman S, Frankel SA (1957). Colorimetric method for the determination of serum glutamic oxalacetic and glutamic pyruvic transaminases. Am. J. Clin. Pathol. 28(1):56-63.

Rice-Evans C, Miller NJ, Paganga G (1997). Antioxidant properties of phenolic compounds. Trends Plant Sci. 2:152-159.

Sharpe P, Liu W, Ytiek I (1998). Glucose induces oxidative damage in vascular contractile cells. Comparison of aortic smooth muscle cells and retinal pericytes. Diabetes 47:801-809.

Shiefler W.C (1980). Statistics for biological science, 2nd edition. Addison, Wesley, Pub. Co., London. 121 p.

Singh A, Handa SS (1995). Hepatoprotective activity of *Apium graveolens* and *Hygrophila auriculata* against paracetamol and thioacetamide intoxication in rats. Ethanopharmacol. 49(3):119-126.

Swei A, Suzuki H, Parks DA, Delano FA, Schmid-Schonbein GW (1998). Mechanism of oxygen free radical formation in experimental forms of hypertension. INABIS 1:837.

Tsi D, Benny KH (1999). The mechanism underlying the hypocholesterolemic activity of aqueous celery extract, its butanol and aqueous fraction in genetically hypercholesterolemic RICO rats.

Venkateswaran S, Pari L (2002). Antioxidant effect of *Phaseolus vulgaris* in STZ induced diabetic rats. Asia Pac. J. Clin. Nutr. 11:206-209.

Vucic M, Gavella M, Bozikov V, Ashcroft SJ, Rocic B (1997). Super-oxide Dismutase activity in Lymphocytes and polymorphonuclear cells of Diabetic patients. Eur. J. Clin. Chem. BioChem. 35:517-521.

Winterbourn CC, Hawking RE, Brain M, Carrel RW (1975). Deter-mination of Superoxide Dismutase. J. Lab. Clin. Med. 2:337-341.

Wolff SP, Jiang ZY, Hunt JV (1991). Protein glycation and oxidative stress in diabetes mellitus and ageing. Free Radic. Biol. Med. 10:339-352.

Wright JR, Abraham C, Dickson BC, Yang H, Morrison CM (1999). Streptozotocin dose-response curve in tilapia, a glucose–responsive teleost fish. Gen. Comp. Endocrinol. 114:431-440.

Wu X, Beecher GR, Holden JM, Haytowitz DB, Gebhardt SE, Prior RL (2004). Hydrophilic antioxidant capacities of common foods in the United States J. Agric. Food Chem. 52(12):4026–37.

26

Histopathological examination of formulated drugs against typhoid

S. S. Haque*, A. Sharan and U. Kumar

Department of Clinical Biochemistry, Indira Gandhi Institute of Medical Sciences Patna-14, India.

Typhoid fever (TF) is a systemic bacterial infection caused by *Salmonella typhi*, a facultative and gram negative rods. The infection is usually acquired through the ingestion of contaminated water or food. Almost 80% of cases and deaths occur in Asia. The attack rate as high as 1100 cases per 100000 populations have been documented in developing countries. In typhoid fever, various organs can be involved leading to a wide range of presentation, from uncomplicated to a complicated one involving multiple organs. Histopathological derangements are common in typhoid fever, whereas, hepatic dysfunction has been reported variably from less than 1% to as high as 26%. Nitric oxide (NO•) is synthesized in endothelial cells, from the terminal guanidine nitrogen atom of L-Arginine by means of NO-synthase (NOS). NO• may regulate hepatic metabolism directly by causing alterations in hepatocellular metabolism and function, or indirectly as a result of its vasodilator properties. In this study we evaluated the liver tissues by carrying out a histological examination. We found that extensive tissue with cords of hepatocytes consisting of neutrophils and macrophages, had granulomatous lesions and mild necrosis before and after treatment with the formulated drugs that is L-arginine and ciprofloxacin.

Key words: Histopathology of liver tissue, typhoid, nitric oxide.

INTRODUCTION

Typhoid fever is an important health concern in developing countries (including those in Central and South America, Asia, Indian Subcontinent, Africa and the Caribbean), where hand washing and other such hygienic practices may be less frequent, and where water may be contaminated with sewage. Thus, travelers to these countries are most at risk. In addition, carriers or those who have recovered from typhoid fever may still shed the bacteria. For developed countries such as the United States, the chances of *S. typhi* transmission are very low because of high hygienic standards. *S. typhi* targets intestinal epithelial cells (enterocytes), causing the inflammation of other cells in the intestinal Payer's patches and subsequently the mesenteric lymph nodes, spleen and bone marrow associated with typhoid fever (Ohl et al., 2001). The mechanism by which *S. typhi* attaches to host cell is common among bacteria, which utilizes long, hair-like filaments known as fimbriae that are coated with receptor specific adhesins that recognize and bind to specific types of sites on the surface of target cells (Baulmer et al., 1996). Until 1980s, chloramphenicol was the undisputed first-line drug for the treatment of typhoid. Since 1970, multiple resistant *Salmonella* have caused extensive outbreaks in many developing countries. Third generation cephalosporin and fluoroquinoles have been found effective in treatment of these cases (Manchanda et al., 2006). However, isolates of *S. typhi* with reduced susceptibility to flouroquinoles (as indicated in the laboratory by resistance to nalidixic acid) have now appeared in the Indian subcontinent and other regions. These nalidixic acid resistant but ciprofloxacin sensitive strains have increased MIC (minimum inhibitory concentration) for ciprofloxacin although they are still within the current NCLLS (National Committee for Clinical Laboratory Standards) range for susceptibility (0.125 to 0.5 mg/ml) (Rowe et al., 1995; Brown et al., 1996; Jesudason et al., 1996; Chitnis et al., 1999; Kapil et al., 2002).

Nitric oxide is a highly reactive gas that participates in many biochemical reactions. During the last few years

*Corresponding author. E-mail: sshaq2002@yahoo.co.in.

Table 1. Treatments schedule.

Groups	Treatments
1	Negative control (normal saline)
2	Positive control (S. typhimurium(0.6 x LD$_{50}$)+ saline
3	S. typhimurium (0.6 × LD$_{50}$) + Ciprofloxacin (400 mg per kg b. wt)
4	S. typhimurium (0.6 × LD$_{50}$) + Arginine (1000 mg per Kg b.wt)
5	S. typhimurium (0.6 × LD$_{50}$)+Arginine (500 mg per kg b. wt) + Ciprofloxacin (200 mg per kg b. wt)
6	S. typhimurium (0.6 × LD$_{50}$) + Arginine (250 mg per kg b. wt) + ciprofloxacin (200 mg per kg b. wt)

the role of NO in health and diseases has been further understood (Nathan, 1997; Fang, 1997). The role of NO in biological system was first reported by Gruetter et al. (1979), he bathed the isolated pre-contracted strips of coronary artery in Krebs' bicarbonate buffer bubbled with NO gas and marked relaxation response in pre-contracted strips of coronary artery was observed. NO is synthesized within cells by an enzyme NO synthase (NOS). NOS produce NO from arginine with the aid of molecular oxygen and NADPH. NO diffuses freely across cell membranes. Since there are so many other molecules, with which it can interact, it is quickly consumed close to where it is synthesized. Key discoveries in 1987 included reports that arginine is the precursor for mammalian nitrite/nitrate synthesis (Hibbs et al., 1987a) and that NO is an endothelium derived relaxing factor (Palmer et al., 1987; Ignarro et al., 1987b). Ciprofloxacin, ofloxacin, perfloxacin and fleroxacin are common fluoroquinolones proved to be effective against typhoid. In children, the first two are only used in our country and there is no evidence of superiority of any particular fluroquinolones. Many studies have suggested that patients in Indian subcontinent or with the history of travel to the Indian subcontinent should receive ciprofloxacin as first line therapy (Rowe et al., 1995; Gulati et al., 1992). Physiological arginine concentrations may be limiting for cellular NO synthesis as plasma concentrations of arginine are typically found in the range of 80 to 110 μM. It has been reported that NO plays a protective role in the liver in septic and inflammatory conditions (Harbrecht et al., 1992, 1994).

The aim of this work was to evaluate histopathogical results to establish the therapeutic effect of L-arginine and ciprofloxacin against typhoid.

MATERIALS AND METHODS

Dose and dosage

Animals

Swiss albino mice (25 to 30 g), 6 to 8 weeks old were obtained from the central animal house of Hamdard University, New Delhi, India. The animals were kept in Poly-propylene cages in an air-conditioned room at 22/25°C and maintained on a standard laboratory feed (Amrut Laboratory, rat and mice feed,

Navmaharashtra Chakan Oil Mills Ltd, Pune) and water *ad libitum*. Animals were allowed to acclimatize for one week before the experiments under controlled light/dark cycle (14/10 h). The studies were conducted according to ethical guidelines of the "Committee for the purpose of control and supervision of experiments on animals (CPCSEA)" on the use of animals for scientific research.

Bacteria

In this experiment only, *Salmonella typhimurium* (wild) was used. The standard strain of this pathogen was obtained from the National Salmonella Phage Typing Centre, Lady Harding Medical College, New Delhi, India. This bacterial strain was further confirmed by the Department of Microbiology, Majeedia Hospital, New Delhi, India. The drug was administered orally and *S. typhimurium* intraperitoneally. Animals were divided into six groups. Each group comprised of six animals. The treatments followed the schedule indicated in Table 1.

Histopathological studies

Animals were sacrificed by cervical dislocation. The liver tissues were immediately removed and fixed for the histopathological studies. The steps involved were as follows:

Fixation and processing

The tissues were fixed immediately after dissection in 10% phosphate buffered formaldehyde solution, pH of 7. The tissues were cut into 2 to 4 mm thick sections to ensure that the fixative readily penetrated throughout the tissues. Processing involved dehydration and clearing of tissues as well as their infiltration with paraffin. The tissue block was passed through the series of steps as per the processing schedule, allowing 1 h at each stage. They were dehydrated through graded solutions of alcohol ending in two changes of absolute alcohol for 2 h each. They were cleared 2 changes of xylene, infiltrated in 2 changes of paraffin wax for 2 h each using the automatic tissue processor. During the process of embedding, the tissue blocks were oriented in such a way that sections were cut in a desired plane of tissues. Two L-shaped metal moulds were laid on metal plate so as to enclose a square or a rectangular space. It was then partially filled with melted paraffin and allowed to cool until reasonably firm. The set block of paraffin with tissue was removed from moulds and then trimmed to suitable sizes and fixed on a metal object holder. The block was further trimmed and kept at 0°C.

Section cutting

The sections of 4 to 6 μm thickness were cut on albuminized slides.

Table 2. Staining (hematoxylin and eosin).

Reagent	Amount used
Harris hematoxylin stain	5 g
Ammonium/potassium alum	100 g
Hematoxylin crystal	5 g
Alcohol (100%)	50 ml
Distilled water	1000 ml

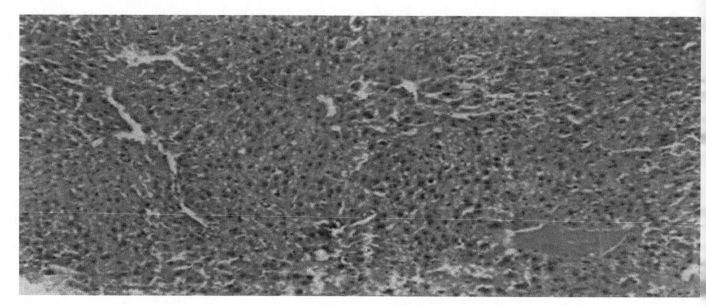

Figure 1a. Histopathological changes in liver. Normal liver section of control mice. Hepatocytes are arranged in columns. No pathological lesions were observed.

The sections were drained with water and dried on a hot plate at about 50°C for 30 min before staining (Table 2). The hematoxylin crystals were dissolved in alcohol and alum in water by the aid of heat. It was then heated to simmer until it became dark purple. The solution was removed from heat immediately and was plunged into basin of cold water until it cooled. Finally, 2 to 4 ml of glacial acetic acid was added (which increases the precision of nuclear stain). The stain was filtered before each use.

Eosin phloxine stain

Eosin (1.0 g) was dissolved in 100 ml of distilled water and 10 ml. 1% phloxine solutions were added. Finally, 780 ml of 95% alcohol and 4 ml of glacial acetic acid was added to it. It was filtered before use.

Procedure

Sections measuring approximately 0.2 x 0.2 cm were taken from the liver of mice. They were dehydrated through graded solutions of alcohol ending in two changes of absolute alcohol for 2 h each. They were cleared in 2 changes of xylene, infiltrated in 2 changes of paraffin wax for 2 h each using the automatic tissue processor and embedded in molten paraffin wax (DPX). Finally the slides were observed for histopathological changes.

RESULTS

Histopathological examination of liver

Histopathological examination of uninfected mice liver showed cords of hepatocytes arranged in columns with central veins and portal triads (Figure 1a). Infection with $0.6 \times LD_{50}$ of *S. typhimurium* showed multiple lesions of nodular microabsces or granulomatous lesions that were composed of degenerated hepatocytes with variable degree of central necrosis surrounded by the sheets of neutrophils and macrophages, and severe necrosis were observed (Figure 1b). In contrast, liver sections of L-arginine treated mice showed tissue with cords of hepatocytes consisting of neutrophils and macrophages, showing granulomatous lesions and mild necrosis were seen (Figure 1c). In ciprofloxacin treated mice infected with $0.6 \times LD_{50}$ of *S. typhimurium,* no significant pathological changes in liver were observed. Sections showed that the liver tissue was comprised of cords of hepatocytes showing mild fatty changes and extensive focal neutrophilic infiltrate consisting of granuloma. No area of necrosis was seen (Figure 1d). Similarly,

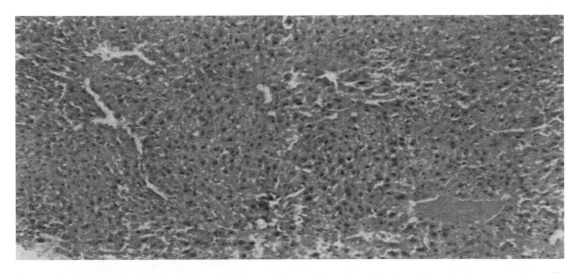

Figure 1b. Histopathological changes in liver. Normal liver section of control mice. Hepatocytes are arranged in columns. No pathological lesions were observed.

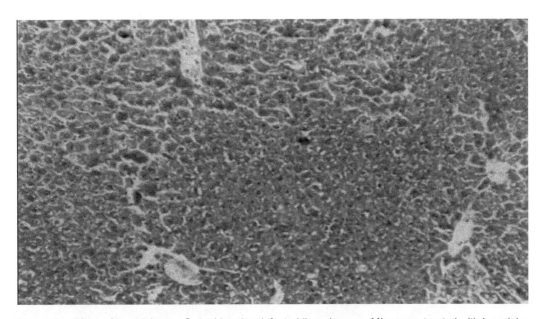

Figure 1c. Effect of L-arginine on *S. typhimurium* infected liver damage. Mice were treated with L-arginine (1000 mg per kg b. wt) after infection with challenge dose of 0.6 x LD$_{50}$ *S. typhimurium*. At day 14, liver section were examined histopathologically which revealed that cords of hepatocytes showing focal granulomatous collection of neutrophils and macrophages (G) and there is mild sign of necrosis (N).

treatment with drugs in combination that is 1/2 Arginine + 1/2 Ciprofloxacin showed less significant pathological changes in the liver, and maximum decreases in the level of granulamatous lesion and necrosis (Figure 1e).

DISCUSSIONS

Histopathological examination of the liver

Histopathological examination of paraffin sections prepared from normal mice showed normal architecture of hepatocytes and infection with 0.6 x LD$_{50}$ of *S. typhimurium* showed multiple lesions of nodular microabscess or granulomatous lesions thatwere composed of degenerated hepatocytes with variable degree of central necrosis surrounded by the sheets of neutrophils and macrophages, and severe necrosis were observed (Figures 1a and b). In *S. typhimurium*, infected mice treated with L-Arg, and sacrificed on day 14, the liver tissue was found to have extensive cords of hepatocytes consisting of neutrophils and macrophages,

154

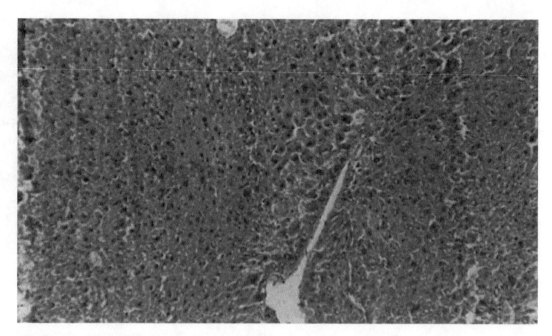

Figure 1d. Effect of ciprofloxacin on *S. typhimurium* induced liver damage. Mice were treated with ciprofloxacin (400 mg per kg b. wt) after infection with challenge dose of 0.6 x LD$_{50}$ *S. typhimurium*. At day 14, liver section were examined histopathologically which revealed that cords of hepat ocytes showing focal granulomatous collection of neutrophils and macrophages (G) and there is no sign of necrosis (N).

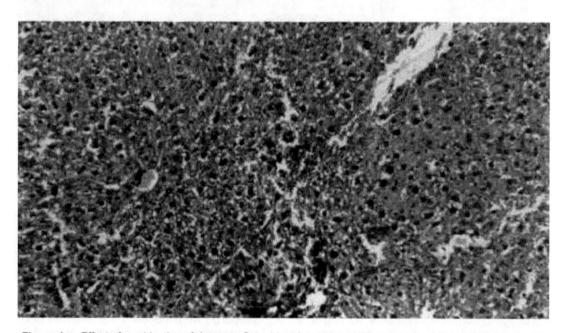

Figure 1e. Effect of combination of drugs on *S. typhimurium* induced liver damage. Mice were treated with B+1/2 Arg+1/2 Cip after infection with challenge dose of 0.6 x LD$_{50}$ *S. typhimurium*. At day 14, liver section were examined histopathologically which revealed that cords of hepatocytes showing focal granulomatous collection of neutrophils and macrophages (G) and there is less sign of necrosis (N).

showing granulomatous lesions and mild necrosis (Figures 1c and d). In ciprofloxacin treated mice, no significant pathological changes in liver were observed.

Conclusion

This study confirms that formulated drugs have significant

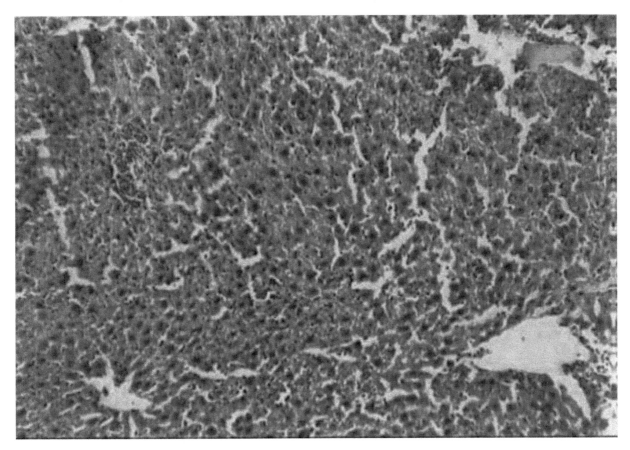

Figure 1f. Effect of combination of drugs on *S. typhimurium* induced liver damage. Mice were treated with B+1/4Arg+1/2Cip after infection with challenge dose of 0.6 x LD$_{50}$ *S. typhimurium*. At day 14, liver section were examined histopathologically which revealed that cords of hepatocytes showing focal granulomatous collection of neutrophils and macrophages (G) and there is mild sign of necrosis (N).

role on typhoid and we have corroborated these findings with normal histopathological observations. Our results are consistent with the earlier reports (Umezawa et al., 1997; MacFarlane et al., 1999; Mastroeni et al., 2000). It was found that when the mice were treated with combination, this combination (B+1/2 Arg+1/2 Cip) caused less granuloma or no necrosis with other combination of drugs (Figures 1e and f).

REFERENCES

Baumler AJ, Tsolis RM, Heffron F (1996). The lpf fimbrial operon mediates adhesion of *Salmonella typhimurium* to murine Peyer's patches. Proc. Natl. Acad. Sci. US A. 9: 279-283.

Brown JG, Brooks BW, Blais BW, Yamazaki H (1996). Application of cloth-based enzyme immunoassay for the characterization of monoclonal antibodies to Salmonella lipopolysaccharide antigens. Immunol Invest. 25(4): 369-381.

Chitnis V, Chitnis D, Verma S, Hemvani N (1999). Multidrug-resistant *Salmonella typhi* in India. Lancet. 7: 354(9177): 514-515.

endotoxemia promotes intrahepatic thrombosis and an oxygen radical-mediated hepatic injury. J. Leukocyte Biol. 52: 390-394.

Fang FC (1997). Perspectives series, host/pathogen interactions. Mechanisms of nitric oxide-related antimicrobial activity. J. Clin. Invest. 99: 2818-2825.

Gruetter CA, Barry BK, McNamara DB, Gruetter DY, Kadowitz PJ,

Ignarro LJ (1979). Relaxation of bovine coronary artery and activation of coronary arterial guanylate cyclase by nitric oxide, nitroprusside and a carcinogenic nitrosoamine. J. Cyclic Nucleotide Protein Phosphor. Res. 5: 211-214.

Gulati S, Marwaha RK, Singhi S, Ayyagari A, Kumar L (1992). Third generation cephalosporins in multi-drug resistant typhoid fever. Indian Pediatr. 29(4): 513-516.

Harbrecht BG, Billair TR, Stadler J, Demetris AJ, Ochoa J, Curran RD , Simmons RL (1992). Inhibition of nitric oxide synthesis during

Harbrecht BG, Stadler J, Demetris AJ, Simmons RL, Billiar TR (1994). Nitric oxide and prostaglandins interact to prevent hepatic damage during murine endotoxemia. A. J.

Hibbs JB Jr, Taintor RR, Vavrin Z. (1987a). Macrophage cytotoxicity, Role for L-arginine deiminase and imino nitrogen oxidation to nitrite. Sci. 235: 473-476

Ignarro LJ, Byrns RE, Buga GM, Wood KS (1987b). Endothelium-derived relaxing factor from pulmonary artery and vein possesses pharmacologic and chemical properties identical to those of nitric oxide radical. Circ Res. 61: 866-879.

Jesudason MV, John R, John TJ (1996). The concurrent prevalence of chloramphenicol-sensitive and multi-drug resistant *Salmonella typhi* in Vellore, S. India Epidemiol. Infect. 116: 225-227.

MacFarlane AS, Schwacha MG, Eisenstein TK (1999). *In vivo* blockage of nitric oxide with aminoguanidine inhibits immunosuppression induced by an attenuated strain of *Salmonella typhimurium*, potentiates *Salmonella* infection, and inhibits macrophage and polymorphonuclear leukocyte influx into the spleen. Infect. Immun. 67: 891-898.

Manchanda V, Bhalla P (2006). Emergence of non-ceftriaxone-susceptible Neisseria meningitidis in India. *J. Clin Microbiol.* 44(11):4290-1. Epub 2006 Sep 27.

Nathan C (1997). Perspectives series: nitric oxide and nitric oxide synthases. J. Clin. Invest. 100: 2417-2423.

Ohl ME, Miller SI (2001). Salmonella: a model for bacterial pathogenesis. Annu. Rev. Med. 52: 259-74.

Rowe B, Ward LR, Threlfall EJ (1995). Ciprofloxacin-resistant Salmonella typhi in the UK. Lancet. Sci. 11:346 (8985): 1302. 235: 473-476.

Umezawa K, Akaike T, Fujii S, Suga M, Setoguchi K, Ozawa A, Maedia H (1997). Induction of nitric oxide synthesis and xanthine oxidase and their roles in the antimicrobial mechanism against *Salmonella typhimurium* infection in mice. Infect. Immun. 65, 2932-2940.

27

The effect of indole – 3 – butyric acid (IBA), indole – 3 – pyruvic acid (IPA) and their synergetic effects on biochemical contents on the silkworm, *Bombyx mori*

A. Bhattacharya, S. Chakrabarty and B. B. Kaliwal*

Post graduate Department of Studies in Biotechnology and Microbiology, Karnataka University, Dharwad- 580 003, India.

Topical application with indole – 3 – butyric acid (IBA) showed a significant increase in glycogen, protein and total lipids in the body fat and trehalose and protein contents in the haemolymph in all the groups of the silkworm, *Bombyx mori*. Topical application with indole – 3 – pyruvic acid (IPA) showed a significant increase in glycogen, protein and total lipids in the body fat and trehalose and protein contents in the haemolymph in all the groups except 100 and 150 µg/ml glycogen and 100 µg/ml protein in the body fat of the silkworm, *B. mori*. Topical application with mixture of IBA and IPA showed a significant increase in the glycogen, protein and total lipids in the body fat and trehalose and protein contents in the haemolymph in all the groups except 100 µg/ml proteins in the haemolymph of the silkworm, *B. mori*.

Key words: Biochemical contents, indole – 3 – butyric acid (IBA), Indole – 3 – pyruvic acid (IPA), silkworm.

INTRODUCTION

Insects are unique in having morphological and physiological features manifested for adopting themselves to varied environment. One of the important adaptative responses in insects is mainly achieved by altering the metabolic process. The silkworm is entirely dependent on mulberry leaves as a food source and the protein content of the leaves play an important role in the silk production. There is evidence that the plant growth regulators may act through their effect on the insect's neuroendocrine system or perhaps directly on insect cells (Osborne et al., 1968). It has been reported that the plant growth regulators mimic the moulting hormone ecdysone and restricts the insect growth of *Drosophila hydei*

(Alonso, 1971; Neumann, 1980, 1982). It has been reported that the reduced reproduction effected by low concentrations of ABA and GA$_3$ added to host grass may mean that these compounds act on insects metabolism via its hormone pathways, they serve as biochemical signals to regulate growth of insects, Deoxyribonucleic acid (DNA) synthesis and reproduction of *Aulocare ellitt*, since ABA, GA$_3$ and JH-III are biochemically similar trepenoid compounds derived from mevalonate. DeMan et al. (1981) have suggested that dietary supplementation with plant growth regulators may stimulate the insect growth and reproduction by altering the rate of DNA synthesis and/or the rate of synthesis of the insect moulting hormone. There are a number of reports regarding the supplementation of various plant growth regulators that affect the physiological processes, growth and development in different insects (Edwards, 1966; Osborne et al., 1968; Gurra, 1970; Becker and Roussaux, 1980; Neumann, 1982; Chrominiske et al., 1982; Bur, 1985). It has been reported that supplementation with plant hormones influences on the physiological process, growth and development of silkworm *Bombyx mori* L (Kochi and Kaliwal, 2005;

---

*Corresponding author. E-mail: b_kaliwal@yahoo.com.

Abbreviations: IBA, Indole – 3 – butyric acid; IPA, indole – 3 – pyruvic acid; DNA, deoxyribonucleic acid; PABA, paraminobenzoic acid; TCA, trichloroacetic acid; BSA, serum albumen; CRBD, complete randomized block design; LSD, least significant difference; NOA, naphthoxy acetic acid.

158 Pharmaceutical Biotechnology

Etebari et al., 2004). It has been reported that the dietary supplementation with paraminobenzoic acid (PABA) affects proteins profile in the haemolymph and silkgland (Pramodkumari, 1990). Rup et al. (1997) have reported that the qualitative changes in the protein, lipid and carbohydrate contents under the influence of GA$_3$ in *Zaprinus paravittigeal*. Hugar and Kaliwal (1997) have reported that the topical application with BAP and IAA increases the body fat glycogen, protein and haemolymph protein where as haemolymph trehalose decreases. Goudar and Kaliwal (2001) have reported that 2– 4 D and NOA increases the body fat glycogen, haemolymph trehalose and body fat protein. It was showed that the plant growth regulators viz., IBA, IPA and their mixtures enhances the larval weight, silk gland weight, female cocoon weight, shell weight, filament length, weight and denier, fecundity, hatching percentage and eggs per ovariole in the silkworm, *B. mori*. Plant hormones play a very important role in the growth of plants which is a source of food and also helps in enhancing the metabolism of silk worm which in turn helps in the production of silk. Therefore, the present study was undertaken to find out the effects of IBA, IPA and their synergetic effects on the glycogen, protein and total lipids in the body fat, trehalose and protein in the haemolymph of the silkworm, *B. mori*.

MATERIALS AND METHODS

Animals

In the present study the commercially exploited bivoltine crossbreed silkworm race CSR$_2$ x CSR$_4$ was selected. The race was procured from Rayapur grainage center, Dharwad, Karnataka, India. Leave variety is S$_{36}$.

Test material

The plant growth regulators IBA and IPA were procured from the Central Drug House, New Delhi and Hi Media chemical Company Pvt. Limited., Mumbai, India.
The fifth in star larvae were selected randomly and grouped into different batches for the experiment. Each group consists of five replications each with 20 worms. The IBA and IPA was individually dissolved completely in distilled water and diluted to form 100, 150 and 200 µg/ml. The dietary supplementations of these chemicals started from the beginning of V stadium to the maturation of silkworm larvae. The regulators are topically used on the silkworm body. Amongst the four feedings per day, feeding of treated leaves was alternated with feeding of untreated leaves (Kochi and Kaliwal, 2006).

Tissue preparation

The silkworm *B. mori* larvae were dissected in *Bombyx saline* at pH 6.5 on 6th day of V in star. The body fat was immediately collected and used for the glycogen and protein estimation. The haemolymph was collected by amputating one of the larval thoracic legs in pre-chilled centrifuge tube. The haemolymph collected from 2 to 3 silkworms was used almost immediately for trehalose and protein estimation (Kochi and Kaliwal, 2006).

Glycogen estimation

Anthrone method of Sciefter et al. (1950) was used to determine the body fat glycogen. A known quantity of body fat was homogenized with 2 ml of 20% potassium hydroxide. The glycogen was precipitated by adding equal volume of 80% ethanol and incubated overnight at room temperature. It was centrifuged at 3000 rpm for 15 min and the supernatant was discarded. The residue was dissolved in a known volume of distilled water. Glycogen content was estimated with known aliquots in triplicate by the Anthrone method. Glucose-D was used as the reference standard and the intensity of the colour was read on the spectrophotometer at 620 nm.

Trehalose estimation

The estimation of haemolymph trehalose was carried out according to the method of Roe (1955). Known quantity of haemolymph was collected in each test tube, and added 0.5 ml of 2% of sodium hydroxide to each test tube. After shaking, the tubes were kept in boiling water for 10 min and then the tubes were cooled in an icebox. Then 5 ml of anthrone reagent (0.05% anthrone in 70% sulphuric acid) was added to the tubes, and they were again kept in boiling water for 15 min for the development of colour. Then the tubes were cooled to room temperature. Then the colour intensity was read on spectrophotometer at 620 nm. For the reference standard the trehalose (Sigma, USA) was used. Anthrone positive carbohydrate in the haemolymph is considered as trehalose.

Protein estimation

The method of Lowry et al. (1951) was used for the total protein estimation. The tissue protein was precipitated by the addition of 1 ml of 30% trichloroacetic acid (TCA) solution followed by centrifugation at 3000 rpm for 30 min. It was repeated twice, and then the precipitate was dissolved in 1 ml of 0.1 N sodium hydroxide. A known aliquot of this solution was then mixed with 5 ml of alkaline copper reagent (20% sodium carbonate prepared in 0.1 N sodium hydroxide containing sodium potassium tartrate and 1% copper sulphate). After 10 min 0.5 ml of Folin Ciocalteu's reagent was added to the tubes and the tubes were shaken thoroughly. Then the tubes were kept for 20 min for colour development. The readings were taken on the spectrophotometer at 650 nm. The total haemolymph protein estimation was also carried out. A known quantity of haemolymph was diluted with 0.5 ml of distilled water. A known aliquates of this solution was added with 5 ml of alkaline copper reagent. After 10 min 0.5 ml of Folin Ciocalteu's reagent was added and were mixed thoroughly, then kept for 20 min until the colour develops. The readings were taken on the spectrophotometer at 650 nm. For the reference, standard Bovine Serum Albumen (BSA) (Fatty acid free) was used.

Extraction and estimation of lipids

The method of Folch et al. (1957) was used for the lipid estimation, using chloroform: methanol mixture (2:1 V/V). First, all of the body fat was homogenized with appropriate volume of chloroform: methanol mixture (1:10). The homogenate was then quantitatively transferred to a 50 ml separating funnel and then added similar volume of chloroform. The two solvents were partitioned by the addition of 0.2 volume of water. After the funnel was shaken, the mixture was allowed to stand overnight. The lower chloroform layer containing lipids was drawn off. The lipids sample was kept in vacuum desiccators until constant weight was obtained.

Statistical analysis

The experiments were designed by complete randomized block design (CRBD) method. The date collected were fed to the computer for statistical analysis by using the software SPSS version 6, to study the significance of variance among the treatment groups (one way variance test 'F'). To determine the significant difference among the treatment groups, the least significant difference test (LSD) was carried out. The percentage values were transferred into sine angular values only (Snedecor and Cochran, 1967; Raghava, 1983).

RESULTS

The results on the effects of topical application with different concentrations that is, 100, 150 and 200 µg/ml of plant growth hormones viz. IBA, IPA and their synergetic effects on glycogen, protein and total lipids content in the body fat and protein contents in the haemolymph of CSR_2 x CSR_4 crossbreed race of the silkworm, B. mori are presented in Tables 1 to 3.

Fortification of IBA on the biochemical contents of the silkworm, B. mori

Topical application with 100 µg/ml IBA to silkworm larvae resulted in an increase of 37% glycogen, 28% protein and 4% total lipids in the body fat and 1% protein, 25% trehalose in the haemolymph when compared with those of the corresponding parameters of the carrier control. The increase in glycogen, protein, and total lipids in the body fat and protein and trehalose contents in the haemolymph were statistically significant. Topical application with 150 µg/ml IBA to silkworm larvae resulted in an increase of 40% glycogen, 29% protein and 7% body fat total lipids in the body fat and 8% protein, 41% trehalose in the haemolymph when compared with those of the corresponding parameters of the carrier control. The increase in glycogen, protein and total lipids in the fat body and protein and trehalose contents in the haemolymph were statistically significant. Topical application with 200 µg/ml IBA to silkworm larvae resulted in an increase of 44% glycogen, 32% protein and 10% body fat total lipids and 16% protein, 52% trehalose in the haemolymph when compared with those of the corresponding parameters of the carrier control. The increase in glycogen, protein and total lipids in the body fat and protein and trehalose contents in the haemolymph were statistically significant (Table 1).

Fortification of IPA on the biochemical contents of the silkworm, B. mori

Topical application with 100 µg/ml IPA to silkworm larvae

resulted in an increase of 2% glycogen, 22% protein and 8% total lipids in the body fat and 11% protein, 15% trehalose in the haemolymph when compared with those of the corresponding parameters of the carrier control. The increase in total lipids in the body fat and protein and trehalose contents in the haemolymph was statistically significant. Topical application with 150 µg/ml IPA to silkworm larvae resulted in an increase of 6% glycogen, 28% protein and 20% total lipids in the body fat 13% protein, 16% trehalose contents in the haemolymph when compared with those of the corresponding parameters of the carrier control. The increase in protein and total lipids in the body fat and protein and trehalose contents in the haemolymph was statistically significant. Topical application with 200 µg/ml IPA to silkworm larvae resulted in an increase of 19% glycogen, 31% protein and 56% total lipids in the body fat and 18% protein, 26% trehalose contents in the haemolymph when compared with those of the corresponding parameters of the carrier control. The increase in glycogen, protein, total lipids in the body fat and protein and trehalose contents in the haemolymph were statistically significant (Table 2).

Synergetic effects of IBA and IPA on the biochemical contents of the silkworm, B. mori

Topical application with 100 µg/ml IBA and IPA mixture to silkworm larvae resulted in an increase of 39% glycogen, 16% protein and 11% body fat total lipids in the body fat and 8% protein and 23% trehalose contents in the haemolymph when compared with those of the corresponding parameters of the carrier control. The increase in glycogen, protein and total lipids in the body fat and trehalose contents in the haemolymph were statistically significant. Topical application with 150 µg/ml IBA and IPA mixture to silkworm larvae resulted in an increase of 48% glycogen, 22% protein and 11% body fat total lipids in the body fat and 11% protein and 25% trehalose contents in the haemolymph when compared with those of the corresponding parameters of the carrier control. The increase in glycogen, protein and total lipids in the body fat and protein and trehalose contents in the haemolymph were statistically significant. Topical application with 200 µg/ml IBA and IPA mixture to silkworm larvae resulted in an increase of 91% glycogen, 41% protein and 16% body fat total lipids in the body fat and 32% protein and 26% trehalose contents in the haemolymph when compared with those of the corresponding parameters of the carrier control. The increase in glycogen, protein and total lipids in the body fat and protein and trehalose contents in the haemolymph were statistically significant (Table 3).

DISCUSSION

The last penultimate in star is the most active feeding

Table 1. Effect of Indole-3-butyric acid (IBA) on biochemical contents in the body fat and haemolymph of the silkworm, *B. mori.*

Treatment	Dose µg/ml	Body fat (µg/mg)			Haemolymph (µg/ml)	
		Glycogen	Protein	Total lipid	Trehalose	Protein
IBA	100	9.866 * (137)	59.99 * (128)	313.3 * (104)	390.90 * (125)	2869* (101)
IBA	150	10.133 * (140)	60.40 * (129)	323.3* (107)	440.90 * (141)	3101* (108)
IBA	200	10.399 * (144)	62.00 * (132)	330.0* (110)	472.50 * (152)	3320* (116)
Carrier control	distilled water	7.199 (100)	46.66 (100)	300.0 (100)	310.80 (100)	2854 (100)
Normal control	-	7.133 (99)	48.99 (104)	293.3 (97)	300.30 (97)	2200 (77)
		(S)	(S)	(S)	(S)	(S)
S.Em± CD at 5%		1.166 2.438	3.06 8.76	4.172 9.304	12.20 34.87	3.494 11.785

* - Significant increase/decrease at 5%, S.Em ± - standard error mean, CD- critical difference, S - significant percentage increase/decrease over that of the carrier controls in parenthesis.

Table 2. Effect of Indole-3-pyruvic acid (IPA) on biochemical contents in the body fat and haemolymph of the silkworm, *B. mori.*

Treatment	Dose µg/ml	Body fat (µg/mg)			Haemolymph (µg/ml)	
		Glycogen	Protein	Total lipid	Trehalose	Protein
IPA	100	17.60 (102)	24.66 (122)	280* (108)	290 * (115)	3714* (111)
IPA	150	18.26 (106)	25.86 * (128)	310*(120)	294 * (116)	3774 * (113)
IPA	200	20.46* (119)	26.46* (131)	402* (156)	318 * (126)	3939* (118)
Carrier control	distilled water	17.13(100)	20.13 (100)	257 (100)	252 (100)	3324 (100)
Normal control	-	16.59 (96)	19.06 (94)	140 (54)	264 (104)	3576 (107)
		(S)	(S)	(S)	(S)	(S)
S.Em± CD at 5%		1.12 2.27	2.639 5.571	3.334 9.976	1.401 4.327	128.90 366

* - Significant increase/decrease at 5%. S.Em ± - standard error mean, CD - critical difference, S – significant, percentage increase/decrease over that of the carrier controls in parenthesis.

stage during which the larvae accumulate large quantity of fuel reserves in various tissues and is endowed with unique biochemical adaptations to conserve nutritional resources available during active larval stage of the silkworm, *B. mori.* Chapman (1998) has suggested that insects have adapted to a range of strategies in order to derive and store adequate energy nutrients and water from the food they consumed. The carbohydrates,

protein and lipids biomolecule are supplied by feeding on mulberry leaves. Although the mulberry leaves are complete diet for silkworm it is possible that some deficiencies occur for different reasons (Etebari et al., 2004). Hence, dietary supplementation of plant hormones may influence on the biochemical contents of the silkworm, *B. mori.* The biomolecules are stored in the body fat and haemolymph during the fifth in

star stage. It is well demonstrated that carbohydrates are stored in the body fat as glycogen, which is converted into trehalose in the body fat before it is released into the haemolymph for its utilization. Body fat, apart from converting stored glycogen into trehalose, is a major site of protein synthesis, which is essential for the maintains of the growth and reproduction. Hence, body fat in insects plays an important role

Table 3. Synergetic effects of Indole-3-butyric acid (IBA) and Indole-3-pyruvic acid (IPA) on biochemical contents in the body fat and haemolymph of the silkworm, *B. mori.*

Treatment	Dose μg/ml	Body fat (μg/mg)			Haemolymph (μg/ml)	
		Glycogen	Total lipid	Protein	Trehalose	Protein
IBA + IPA	100	22.90 * (139)	360.0 * (111)	84 * (116)	616.35 * (123)	3158 (108)
IBA + IPA	150	24.24 * (148)	360.0 * (111)	88* (122)	627.05 * (125)	3266 * (111)
IBA + IPA	200	31.25 * (191)	376.6 * (116)	102 * (141)	630.00 * (126)	3858 * (132)
Carrier control	distilled water	16.36 (100)	323.3 (100)	72 (100)	497.70 (100)	2922 (100)
Normal control	-	11.22 (68)	320 (99)	64.8 (90)	502.95 (101)	2900 (99)
		(S)	(S)	(S)	(S)	(S)
S.Em± CD at 5%		0.745 2.332	6.610 14.742	0.989 3.133	28.72 60.32	154.92 323.78

* - Significant increase/decrease at 5%, S.Em ± - standard error mean, CD - critical difference, S – significant percentage increase/decrease over that of the carrier controls in parenthesis.

in the synthesis of proteins and trehalose and that haemolymph serves as a vehicle for the transportation of these substances for their utilization in the body. Lipids are important constituents of cuticle and help in acylation of glucose-6-phosphate during chitin synthesis (Wyatt, 1967). The lipid in the body fat is an energy resource which can be mobilized rapidly during starvation, oogenesis, embryogenesis and moulting and is used to sustain continuous muscular activity (Gilbert and Chino, 1974). It has showed that the plant growth regulators affect the economic parameters of the silkworms, it is likely that they may also affect the synthesis, storage and release of the biological molecules from the body fat to the haemolymph which will help for the growth and development of silkworm, *B. mori.* As we have observed in earlier reports that dietary supplementation with plant growth regulators influences the glycogen, protein and total lipids in the body fat and trehalose and protein in the haemolymph of the silkworm, *B. mori* (Bur, 1985; Pramadokuimari, 1990; Rup et al., 1997; Hugar and Kaliwal, 1997; Goudar and Kaliwal, 2001; Kochi and Kaliwal, 2005; Etebari et al., 2004). In the present study, therefore, the effects of topical

application with IBA, IPA and their mixture on biochemical contents were studied.

Effects of IBA, IPA and their mixture on glycogen in the body fat and trehalose in the haemolymph of the silkworm, *B. mori*

The results of this present study showed that there was a significant increase in the glycogen and the body fat in all the treated groups with IBA, IPA and their mixture. The results obtained in the present study are in agreement with the reported of the bivoltine silkworm, *B. mori* after the treatment with BAP and IAA (Hugar and Kaliwal, 1997). Goudar and Kaliwal (2001) have also reported an increase in glycogen in the body fat of the silkworm treated with NOA and 2, 4 – D. The increase in glycogen in the body fat might be due to the stimulatory effect of these plant growth regulators on glycogenesis reported to increase during feeding period (Pant and Morris, 1969). Wyatt (1967) reported that the quantity of these biomolecules in insect tissue depends on quantum of food intake and variation in their levels, due to the utilization during growth and

metamorphosis. Siegert and Ziegler (1982) have reported decreased metabolism in *Menduca sexta* at the end of last larval in star and further the sugar in the haemolymph and glycogen in the body fat decreased during moulting and increased at the resumption of feeding. It is reported that the homeostatic of trehalose in the haemolymph is maintained through hormonal regulation at the expense of glycogen in the tissue probably from the body fat (Saito, 1963). In the present results, there was a significant increase in trehalose in the haemolymph in all the groups treated with IBA, IPA and their mixture. Hugar and Kaliwal (1997) have reported that there was a significant increase in trehalose in the haemolymph in BAP and IAA treated groups might possibly be due to the conversion of glycogen into trehalose and it's subsequent release into the haemolymph by the fat body (Hugar and Kaliwal, 1997). The results are also in agreement with that reported for the silkworm, *B. mori* after the treatment with NOA, PABA and 2, 4 – D (Goudar and Kaliwal, 2001). There was an increase in glycogen in the body fat and trehalose in the haemolymph as it may be utilized as additional source of fuel or energy required during the pupal and adult transformation. However, the mechanism of action of these plant growth regulators on the body fat synthetic activity and trehalose in the haemolymph is not known. Hence, further investigation is essential in this regard.

Effects of IBA, IPA and their mixture on protein contents in the body fat and haemolymph of the silkworm, B. mori

It is well known that the body fat of an insect is regarded as liver of vertebrate in carrying out intermediary metabolism as well as protein synthesis and its storage (Wigglesworth, 1972). Therefore, body fat is an important organ in the insects, which plays an important role in anabolic as well as catabolic activities of insects. The results of the present study indicated that there was significant increase in protein in the body fat and haemolymph in all the groups treated with IBA, acid IPA and mixtures. The results obtained in the present study support the views of Hugar and Kaliwal (1997) where the body fat protein and haemolymph protein increased significantly in the groups treated with BAP and IAA. Similar results were also obtained by Goudar and Kaliwal (2001) in the silkworm, B. mori treated with PABA, 2, 4 – D and NOA. The increased of protein contents in the body fat and haemolymph protein may possibly be due to the stimulatory effects of the plant growth regulators at a given concentration on the synthetic activity of the body fat and the increased haemolymph protein might be due to the release of excess of protein by the body fat into the haemolymph and at the same time the weight of the silk gland has also increased significantly. This also coincides with the subsequent increase in the cocoon weight and its shell weight of the silkworm, B. mori.

Effects of IBA, IPA and their mixture on total lipids content in the body fat and haemolymph of the silkworm, B. mori

In the present study, the total lipids in the body fat are increased in all the groups treated with IBA, IPA and their mixtures. Similar results have been reported that the body fat total lipids, phospholipids and neutral lipids in the body fat were increased in all the groups treated with 2, 4- dichlorophenoxy acetic acid (2, 4 – D) and naphthoxy acetic acid (NOA) may be due to the stimulatory effect on the synthetic activity in the body fat (Goudar and Kaliwal, 2001). Increase in the total lipids in the body fat might possibly be due to stimulatory effect of IBA, IPA and their mixtures at a given concentration on the body fat synthetic activity and ovarioles might have not sequestered the lipids from the body fat in excess of its requirements, so, the accumulation of total lipids was seen. Moreover, there was significant increase in fecundity might possibly suggest that the ovariole might have sequestered the lipids from the body fat to the eggs

but the ovariole has not sequestered the lipids from the body fat in excess of its requirements, hence, there was an accumulation of total lipids in the body fat. Guerra (1970) citing the references of Harper (1963) have quoted, that the metabolic processes taking place within the living organism are nearly the reflection of the chemical composition of the body.

Since, the concentration of the most chemical substances in the body fluids varies within rather narrow limits, significant changes in the normal metabolism which are detrimental to insect development and/ or reproduction could be produced by inducing an excess or a deficiency of essential metabolites. The sensitive and efficient regulation of the rates of metabolic processes controlling life is made possible by several known mechanism. These are the nervous system, hormones, the stimulation or inhibition of enzyme activity, feedback inhibition and the induction or suppression of enzyme synthesis whether the increase/decrease in glycogen, protein and total lipids in the body fat and trehalose and protein contents in the haemolymph after treatment with all these plant growth regulators in the present study, may be due to their influence on nervous system or hormones or the stimulation or inhibition of enzymes activity or the induction or suppression of enzyme synthesis were not known. Hence, further investigation on mechanisms of plant growth regulators on the biochemical contents of the silkworm is necessary. In the present study the plant growth hormones that are IBA and IPA and their mixtures affect the biochemical contents such as glycogen, protein and total lipids in the body fat and trehalose and protein contents in the haemolymph thus affecting the physiological process of the silkworm, B. mori. The contents were dose dependent. The mulberry leaf itself has different levels of plant growth hormones but dietary supplementation of plant hormones alters the levels of biochemical contents leading to variations in physiological activities, either improving or reducing the economic traits of the silkworm, B. mori. However, the exact effects of these hormones on the body fat and haemolymoh are essential in the silkworm, B. mori.

ACKNOWLEDGEMENT

We thank the UGC for the financial assistance and Chairman, Post graduate Department of Studies in Zoology, Karnatak University, Dharwad for providing research facilities.

REFERENCES

Alonso C (1971). The effect of gibberelic acid upon developmental processes in Drosophila hydei. Entomology Experimental and Application. 14: 73-82.
Becker JL (1975). Role of vitamin B12 in the reduction of ribonucleotides into deoxyribonucleotides in Drosophila cells grown in

vitro. Biochemical, 58: 427-430.

Bur M (1985). Influence of plant growth hormones on development and reproduction of Aphids. (Homoptera: Aphidiae- Aphidadae). Entomol. Gene., 10: 183-200.

Chapman RF (1998). The insect structure and function, Cambridge University Press, Cambridge.

Chrominiske A, Neumann SV, Jurenka R (1982). Exposure to ethylene changes on nymphal growth rate and females longevity in the grass hopper, Melanoplus sanguinipes. Naturwissen Schofte, 69: 45.

DeMan W, De Loof A, Briers T, Huybrechts R (1981). Effect of abscisic acid on vitellogenesis in Sarcophaga bullata. Entomol. Exp. Appl., 29: 259-267.

Edwards LJ (1966). Growth inhibition of the house cricket with with ethylene. J. Econ. Entomol., 59: 1541-1542.

Etebari KE, Matindoost L (2004). Effect of feeding mulberry enriched leaves with ascorbic acid on some biological, biochemical and economical characteristics of silkworm, *Bombyx mori* L. Int. J. Indust. Entomol., 7: 81-87.

Folch J, Lees M, Stanley SGH (1957). A simple method for isolation and purification of total lipids from animal tissue. J. Biol. Chem., 226: 497-509.

Gilbert LJ, Chino P (1974). Transport of lipids in insects. J. Lipid Res., 15: 439-456.

Goudar KS, Kaliwal BB (2001). Effect of naphthoxyacetic acid on the economic parameters of the silkworm, *Bombyx mori* L. Indust. Entomol., 3(2): 157-162.

Gurra AA (1970). Effect of biologically active substances in the diet on development and reproduction of Heliothes sps. J. Econ. Entomol., 63: 1518-1521.

Harper HA (1963). Enzymes chapter 7 In: Review of physiological chemistry, 9th ed. Long Medical Publications, Los Altos Calif.

Hugar II, and Kaliwal BB (1997). Effect of phytohormone, indole-3-acetic acid (IAA) on the economic parameters of the bivoltine silkworm, *B. mori* L. Bull. Seric. Res., 8: 67-70.

Kochi SC, Kaliwal BB (2005). Effect of sialic acid on commercial triats of the bivoltine crossbreed races of the silkworm, *Bombyx mori* L. Caspian. J. Environ. Sci., 3: 107-115.

Kochi SC, Kaliwal BB (2006). The effects of potassium bromide on biochemical contents of the fat body and heamolymph of crossbreed races of the silkworm, *Bombyx mori* L. Caspian. J. Environ. Sci., 4: 17-24.

Lowry H, Rosebrough NL, Far AL, Randalll RJ (1951). Protein measurement with folin phenol reagent. J. Biol. Chem., 193: 265-275.

Neumann SV (1980). Regulation of grasshopper fecundity, logivity and egg viability by plant growth hormone. Experimentia, 36: 130-131.

Neumann SV (1982). Plant growth hormones affect grasshopper growth and reproduction. Proceeding 5th International Symp. on insect plant relationships, (Ed. J. H. Visser, A. K. Mille). pp. 57-62.

Osborne DJ, Carlisle DB, Ellis PE (1968). Protein synthesis in the fat body of female desert locus Schistocerca gregaria Fork in relation to maturation. Gen. Comp. Endocr., 11: 347-354.

Pramodkumari J (1990). On quantitative increase of silk production by the administration of Para aminobenzoic acid. Recent trends in Sericulture. pp. 164-178.

Raghava RD (1983). 'Statistical techniques in agricultural and biological research', Oxford and IBH Publishing Co. New Delhi.

Roe JH (1955). The determination of sugar in blood and spinal fluid with anthrone reagent. J. Biol. Chem., 242: 424-428.

Rup PJ, Kaur P, Sohal SK (1997). Influence of coumarin (a secondary plant compound) on the morphology and biochemistry of the mustard aphid Lipaphiserysimi (Kalt). J. Environ. Biol., 251-257.

Saito S (1963). Trehalose in the body fluid of the silkworm, Bombyx mori L. J. Insect. Physiol., 9: 509-519.

Sciefter S, Dayton S, Novic B, Myntiyer E (1950). The estimation of glycogen with anthrone reagent. Arch. Biochem., 25-191.

Siegert K, Ziegler R (1982). Role of Corpora curdiaca in starvation induced activation of fat body glycogen phosphorylase in larvae of the tobacco hornworm Manduca sexta (Lepidoptera: Sptingidae). Gen. Comp. Endocrinol., 46: 382.

Snedecor GW, Cochran WG (1967). Statistical methods. Oxford and IBH Publishing Co., New Delhi, India.

Wigglesworth VB (1972). The principles of insect physiology. 7th ed. Chapman Hall, London.

Wyatt GR (1967). The biochemistry of sugars and polysaccharides in insects. Adv. Insect. Physiol. 4: 287-360.

28

Synthesis, characterization and biological activity of 2-Aryl -2, 3-dihydro-1*H*-perimidine

Hashim J. Azeez[1] and Kezhal M. Salih[2]

[1]Department of Chemistry, College of Education, Salahaddin University, Erbil, Iraq.
[2]Department of Pharmaceutical Chemistry, College of Pharmacy, Hawler Medical University, Erbil, Iraq.

A series of new 2-Aryl-2,3-dihydro-1*H*-perimidine, derivatives (3a - j) were synthesized under reflux and at room temperature by condensation reaction of 1,8-diaminonaphthalene (2) with various substituted benzaldehyde using glacial acetic acid a catalyst. The synthesized compounds were characterized by spectroscopic methods, infrared (IR), proton nuclear magnetic resonance (^{1}H-NMR), carbon nuclear magnetic resonance (^{13}C-NMR) and carbon nuclear magnetic resonance-distortionless enhancement by polarization (^{13}C-NMR-DEPT). The synthesized compounds were screened for their biological activity against the Gram-positive bacteria *Staphylococcus aureus* and the Gram-negative bacteria *Escherichia coli*. The results showed that 89% of the synthesized compounds were not active against *S. aureus*, while *E. coli* showed 100% sensitivity to the mentioned compound. These results illustrate the marked bactericidal effect of all the synthesized compounds.

Key words: 1, 8-Diaminonaphthalene, 2,3-dihyroperimidin, perimidine.

INTRODUCTION

The derivatives of perimidine described as DNA–intercalating antitumoral agents against carcinogenic lines, a small number of DNA-binding ligands, were assumed to have an important role in cancer chemotherapy such as adriamycin, actinomycine, amsacrine and mitoxantrone. A large number of studies on the structure activity relationships of these compounds have demonstrated the requirement for intercalative binding to DNA for biological activity which has led researcher to design new compounds which have generally been tricyclic or tetracyclic moieties in order to maximize the strength binding to DNA (Ihan et al., 2008; John, 1987). There are several preparative methods for the synthesis of perimidine derivatives. The most commonly method for the preparation of perimidines is the condensation reaction of 1,8-diaminonaphthalene with a carbonyl group which needs special reagent or several reaction conditions (Varsha et al., 2010).

The perimidines have a wide application in industrial field; they are used as dyes (Kazuhoki et al., 2010). Their famous 2,3-Dihydro-1*H*-perimidine (1) (Figure 1) is a saturated form of perimidine at positions 2 and 3 which is a synthetic tricyclic compounds including two nitrogen atoms. Heterocyclic compounds such as perimidine are of a wide interest because they exhibit diverse range of biological activities (Kang and Hsiu, 1984).

Small ring heterocyclic compounds containing nitrogen have been investigated for a long time because of their

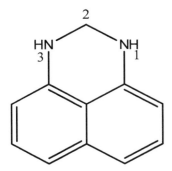

Figure 1. 2,3-Dihydro1*H*-perimidine compound

important medical properties; among these types of molecules is perimidine ring. The biological activities of these types of compounds against some microorganisms were reported in the literature (Kang and Hsiu, 1984).
Their famouse dyes were reported in the literature as solvent black 3. The perimidine derivatives have different uses and importance; they were used as an intermediate inorganic synthesis (Kang and Hsiu, 1984, 1985). Different routs were used in the synthesis of perimidine derivatives, such as microwave irradiation method (Cado and Stephen 1996). 2-Methyl-2-(4-biphenyl) perimidine and 2,2-dimethylperimidine served as an odor sensor which may be useful for discriminating between the odor of human or other mammalian individuals, and they found out that the perimidine monomers and polymers were used in the manufacture of the sensor (Gibson et al., 1999). Corn (1990) investigate novel near infrared absorbing dyes of perimidine and dihydroperimidine. Other spiroperimidine were reported as a photochromic compounds (Davis et al 2005). Herein, the synthesis spectral data biological studies against. Gram-positive bacteria *Staphylococcus aureus* and Gram-negative bacteria *Escherichia coli* and their comparison with gentamicin of new compounds (3a - j) were achieved. The similar mechanism of action between gentamicin and streptomycin with other aminoglycosides has been approved by many researchers (Jacquelyn, 2008). The bactericidal action of gentamicin was accompanied by inhibition of growth, their results showed that the protein biosynthesis fails within minutes after addition of gentamicin to cultures susceptible bacteria for example Gram-negative bacteria *E. coli*. The mechanism of action of antibiotic on the biosynthesis of DNA and RNA in the Gram-negative bacteria *E. coli* was reported by several investigators, measuring the ^{14}C-labeled thymidine to the DNA of *E. coli* and measuring the incorporation of ^{14}C-labeled uracil in the global RNA of the same bacteria. Their result showed the less effect of the antibiotic on the RNA biosynthesis. They found out that nucleic acid biosynthesis is relatively unaffected by gentamicin and

they concluded that the gentamicin is a specific inhibiter of protien biosynthesis in susceptible bacteria; gentamicin inhibited the polymerization of phenylalanine in a standard ribosome poly U cell-free system (Fred et al, 1969).

MATERIALS AND METHODS

Measurement

Melting points were determined by open capillary method and are uncorrected. The infra red (IR) spectra in (KBr pellets) were recorded on a thermo mattson IR 300 Spectrophotometer and Bio-rad Merlin FTIR spectroscopy, Mod FTS 3000. The nuclear magnetic resonance (^{1}H-NMR and ^{13}C-NMR) spectra were recorded on Brucker (300 MHz) at Al-Albayt University-Jordon. Mass spectra (MS) were recorded on High resolution mass Bruker Daltonics Data Analysis 3.4, and the gas chromatography-mass spectrometry (GC-MS) (EI), Shimatzu, Japan, at Al-Albayt University-Jordon. Thin layer chromatography (TLC) was carried out using silica gel coated aluminium sheets DC-Aloufoline 20 × 20 cm Kieseigel 60 F$_{254}$ pre-coated Germany Merck.

Synthesis of 2-Aryl-2, 3-dihydro-1H-Perimidine (3 a-e)

1,8-Diamino naphthalene (1.5820 g, 0.01 mole) was dissolved in 10 ml absolute ethanol. The soluble appropriate aldehydes (0.02 mole) in 10 ml absolute ethanol when added is followed by the addition of few drops of glacial acetic acid. The reaction mixture was stirred for 24 h at room temperature. The products were filtered, washed with cold absolute ethanol, recrystallized from absolute ethanol. The physical properties and yield percent are recorded in Table 3.

Synthesis of 2-Aryl-2, 3-di hydro-1H-Perimidine (3f-j)

The same procedure as described earlier was carried out under reflux for (1 to 3 h). Progress of the reaction was monitored by TLC (chloroform). At completion, the mixture was cooled to room temperature and filtered. The solid products were washed with ethanol and dried in an oven at 60°C. The products were filtered and recrystallized from appropriate solvent. The physical properties are listed in Table 3.

Biological study

The sensitivity of 2-Aryl-2,3-dihydro-1H-perimidine (3 a to j) were carried out against two kinds of bacteria, Gram-positive *S. aureus* and Gram-negative bacteria *E. coli* using disc agar diffusion method (Shakhawan 2001). The tests were performed using Muller Hinton agar, the medium was prepared using nutrient agar for preservation of pure culture, then sterilized by autoclave, and poured in Petri dish to a depth of 4 mm. Activation of each type of bacteria Gram-positive (*S. aureus*) and Gram-negative (*E. coli*) was done before culturing on the nutrient agar in a nutrient broth which was used for dilution of bacterial and cultivation of culture isolates for 24 h in 37°C, then inoculation of the plates. The discs of the synthesized compounds were prepared by mixing a compound with KBr powder (1:3). The mixture was pressed under pressure KBr which has been used as a blank disc. The dried surface of the Muller Hinton agar plate was streaked; five dried discs were placed on the surface of the cultured media per petri dish. The plates were then incubated at 37°C for 18 to 24 h. Microbial growth was indicated by measuring the diameter of the zone of inhibition.

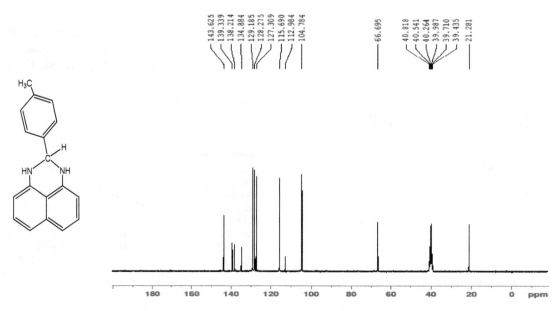

Figure 2. ^{13}C-NMR spectrum of compound (3e).

RESULTS AND DISCUSSION

The reaction of substituted benzaldehydes with primary diamines (2) afforded 2-Aryl-2,3-dihydro-1H-Perimidine (3a - j). The desired compounds prepared in different conditions while no analogues reactions using room temperature have yet been described. Thus 1,8-diaminonaphthalene was allowed to react with various substituted benzalaldehydes in absolute ethanol using glacial acetic acid as a catalyst for 24 h at room temperature. The rapid condensation was monitored by TLC using (chloroform as eluent), while the substituted benzaldehydes (f - j) did not react at room temperature. Therefore the desired compounds were prepared by condensation reaction under reflux for 1 to 3 h.

The possible mechanism of this reaction first involves the formation of azomethine bond followed by nucleophilic attack by the basic nitrogen of the second free amino group. Cyclization takes place with the formation of the final product. The structure of the title compounds were characterized based on their physical, analytical and spectral data. From the IR spectra of compounds 3a to j, a new sharp N - H stretching bands were observed at 3401 to 3364 cm^{-1}. The existence of the N - H stretching bands confirmed the cyclization at the positions 1, 2, 3 and the disappearance of four bands belong to two NH$_2$ stretching for symmetric and asymmetric vibration of the NH$_2$ groups at 3412, 3386, 3332, 3304 cm^{-1} in IR spectrum of 1, 8 to diaminonaphthalene which supported the formation of the products (Table 4). The position of the bond was also confirmed by the ^{1}H - NMR spectra of the compounds (Table 5). The singlet at δ 5.35 to 6 ppm in the spectrum of 3a - j showed the C-H proton supported by observation of a signal in the ^{13}C - NMR at δ 61.378 - 66.628 ppm (Akbar et al., 2009). In addition, the appearance of multiplets signals at δ 6.6 - 8.1 ppm for ten protons belongs to phenyl and naphthyl rings, which were recorded as 10 signals in ^{13}C - NMR spectrum (Figure 2). The singlet signal belongs to two N - H of perimidine moiety seen at δ 7.4 ppm in ^{1}-HNMR spectrum (Table 5). The ^{13}C-NMR-DEPT-135 spectrum showed 8 signals assigned to protonated carbon for compound (3h) and both compounds (3e and i) showed 5 signals for 5 protonated carbon and the CH$_3$ carbon was observed at δ 21.263 ppm (Table 5).

The electron ionization mass spectrometry (EIMS) of 2 compounds, 3e and 3h, which were chosen as prototypes, were obtained. The MS of the compound 3e showed a molecular ion peak(M$^+$) with high intensity at m/z 259%, other peaks were observed due to fragments as a result of loss of protons, CH$_3$, C$_6$H$_3$, H$_2$ molecules, followed by loss of CH and N atom. C$_2$, which is another fragmentation, was recorded from the origin compound while the MS of compound 3h was calculated from molecular ion peak m/z 290.1 and showed peaks due to fragments, supporting the expected structures.

Antimicrobial activities

Experiments were performed to evaluate the activities of the synthesized compounds against two species of bacteria S. aureus and E. coli. Anti-microbial study was assessed by measuring the minimum inhibitory zone (using disk agar diffusion method) and the results were

Table 1. Perimidine's antibacterial activity measured by the disc diffusion method.

Compound	R	*S. aureus* (mm)	*E. coli* (mm)
3a	-H	20	25
3c	4-OCH$_3$	NIZ	40
3d	2-Br	NIZ	42
3e	4-CH$_3$	NIZ	26
3f	4-Br	NIZ	42
3g	2-OH	NIZ	44
3h	2-NO$_2$	NIZ	40
3i	4-NO$_2$	NIZ	40
3j	4-Cl	NIZ	40
Gentamicin			26

Values are represented as mean inhibition zone (mm), highly reactive (Inhibition zone > 24 mm), Active (inhibition zone 20 to 24 mm), NIZ = no inhibition zone.

represented in Table 1. The biological interest of perimidine derivatives were recorded in the literatures (Kang and Hsiu, 1984). Therefore the antibacterial study was done and the activity was determined by the disc diffusion method at the concentration of 50 µg per disk. All the synthesized used compounds were tested for their antibacterial activity against both bacteria *S. aureus* and *E. coli*. The gentamicin was chosen as a standard antibacterial agent. The synthesized compounds were more active against *E. coli* and showed negative effect against *S. aureus*. The compound 3a was moderately active against both the gram-positive and the gram-negative tested bacteria, whereas the most effective compound of perimidine derivatives was (3g) against *E. coli* indicating that the presence of (OH) group in 3g caused potential antibacterial activity, while both compounds (3a and 3e) were compared to (3g), they showed the lower activity against *E. coli*. Compounds 3a - j were found to exhibit more activity than the standard drug gentamicin that has a wide effect on the *E. coli*.

The results showed the effect of substituents on the activity of perimidine derivatives against both bacteria. Gram-positive bacterial cell walls contain peptidoglycan and teichoic or teichuronic acid, and the bacterium may or may not be surrounded by a protein or polysaccharide envelope. Gram-negative bacterial cell walls contain peptidoglycan, lipopolysaccharide, lipoprotein, phospholipid and protein. The critical attack site of anti-cell-wall agents is the peptidoglycan layer. This layer is essential for the survival of bacteria in hypotonic environments; loss or damage of this layer destroys the rigidity of the bacterial cell wall, resulting in death (Harold et al 1996). Gentamicine is a type of antibacterial agent that inhibits protein synthesis, the aminoglycosides irreversibly bind to the 30S ribosome and freeze the 30S initiation complex (30S-mRNA-TRNA) so that no further initiation can occur, the aminoglycosides also slows down

Table 2. The percentage of the active compounds against *S. aureus* and *E. coli* susceptibility.

Types of bacteria	Sensitive (%)	Resistance (%)
S. aureus	11	89
E. coli	100	0

protein synthesis that has already initiated and induced misreading of the mRNA (David et al., 2007; Marie-Paule et al., 1999; Davis, 1987). It may also destabilize bacterial membranes, inhibit the polymerization of phenyl alanine in a standard ribosome polymerization. Fragoso and Ciferri have been concerned with gentamicin-induced misreading of RNA code words as indicated by stimulations of ambiguous incorporation of certain amino acids in cell-free system, employing synthetic polyribonucleotides as model messenger RNAs (Fred et al, 1969). The increased activity may be attributed to enhancement of lipophilicity due to incorporation of aromatic benzene ring and substituent NO$_2$, CH$_3$ groups at meta and para positions with the presence of two N-H groups; these compounds tend to be highly bound to plasma protein, the more lipophilic compound the greater compound the greater binding. Table 2 investigates the percentage of sensitivity of the bacteria species under the study which was 11% for *S. aureus* while sensitivity of *E. coli* was 100%.

Conclusion

In the present work, a series of new 2-Aryl-2, 3-dihy dro-1H-perimidines (3a - j) were synthesized and characterized by spectral studies. All the synthesized compounds were evaluated for their antibacterial activities against *S. aureus* and *E. coli* microorganisms by agar diffusion method.

Table 3. Some physical properties of 2-Aryl-2, 3-dihydro-1*H*-perimidines (3a to j).

No.	R	MF	Yield%	MP °C	Color	R_f Chloroform
3a	-H	$C_{17}H_{14}N_2$	52	198-200	Green	0.73
3b	4-F	$C_{17}H_{13}FN_2$	75	180-182	Pale violet	0.89
3c	4-OCH$_3$	$C_{18}H_{16}N_2O$	60	160-162	Pale violet	0.94
3d	2-Br	$C_{17}H_{13}BrN_2$	55	182-184	Pale pink	0.75
3e	4-CH$_3$	$C_{18}H_{16}N_2$	65	161-164	Pale pink	o.64
3f	4-Br	$C_{17}H_{13}BrN_2$	70	108-110	Greenish yellow	o.779
3g	2-OH	$C_{17}H_{14}N_2O$	68	188-191	Yellow	o.5
3h	2-NO$_2$	$C_{17}H_{13}N_3O_2$	60	170-174	Red	o.74
3i	4-NO$_2$	$C_{17}H_{13}N_3O_2$	90	202-204	Orange	o.6
3j	4-Cl	$C_{17}H_{13}ClN_2$	98	167-169	Yellow	0.56

Table 4. Assignments of characteristic frequencies (cm^{-1}) of IR spectra for the prepared 2-Aryl-2, 3-dihydro-1*H*-perimidine (3a to j).

Compounds	N-H str.	C-H str. (aromatic)	C-H str.	N-H Def.	*C=Cstr.*	*o-p-m* Subs.
3a	3368	3024	2987	1602	1490	699, 749
3b	3401	3040, 306	2800	1599	1506	815
3c	3365	3037	2795	1598	1512	813
3d	3380	3054	2800	1602	1589	747
3e	3365	3037, 2915	2795	1598	1483	814
3f	3347	3042	2849	1602	1588	812
3g	3368	3065	-	1602	1489	753
3h	3357	3357	2852	1601	1518	758
3i	3364	3069,3046	2799	1600	1512	815
3j	3379	3049	2800	1589	1488	817

Table 5. Chemical shift of ^{1}H-NMR and ^{13}C-NMR spectra data for some prepared 2-Aryl-2, 3-dihydro-1H-Perimidine (3a-j).Solvent: DMSO d$_6$

Compound	(δ) ppm
3b	^{1}H-NMR s, 1H6.7 (N-H); m, 10H6.5(C-H) Ar.; s, 1H5.4(C-H) Perimidine moiety
3e	^{1}H-NMR s, 1H 6.7(N-H); m,10H 6.4-7.4(C-H)Ar.; s,1H5.3(C-H) Perimidine moiety; s,3H 2.3(CH$_3$). ^{13}C-NMR C$_1$:138.186 C$_{2,2}$:129.66 C$_{3,3}$:127.289C$_4$:143.59C$_5$:66.628 C$_{6,6}$:139.32C$_{7,7}$:104.734C$_{8,8}$:128.252C$_{9,9}$:115.637C$_{10}$:134.846
3h	^{1}H-NMR s,1H 6.8(N-H); m,10H6.5-8(C-H)Ar.; s,1H5.8(C-H) Perimidine moiety. ^{13}C-NMR C$_1$:147.871C$_{2,2}$,127.14 C$_{3,3}$:129.493 C$_4$:150.294 C$_5$:63.359 C$_{6,6}$:142.516 C$_{7,7}$:105.041 C$_{8,8}$:123.855 C$_{9,9}$:116.045 C$_{10}$: 134.751. C$_{11}$:112: 832
3i	^{1}H-NMR s,1H 6.(N-H); m,10H(C-H)Ar.; s,1H5.8(C-H) Perimidine moiety. ^{13}C-NMR C$_1$C$_1$:147.871 C$_{2,2}$,127.14 C$_{3,3}$:129.493 C$_4$:150.294 C$_5$:63.359 C$_{6,6}$:142.516 C$_{7,7}$:105.041 C$_{8,8}$:123.855 C$_{9,9}$:116.045 C$_{10}$: 134.751 C$_{11}$:112: 832

From the results we concluded that most of the synthesized compounds were not effective against *S. aureus*, except the compound 3a which has clear activity against *S. aureus*, while all of the synthesized compounds (100%) showed a wide effect against *E. coli*, as well as the entire synthesized compounds compared to standard drug gentamicin and they showed higher effect than gentamicin.

Conflict of Interests

The author(s) have not declared any conflict of interests.

ACKNOWLEDGEMENTS

Deepest thanks to Mr. Muhannad Muhamad, Water,

Environment and Arid Regions Research Center (WEARRC), Central Labs, for measuring the spectroscopic data of this study, Al-Albayt University-Jordon. I would like to thank the head of Chemistry Department, College of Science and Education, Salahaddin University Erbil, Iraq, for their assistance. Finally, thanks to all staff and members of the College of Pharmacy and to all who assisted in executing this study.

REFERENCES

Akbar M, Naser F, Nemat B (2009). Zeolite catalyzed efficient synthesis of perimidines at room temperature. Turk. J. Chem. 33:555-560.

Cado, F, Di-Martino JL, Jacquault P, Bazureau JP, Hamelin J (1996). Amidine enamine tautomerism: addition of isocynate to 2-subistituted 1H-perimidine. Some synthesis of microwave irradiation. Bull. Soc. Chim. France 133(6):587-595.

Corn SN (1990). Novel near – infrared absorbing dyes. White Rose Etheses Online 1-2.

Davis R, Tamaoki N (2005). Photochromic proheterocyclic Molecules,2,3-Dihydro-2-spiro-7-[8-imino-7`,8`-dihydronaphthalene-1`amine] Perimidine. Org. Lett. 7:1461.

Davis BD (1987). Mechanism of bactericidal action of aminoglycosides. Microbial. Rev. 5(3):341.

David G, Richard S, John P, Mike B (2007). Medical Microbiology, 17th ed. Elsevier. P 57.

Fragoso RG, Ciferri R (1928). Hongos parasitos y saprifitos de la Republica Dominicana. Bull. R. Soc. Espan. Hist. Nat. 28:377-388.

Fred EH, Stefan GS (1969). Mechanism of action of Gentamicin. J. infect. Dis. 119 (4-5):364-369.

Gibson, TD, Puttick P, Hulbert JN, Marshall RW, Li Z (1999). Odor sensor. "5928609". Available at: http://www.freepatentsonline.com/5928609.html"

Harold CN, Thomas DG (1996). Medical Microbiology, 4th edition. University of Texas Medical Branch, Galveston. Chapter 11.

İhan I, Zerrin I, Dilovan Gand Yusuf Ö (2008). Cytotoxic effects of some perimidine derivatives on F2408 and 5Rp7 cell lines. FABAD J. Pharm. Sci. 33:135-143.

John MH, Woodgate PD, Denny WA (1987). Potential antitumor agents. 53. Synthesis, DNA binding properties, and biological activity of perimidines designed as "Minimal "DNA- Intercalating Agents. J. Med. Chem. 30:2081-2086.

Jacquelyn GB (2008). Microbiology, 7th edition. John Wiley & Sons Inc., Asia. P 383.

Kazuhiko H, Kanagawa JP, Kazunori A, Yuka I, Minquan T, Suguru N, Shinji H, Takashi M, Makoto F, Miho W, Tomoko M (2010). Perimidine substituted squarylium dye, dispersion medium, detection medium and image forming materials. Patent application. pp. 1-14.

Kang CL, Hsiu H (1984). Chen reaction of hydrazinoperimidine with Acetylacetone, J. Heterocyclic Chem. 21(3):911-912.

Kang CL, Chen HH (1985). Cyclocondensation of 2-Hydrazine perimidine with diethyl oxalate and ethyl pyruvate. J. Heterocycl. Chem. 22(5):1363-1364.

Marie-Paule ML, Youri G, Paul MT (1999). Aminoglycosides, Activity and Resistance. Antimicrob. Agents Chemother. 43(4):727-737.

Shakhawan ARO (2001). Synthesis of a new series of thiazolidinone derivatives with studying their biological activities. P 30.

Varsha G, Arun V, Robinson P, Manju S, Digna V, Leeju P, Jayachandran VP, Yusuff KKM (2010). Two new fluorescent heterocyclic perimidines: first syntheses, crystal structure and spectral characterization. Tetahedron Lett. pp1-7.

29

Effect of EDTA on the activity of ciprofloxacin against *Shigella sonnei*

Clement Jackson[1*], Musiliu Adedokun[1], Emmanuel Etim[1], Ayo Agboke[1], Idongesit Jackson[1] and Emmanuel Ibezim[2]

[1]Faculty of Pharmacy, University of Uyo, Akwa Ibom, Nigeria.
[2]Faculty of Pharmaceutical Sciences, University of Nigeria, Nsukka, Enugu State, Nigeria.

Ethylenediamine Tetraacetic Acid (EDTA) is a compound predominantly known for its chelating ability. It has also been found that in combination with antibacterial agents like benzakolium and chlorocresol, they were able to kill resistant bacteria. EDTA was used in combination with ciprofloxacin, a fluoroquinolone, against *Shigella sonnei*. This was done by determining their respective and combined Minimum Inhibitory Concentration (MIC) and using their obtained MIC in combination to obtain their fractional inhibitory concentration (F.I.C) in order to determine if their interaction is synergistic, antagonistic or additive. Results obtained using the checkerboard technique showed that combinations of EDTA with ciprofloxacin showed synergy at ratios of 9:1, 8:2, 7:3 and 6:4, and additive effect at ratios of 5:5, 4:6, 3:7 and 2:8.

Key words: EDTA, ciprofloxacin, *Shigella sonnei*, synergy.

INTRODUCTION

Several reasons have been advanced to justify the use of combination of two or more antibiotic treatments (Esimone et al., 2006b; Ibezim et al., 2006). For many years now; combination of two or more antibiotics has been recognized as an important method for, at least, delaying the emergence of bacterial resistance (Chambers, 2006). Besides, antibiotic combinations may also produce desirable synergistic effects in the treatment of bacterial infections (Zinner et al., 1981).

However, methods have been developed to quantify the effect of antimicrobial combinations on bacterial growth *in vitro.* Two very distinct traditional methods of testing *in vitro* antibiotic interaction are the checkerboard technique and the time killing curve method (Eliopoulos et al., 1988).

Ciprofloxacin is a broad-spectrum fluoroquinolone and possesses good activity against *Escherichia coli (E. coli)* and *Staphylococcus aureus*. It is active *in vitro* against *Citrobacter* spp., *Serratia* spp., *Klebsiella* spp., *Salmonella* spp., *Shigella* spp., etc. Recently, there have been reports of resistance to this, hitherto effective group

of antibiotics, by efflux mechanism described in *S. aureus* (De Chene et al., 1990).

It has been shown that chelating agents such as Ethylenediamine Tetraacetic Acid (EDTA) destabilize the outer membrane of gram negative bacteria by sequestering the stabilizing divalent cations. Such destabilization leads to the release of substantial (up to 40%) lipopolysaccharides, release of periplasmic enzymes and cell membrane associated proteins and phospholipids. Thus an EDTA-treated bacterium becomes susceptible to agents that do not normally penetrate the outer membrane and as a consequence do not affect the bacteria (Vaara, 1992). This phenomenon is often referred to as permeabilization.

MATERIALS AND METHODS

Culture media

The media used in the study included nutrient broth (Merck Germany), deoxycholate citrate agar (lab M, England) and nutrient agar (Merck Germany).

Test microorganism

Clinical isolates of *Shigella sonnei* were obtained from a patient

*Corresponding author. E-mail: clementjackson1@yahoo.com.

Table 1. Table of the combined activity of EDTA and ciprofloxacin against *Shigella sonnei*.

Drug ratio EDTA:Cipro 10:0	Mic. Mic EDTA: Cipro 150...	Fic. Fic EDTA: Cipro	FIC index	Activity index	Effect
9:1	33.75:12.5	0.225:0.025	0.25	-0.602	SYN
8.2	30:25	0.200:0.050	0.25	-0.602	SYN
7:3	52.5:75	0.35:0.15	0.50	-0.301	SYN
6:4	30.0:150	0.20:0.30	0.50	-0.301	SYN
5:5	90:200	0.60:0.4	1.0	0	ADD
4.6	75:250	0.50:0.50	1.0	0	ADD
3:7	45:350	0.3:0.70	1.0	0	ADD
2:8	30:400	0.2:0.80	1.0	0	ADD
1:9	15:450	0.1:0.90	1.0	0	ADD
0:10	.... : 500				

Key: SYN = synergism; ADD = addictive; CIPRO = ciprofloxacin; Activity index = Log $_{10}$(FIC index).

with dysentery in the Medical Center, University of Nigeria, Nsukka.

Isolation and identification of test microorganisn

Samples of microorganism on Desoxycholate citrate agar (DCA) incubated in air at 37°C for 24 h formed pale pink colonies of 1 - 2 mm in diameter. This test was used to identify *S. sonnei*.

Antimicrobial agents and disc

Ethylenediaminetetra acetic acid, dipotassium salt (sigma chemicals, USA) and sample of ciprofloxacin hydrochloride extracted from the tablets dosage form (Orange Drugs, Nigeria) were used. These were used to prepare the antibiotic disc using Whatman No. 1 filter paper in accordance with the NCCLS standards (1990).

Preparation of culture media

All culture media were prepared according to the manufacturer's specifications.

Maintenance and standardization of test microorganism

The microorganisms were maintained by weekly subculturing on nutrient agar slants stored at 4°C after previous 24 h incubation at 37°C. Prior to each experiment, the microorganisms were activated by successive subculturing and incubation. 24 h old cultures of the test organism were always used. Standardization of test microorganism was according to previously reported method (Chinwuba et al., 1994; Esimone et al., 1999).

Sensitivity of test microorganism

The sensitivity of test microorganism to EDTA and ciprofloxacin hydrochloride was evaluated by determining the minimum inhibitory concentration (MIC) of the antibiotics using the two-fold broth dilution technique previously described (NCCLS, 1990; Esimone et al., 1999).

Evaluation of combined effects of EDTA and ciprofloxacin

Stock solutions of EDTA (300 mg/ml) and ciprofloxacin (500 mg/ml) prepared in double-strength nutrient broth and autoclaved at 121°C for 15 min, were employed. Thereafter varying proportions of the EDTA and ciprofloxacin (cipro) were prepared according to the continuous variation checkerboard method previously described (NCCLS, 1990). Each proportion of the EDTA/ ciprofloxacin combination was serially diluted (2 fold), inoculated with 0.1 ml of 10^6 CFU/ ml culture of test microorganism and then incubated for 24 h at 37°C. Interaction was assessed algebraically by determining the fractional inhibitory concentration (FIC) indices according to the equations:

$$FIC_{index} = FIC_{EDTA} + FIC_{Cipro} \tag{1}$$

FIC_{EDTA} = Fractional inhibitory concentration of EDTA

$$= \frac{\text{MIC of EDTA in combination with ciprofloxacin}}{\text{MIC of EDTA}} \tag{2}$$

FIC_{cipro} = Fractional inhibitory concentration of ciprofloxacin

$$= \frac{\text{MIC of ciprofloxacin in combination with EDTA}}{\text{MIC of ciprofloxacin alone}} \tag{3}$$

RESULTS AND DISCUSSION

The combined effects of EDTA and ciprofloxacin against *S. sonnei* are presented in Table 1.

Combined drug use is occasionally recommended to prevent resistance emerging during treatment and to achieve higher efficacy in the treatment of infections and diseases. The combination is hoped to achieve a synergistic effect in this study. Results of the systematic and scientific evaluation of the in vitro effects of EDTA and Ciprofloxacin have been presented in this paper.

In the checkerboard technique, the interactions between EDTA and ciprofloxacin against *S. sonnei* indicate additivity at some combination ratios and synergy at other ratios as reflected in Table 1. FIC $_{index}$ values < 1 were considered as synergy and the degree of synergy increases as the value tends towards zero. FIC $_{index}$ values of 1 indicate additive effect, values greater than 1, but less than 2 represent indifference while values greater than 2 show antagonism (Vaara, 1992; Esimone et al., 1999).

Based on these, synergistic effect was obtained by combination of EDTA and ciprofloxacin against in the ratios (9:1, 8:2, 7:3, 6:4) while others (5:5, 4:6, 3:7, 2:8, 1:9) showed additive effect.

These results show that there is minor therapeutic advantage in the use of these agents (EDTA and ciprofloxacin) in combination therapy against infections due to *S. sonnei*. However, further work can be done using other chelating agents/quionolone combinations to see if there will be greater therapeutic benefits.

In conclusion, it may be stated that there is a favorable interaction between EDTA and Ciprofloxacin against *S. sonnei* in some given combination.

ACKNOWLEDGEMENTS

We appreciate the members of technical staff of Department of Pharmaceutics, University of Nigeria, Nsukka for their assistance. We also acknowledge the staff of God's Glory Computers Institute, Uyo, Nigeria for typing the article free, especially Miss Immaculata Idam.

REFERENCES

Chambers HF (2006). General principles of antimicrobial therapy, In Goodman and Gilman's pharmacologiced Basis of Therapeutics, Bruton LL(ed), 11th Ed., mc Graw Hill: USA, pp. 1102-1104.

Chinwuba GN, Chiori GO, Ghobashy AA, Okore VC (1994). Determination of synergy of Antibiotic combination by overlay inoculum susceptibility disc method. Drug Discov. Drug Res., 41: 148 –150.

De chene M, Leying H, Cullman (1990). W. role of the outer membrane for Quinolone resistances in Enterobacteria. Chemotherapy, 36: 13-23.

Eliopoulos GM, Eliopons CT (1988). Antibiotic combinations: should they be tested? Clin. Microbial Rev., 1: 139-156.

Esimone CO, Adikwu MU, Uzuegbu DB, Udeogaranya PO (1999). The effect of ethylenediaminetetraacetic acid on the antimicrobial properties of Benzoic acid and cetrimide. J. Pharm. Res. Dev., 4(1): 1-8.

Esimone CO, Iroha IR, CO Ude IG, Adikwu MU (2006). *In vitro* interaction of ampicillin with ciprofloxacin or spiramycin as determined by the Decimal assay for additivity technique. Niger. J. Health Biomed. Sci., 5(1): 12-16.

Ibezim EC, Esimone CO, Okorie O, Obodo CE, Nnamani PO, Brown SA, Onyishi IV (2006). A study of the *in vitro* interaction of cotrimoxazole and Ampicilin using the checkerboard method. Afr. J. Biotechnol., 5(13): 1284-1288.

National Committee for Clinical Laboratory standards (NCCLS) (1990). Performance standards For Antimicrobial Disc susceptibility test 4th ed.; approved Document M2 – a4 (NCCLS) villanova pa.

Vaara M (1992). Agents that increase the permeability of the outer membrane. Microb. Rev., 56: 395-411.

Zinner SN, Klastersky J, Gaya BC, Riff JC (1981). *In vivo* and *in vitro* studies of three antibiotic combinations against gram negative bacteria and *Staphylococcus aureus*. Antimicrob. Agents chemother., 20: 463-469.

30

Pharmacognostic evaluation of the *Amaranthus viridis* L.

Musharaf Khan[1]*, Shahana Musharaf[2], Mohammad Ibrar[1] and Farrukh Hussain[1]

[1]Department of Botany, University of Peshawar, Pakistan.
[2]Chemistry Government Girls Degree College, Sheikh, Malton Mardan, Pakistan.

The *Amaranthus viridis* Linn. (Family Amaranthaceae) plant was studied to determine the various parameters for pharmacognostical standards. The present investigation deals with the report on macro and microscopical, vein islet and vein termination numbers, palisade ratio, stomatal index (upper and lower surfaces of the leaf) and different chemical parameters have been determined. These findings will be useful towards establishing pharmacognostic standards on identification, purity, quality and classification of the plant, which is gaining relevance in plant drug research.

Key words: *Amaranthus viridis* Linn., pharmacognostical standards, macro and microscopical, chemical parameters.

INTRODUCTION

Amaranthus viridis Linn. is an annual herb, erect, 10 to 75 (-100) cm stem; slender, branched, angular, glabrous leaves; glabrous, long petiolate, 10 cm, lamina deltoid-ovate to rhomboid-oblong, 2 to 7 × 1.5 to 5.5 cm flowers; green, axillary or terminal, often paniculate spikes, 2.5 to 12 cm long and 25 mm wide. Bracts and bracteoles ovate to lanceolate-ovate, whitish, pale or reddish awn, bracteoles shorter than the perianth (1 mm); Perianth, male flowers, oblong-oval, acute, concave, 1.5 mm, female flowers narrowly oblong to narrowly spathulate, finally 1.25 to 1.75 mm, midrib green and thickened above. Stigmas 2 to 3, short, erect. Capsule subglobose, 1.25 to 1.5 mm. Seed, 1 to 1.25 mm, round, compressed, dark brown to black, reticulate. Flowering summer-fall (Ali and Qaiser (eds) 1995-2004). A decoction of the entire plant is used to stop dysentery and inflammation (Duke and Ayensu, 1985). The plant is antidiabetic, antihyperlipidemic and antioxidant (Ashok et al., 2010). The plant has antiproliferative and antifungal lectin (Kaur et al., 2006). The plant is emollient and vermifuge (Duke and Ayensu, 1985; Chopra et al., 1986). The root juice is used to treat inflammation during urination and constipation (Manandhar, 2002). The process of standardization can be achieved by stepwise pharmacognostic studies (Ozarkar, 2005). These studies help in identification and authentication of the plant material. Correct identification and quality assurance of the starting materials is an essential prerequisite to ensure reproducible quality of herbal medicine which will contribute to its safety and efficacy. Simple pharmacognostic techniques used in standardization of plant material include its morphological, anatomical and biochemical characteristics (Anonymous, 1998). However, *A. viridis* is a common plant in certain parts of Asia especially Pakistan, where it is consumed as a leafy vegetable but there is very less information is available about the pharmacognostic parameters of this plant and therefore study is designed for pharmacognostical evaluation of *A. viridis* aiming towards standardization and correct identification of this species and differentiate it from the other species. The objective of the present study is to evaluate various pharmacognostic standards like macroscopy and microscopy of *A. viridis* and microscopical characteristics of powdered plant specie.

MATERIALS AND METHODS

The first step in standardization of herbal drugs is the correct identification of plant macroscopic and microscopic characters. The fresh specimens of the plants were collected from the Department of Botany, University of Peshawar, Pakistan. The taxonomic identity of the plant was confirmed by Department of Botany Peshawar,

---
*Corresponding author. E-mail: k.musharaf@gmail.com.

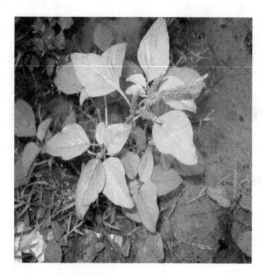

Figure 1. *A. viridis* L.

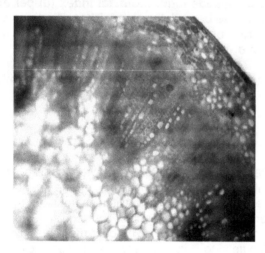

Figure 2. Transverse section of stem shows xylem and phloem.

University, Pakistan. A voucher specimen has been deposited in department herbarium. The specimen was cleaned, washed and air dried for 15 days and was used for different tests, that is, microchemical tests. These entire specimens were ground with the help of electric grinder and were preserved in airtight bottles to combat climatic conditions and moisture. Some fresh specimens were used to study morphological characters and anatomical parameters.

Macroscopy

The following macroscopic characters for the fresh parts of plant were noted: Size and shape, colour, surfaces, venation, the apex, margin, base, lamina, texture, odour and taste (Wallis, 1985; Evans, 2002).

Microscopy

The anatomies of the root, stem and leaf were determined by a

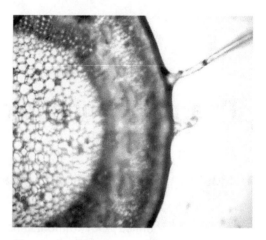

Figure 3. Transverse section of root show pericycle, cortex etc.

standard method (Wallis, 1985; Evans, 2002). The outer epidermal membranous layer of leaf (in fragments) were cleared in chloral hydrate, mounted with glycerin and observed under a compound microscope. The presence/absence of epidermal cells and stomata (type and distribution) were observed. The transverse sections of the fresh leaf, stem and root as well as a small quantity of the powdered plant were also cleared, mounted and observed under a compound microscope (Clark, 1960; Bokhari, 1971; Cotton, 1974; African Pharmacopoeia, 1986; Subrahmanyam, 1996).

Chemomicroscopic examination

Examination of the powder for starch grains, lignin, mucilage, calcium oxalate crystals, cutin and suberin were carried out using standard techniques (Evans, 2002).

Phytochemical investigation

Chemical tests were employed in the preliminary phytochemical screening for various secondary metabolites such as tannins, cardiac glycosides, alkaloids, saponins, anthracene derivatives and cyanogenetic glycosides (Johansen, 1940; Brain and Turner, 1975; Ciulei, 1981; Harborne, 1992; Evans, 2002).

Quantitative investigation

Quantitative leaf microscopy to determine palisade ratio, stomata number, stomata index, vein – islet number and veinlet termination number were carried out on epidermal peelings (British Pharmacopoeia, 1980).

RESULTS AND DISCUSSION

A. viridis is currently being used in the treatment of various disease conditions without standardization. The standardization of a crude drug is an integral part of establishing its correct identity. Before any crude drug can be included in a herbal pharmacopoeia, pharmacognostic parameters and standards must be established (Figures 1-5). *A. viridis* is a plant that has

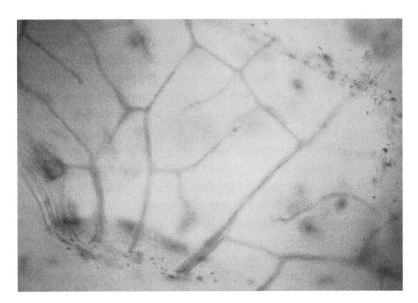

Figure 4. Lower side of leaf vein islet number and vein termination number.

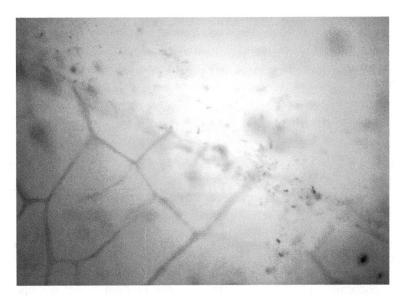

Figure 5. Upper side of leaf vein islet number and vein termination number.

been confused with other species due to their relative similarities. The results of these investigations could, therefore, serve as a basis for proper identification, collection and investigation of the plant. The macro – and micro – morphological features of the plant described, distinguishes it from other members of the genera. Chemomicroscopy, numerical data and quantitative plant microscopy are parameters that are unique to the plant and are required in its standardization.

Colour of the upper surface of the leaf is dark green and that of the lower surface is light green in fresh while in dry form both surfaces are light green in colour. Venation of the leaf was reticulate and unicostate. In both fresh and dry forms of the leaf; shape was cordate,

composition was simple, margin was entire and apex was obtuse. In both fresh and dry forms of the stem: Kind was herbaceous, colour was light green, shape was cylindrical, direction of the growth was upright, fracture was fiberous, surface was smooth and phyllotaxis was opposite while odour was irritating in fresh and indistinct in dry form. In both fresh and dry forms of the root, the colour was whitish, shape was cylindrical, rootlets were present, direction of growth was horizontally downward, fracture was fibrous and texture was smooth while odour was pungent in fresh and indistinct in dry form (Table 1).

Leaf epidermal cells, both sides with polyhedral to hexagonal shaped of smooth walls. Size of epidermal cells; adaxail -137 × 45 µm. Stomata of anisocytic to

Table 1. Macroscopical features of the different parts of *A. viridis* L.

Plant part	Parameter	Fresh plant	Dry plant
Leaf	Colour	Upper surface dark green; lower surface light green	Both surface light green
	Composition	Simple	Simple
	Venation	Reticulate; unicostate	Reticulate; unicostate
	Margin	Entire	Entire
	Apex	Obtuse	Obtuse
	Shape of leaf	Cordate	Cordate
Stem	Colour	Light green	Light green
	Odour	Irritating	Indistinct
	Shape	Cylindrical	Cylindrical
	Phyllotaxy	Opposite	Opposite
	Kind	Herbaceous	Herbaceous
	Direction of growth	Upward	Upward
	Fracture	Fiberous	Fiberous
	Texture	Smooth	Smooth
Root	Colour	Whitish	Whitish
	Odour	Pungent	Indistinct
	Shape	Cylindrical	Cylindrical
	Rootlets	Present	Present
	Direction of growth	Horizontal downward	Horizontal downward
	Fracture	Fiberous	Fiberous
	Texture	Smooth	Smooth
	Composition	Simple	Simple
	Venation	Reticulate; unicostate	Reticulate; unicostate
	Margin	Entire	Entire
	Apex	Obtuse	Obtuse
	Shape of leaf	Cordate	Cordate

staurocytic type, with the length of 85 μm aperture size 12 μm. Epidermis of the stem is spherical in shape and is compactly packed. The mean length of the epidermis cells, cortical tissue, endodermis, pericycle, xylem, phloem, pith and parenchymatous cells was found to be 25, 13, 16, 15, 29, 20, 14 and 18 μm, respectively while the mean width was found 15, 7, 13, 11, 14, 12, 10 and 12 μm, respectively. Epidermis of the root is rectangular in shape and is compactly packed. The mean length of the epidermis cells, cortical tissue, endodermis, pericycle, xylem, phloem, pith and parenchymatous cells was found to be 34, 25, 19, 10, 14, 18, 34 and 13, respectively while the mean width was found 12, 18, 10, 5, 11, 12, 18 and 9 μm, respectively (Table 2).

Vein termination ranges from 44.65 t0 57.25, vein islet number ranges from 14.56 to 23.57 and the palisade ration ranges from15.62 to 24.42. Stomatal index of the upper surface of leaf is 21.25 to 24.62 and of the lower surface of the leaf of the plant 42.54 to 43.47 (Table 3). Alkaloids (Alk), saponins (Sap), starch (Sta), fat, protein (Pro) and cellulose (Cel) were present in all parts of the plant. Mucilage (Muc) and calcium oxalate (Cao) were present in stem only and were absent from other parts of the plant. Anthraquinon derivatives (Anth) and lignin (Lig) were present in root and stem and were absent from leaf and flower of the plant (Table 4). Yadav et al. (2007) reported flavonoids, saponins, steroids, alkaloids, carbohydrates and proteins in *Chenopodium album* Linn. root. Tannin was absent from all parts of the plant. Cutin was present in stem and leaf and was absent from root and flower. Badami et al. (2007) reported alkaloids, carbohydrates, proteins and amino acids, steroids, glycosides, saponins, tannins and fixed oils in *Caesalpinia sappan*.

A. viridis is a plant which is known to have some ethno pharmacological activities and is being well researched on. The results of these investigations could, therefore, serve as a basis for proper identification, collection and investigation of the plant. These parameters which are being reported for the first time could also be useful in the preparation of the herbal section of the proposed Pakistani Pharmacopoeia. Any crude drug which is

Table 2. Anatomical features of the root and stem of the *A. viridis* L.

Plant cell	Value	Root Length (µm)	Root Width (µm)	Stem Length (µm)	Stem Width (µm)
Epidermis	Minimum	25	10	22	14
	Maximum	43	16	30	18
	Mean	34	12	25	15
Cortex	Minimum	20	15	10	05
	Maximum	28	21	17	09
	Mean	25	18	13	07
Enodermis	Minimum	13	09	19	11
	Maximum	24	12	12	16
	Mean	19	10	16	13
Pericycle	Minimum	07	04	12	09
	Maximum	12	07	19	13
	Mean	10	05	15	11
Xylem	Minimum	12	09	26	12
	Maximum	19	14	34	19
	Mean	14	11	29	14
Phloem	Minimum	15	10	18	10
	Maximum	21	14	25	16
	Mean	18	12	20	12
Pith	Minimum	27	16	12	08
	Maximum	38	22	18	14
	Mean	34	18	14	10
Parenchyma	Minimum	10	07	15	10
	Maximum	17	12	21	15
	Mean	13	09	18	12

Table 3. Microscopic characteristics of the *A. viridis* L. Leaf.

S/No.	Parameter	Value
1	Vein Islet number	14.56 - 23.57/mm^2
2	Vein termination number	44.65 - 47.25/mm^2
3	Palisade ratio	15.62 - 17.42/mm^2
4	Stomatal index (Upper surface)	21.25 - 24.62
5	Stomatal index (Lower surface)	42.54 - 43.47

Table 4. Microchemical screening tests of the different parts of *A. viridis* L.

Plant part	Alk	Muc	Anth	Cao	Sap	Tan	Sta	Fat	Pro	Lig	Cut	Cel
Flower	+	-	-	-	+	-	+	+	+	-	-	+
Leaf	+	-	-	-	+	-	+	+	+	-	+	+
Stem	+	+	+	+	+	-	+	+	+	+	+	+
Root	+	-	+	-	+	-	+	+	+	+	-	+

+: Positive test; - : Negative test; Alk: Alkaloids; Sap: Saponins; Sta: Starch; Prp: Protein; Cel: Cellulose; Muc: Mucilage; Cao: Calcium oxalate; Anth: Anthraquinon derivatives, Lig: Lignin.

claimed to be *A. viridis* but whose characters significantly deviate from the accepted standard aforementioned would then be rejected either as contaminated, adulterated or down right fake.

REFERENCES

African Pharmacopoeia (1986). General methods for Analysis. OAU / STRC Scientific Publications, Lagos, 2(2): 0–5, 137–149, 223-237.

Ali SI, Qaiser M (eds) (1995-2004). Flora of Pakistan, Department of Botany, University of Karachi, Karachi, p. 12.

Anonymous (1998). Macroscopic and microscopic Examination: Quality Control Methods for Medicinal Plant Materials, WHO, Geneva.

Ashok KBS, Lakshman K, Jayaveea KN, Sheshadri SD, Saleemulla K, Thippeswamy BS, Veerapur VP (2010). Antidiabetic, antihyperlipidemic and antioxidant activities of methanolic extract of *Amaranthus viridis* Linn in alloxan induced diabetic rats. Exp. Toxicol. Pathol., Available online 18 July, 2010.

Badami S, Rai SR, Moorkoth S, Rajan S, Suresh B (2007). Pharmacognostic evaluation of *Caesalpinia sappan*. Hamdard Medicus, 50(1): 103–108.

Bokhari MH (1971). Morphology and Taxonomic Significance of Sclereids in *Limonium*. Notes. R. Bot. Gbn. Edin. 30: 43-53.

Brain KR, Turner TD (1975). Practical evaluation of phytopharmaceuticals. Wright – Scientechnica, Bristol. 1st Ed., p. 144.

British Pharmacopoeia (1980). Appendix XI. Her Majesty's Stationery Office,London, A108, 11: A113.

Chopra RN, Nayar SL, Chopra IC (1986). Glossary of Indian Medicinal Plants (Including the Supplement). Council of Scientific and Industrial Research, CSIR Publications, New Delhi.

Ciulei I (1981). Methodology for analysis of vegetable drugs. United Nations Industrial Development Organisation. Romania, pp. 17-25.

Clark J (1960). Preparation of leaf epidermis for topographic study. Stain Technol., 33: 35-39.

Cotton R (1974). Cytotaxonomy of the genus *Vulpia*. *Ph. D Thesis*, University of Manchester, USA.

Duke JA, Ayensu ES (1985). Medicinal Plants of China Reference Publications, Inc., pp. 20-24.

Evans WC (2002). Trease and Evans Pharmacognosy. 13th ec Bailliere Tindall, London, pp. 654–656.

Harborne JB (1992). Phytochemical methods. A guide to moder technique of plant analysis. Chapman and Hill, London, p. 279.

Johansen DA (1940). Plant microtechnique. McGraw Hill Boo Company. New York and London, pp. 189–202.

Kaur N, Dhuna V, Kamboj SS, Agrewala JN, Singh J (2006). A nove antiproliferative and antifungal lectin from *Amaranthus viridis* Lin seeds. Protein Pept. Lett., 13(9): 897-905.

Manandhar NP (2002). Plants and People of Nepal Timber Press Oregon, p. 6.

Ozarkar KR (2005). Studies on anti-inflammatory effects of two herb *Cissus quadrangularis* Linn. and *Valeriana wallichi* DC using mous model. Ph.D. Thesis,University of Mumbai, Mumbai.

Subrahmanyam NS (1996). Labortary Manual of Plant Taxonomy, Vika Publishing house pvt., Ltd., New Delhi, India, pp. 153–156.

Wallis TE (1985). Textbook of Pharmacognosy, 5th Edition. CBS Publishers and Distributors, 485 Jain Bhawan, Shahdara Delhi, pp 252-253.

Yadav N, Vasudeva N, Sharma SK, Singh S (2007). Pharmacognosti and phytochemical studies on *Chenopodium album* Linn., roo Hamdard Medicus, 50(1): 95–102.

31

Instrumental and chemical characterization of *Moringa oleifera* Lam root starch as an industrial biomaterial

Fagbohun Adebisi[1], Adebiyi Adedayo[1], Adedirin Oluwaseye[1], Fatokun Adekunle[1], Afolayan Michael[1], Olajide Olutayo[1], Ayegba Clement[1], Pius Ikokoh[1], Kolawole Rasheed[2] and Aiyesanmi Ademola[2]

[1]Chemistry Advanced Laboratory, Sheda Science & Technology Complex, PMB 186 Garki, Abuja, FCT, Nigeria.
[2]Department of Chemistry, Federal University of Technology, Akure, Ondo State, Nigeria.

Moringa oleifera Lam. (Moringaceae family) is a deciduous plant with tuber-like root at the earlier stage. Starch was isolated from the young tuber of the plant and examined instrumentally for its functional groups, X-ray diffractometer (XRD) profile, elemental analysis and antioxidant activities. The Fourier transform infrared spectroscopy analysis shows that peaks at 3465.23 to 3577.11 cm^{-1} represent OH stretch of alcohol; 3385.18 cm^{-1} represents O-H band of carboxylic acid; 3116.11 cm^{-1} represents =CH stretch of alkenes; 1647.26 cm^{-1} represents C=C stretch of alkenes and 1023.27 cm^{-1} represents C-O stretch. The result of elemental analysis revealed that the starch granules contained: Fe (430.19 ppm), Cu (0.055 ppm) and Zn (0.19 ppm). XRD pattern revealed that the starch granules is an amorphous material and contained iron complex ($C_{24}H_{16}FeN_{10}$). The radical scavenging activity of the plant extract against DPPH (Sigma-Aldrich) was determined by UV-visible spectrophotometer at 517 nm. The result showed higher absorbance of the reaction mixture which indicated lower free radical scavenging activity and the degree of increment in absorbance measurement is indicative of the radical scavenging power of the extract, hence the anti-oxidant capacity and scavenging activity of the starch suspension revealed that it has a very low activity and percentage inhibition when compared with the ascorbic acid standard.

Key words: *Moringa oleifera*, phytochemical screening, antioxidant activity, X-ray diffractometer.

INTRODUCTION

Moringa oleifera Lam. (Moringaceae) is one of the fourteen species of the family Moringaceae, native to India, Africa, Arabia, Southeast Asia, South America and Caribbean Islands (Iqbal et al., 2006). It is commonly called Ben oil tree and locally known as *Zogeli* among the Hausa speaking tribe in Nigeria. Almost every part of *M. oleifera* is useful to man and as forage for livestock.

Recently, starch granules were isolated from the young *M. oleifera* root and physicochemical properties determined (Fagbohun et al., 2013). Some lesser known and unconventional native starch could be good sources of nutrients and industrial biomaterial but the lack of data on the chemical composition and properties of such plants has limited the prospects for their utilization (Viano et al., 1995). Starch is also one of the most widely used biomaterial in the food, textile, cosmetics, plastics, adhesives, paper and pharmaceutical industries. The diverse industrial usage of starch is based on its availability at low cost, high calorific value and inherent excellent physicochemical properties (Omojola et al., 2010). The versatility of starch in industrial applications is clearly defined by its physicochemical properties; therefore, a thorough evaluation of the necessary parameters is important in elucidating its industrial uses.

As a result of the competing demands for starch as food, pharmaceutical and industrial uses coupled with the need to attain self sufficiency in starch production, there is a need to find other high yield sources different from cassava, maize and potato (Gebre-Mariam et al., 2006). Little or no work appears to have been done on the isolation and instrumental characterization of starch from M. oleifera Lam. root. Therefore, the objective of the present study is to isolate starch from M. oleifera root and characterize by Fourier Transform Infrared Spectrophotometer (FTIR), Atomic Absorption Spectrophotometer (AAS), High resolution X-ray Diffractometer (XRD), UV/Visible Spectrophotometer, and Phytochemical Screening.

MATERIALS AND METHODS

Sampling

Two years old M. oleifera was harvested using cutlass from medicinal and botanical gardens located in Sheda Science and Technology Complex (SHESTCO) near Kwali, Abuja (8° 21' N; 6° 25' E) in 2013 and was duly identified in Chemistry Advanced Laboratory of the same organization. Analytical grade reagents were obtained from Chemistry Advanced Laboratory, Sheda Science and Technology Complex, Abuja Nigeria.

Starch isolation

The method of Loss et al. (2012) was adapted with slight modification. Briefly, the fresh roots were peeled and washed thoroughly with water to remove dirt. Peeled tubers (0.944 kg) were chopped into small pieces and wet milled into slurry using a grater and laboratory blender. The paste was dispersed in 3 L of distilled water and filtered through muslin cloth. The filtrate was allowed to stand 24 h. The supernatant was carefully decanted and the mucilage scraped off. This process was repeated three times continuously until a pure starch granule was obtained. The resulting starch was dried in the sun and further dried at 60°C in a hot air oven, pulverized, weighed and stored in sample bottles for instrumental and chemical analysis. The percentage yield was calculated as:

$$\% \text{ Percentage yield} = \frac{\text{Weight of starch granules isolated}}{\text{Weight of peeled tuber chopped}} \times 100 \quad (1)$$

Phytochemical screening

Phytochemical screening was carried out on the starch using methods previously described by Harborne (1973), Trease and Evans (1989) and Sofowora (1993).

Mineral analysis

The following minerals were determined: calcium (Ca), magnesium (Mg), potassium (K), sodium (Na), iron (Fe), zinc (Zn), manganese (Mn), copper (Cu), nickel (Ni), chromium (Cr) and cobalt (Co) using the atomic absorption spectrophotometer (AAS-Shimadzu Japan), as described by the methods of the Association of Official Analytical Chemists (AOAC) (1990). All the determinations were done in duplicates. The concentrations of the mineral content of the starch granule were reported in milligram per gram (mg/g).

Determination of antioxidant activity

The radical scavenging activities of the plant extracts against 2, 2-diphenyl-1-picrylhydrazyl (DPPH) were determined by UV-visible spectrophotometer CECIL, England at 517 nm. Radical scavenging activity was measured by a slightly modified method previously described (Ayoola et al., 2008; Brand-Williams et al., 1995). The following concentrations of the extract were prepared, 0.05, 0.1, 0.2, 0.5, 1.0, 2.0, and 5.0 mg/ml in methanol (Analar grade). Vitamin C (ascorbic acid) was used as the antioxidant standard at concentrations of 0.05, 0.1, 0.2, 0.5, 1.0, 2.0 and 5.0 mg/ml. 1 ml of the extract was placed in a test tube and 3 ml of methanol was added, followed by 0.5 ml of 1 mM DPPH in methanol and thereafter the decrease in absorption was measured on a UV-visible double beam spectrophotometer, CECIL England, ten minutes later. A blank/control solution was prepared containing the same amount of methanol and DPPH. The actual decrease in absorption was measured against that of the control. All test and analysis were run in duplicates and the results obtained were averaged. The radical scavenging activity (RSA) was calculated as the percentage inhibition of DPPH discolouration using the equation below:

$$\% \text{ Inhibition} = \frac{A_b - A_a}{A_b} \times 100 \quad (2)$$

Where Ab is the absorption of the blank sample (without the extract) and Aa is the absorption of the extract.

FT-IR analysis

The FT-IR spectra were obtained using FT-IR-8400S Fourier transform infrared spectrophotometer Shimadzu Japan. The spectra were recorded in transmission mode from 4,000 to 500 cm^{-1} (mid-infrared region) at a resolution of 0.44 cm^{-1}. The sample was mixed with KBr and compressed (1:100, w/w) before acquisition and the background value from pure KBr was acquired before the sample was scanned.

XRD analysis

In order to further characterize M. oleifera root starch, the XRD profile was obtained using high resolution X-ray diffractometer X pert Pro Analytical (Holland) set at the following operating conditions: anode material-copper, original K-Alpha1 wave lenght: 1.54060 Å, used K-Alpha 1 wavelength-1.54060 Å, original K-Alpha2 wavelenght-1.54443 Å, original K-Beta wavelength-1.39225 Å, specimen length 10.00 mm K-A2/K-A1 ratio 0.500, distance

Table 1. The result of Antioxidant activity *of M.oleifera* root starch.

Concentration (mg/ml)	% Inhibition of *Moringa* starch	% Inhibition of Vit. C
5.000	33.86	85.00
3.000	26.06	91.41
2.000	26.09	91.50
1.000	13.13	91.32
0.500	14.61	90.47
0.100	2.080	90.19
0.050	41.13	90.12

Table 2. Phytochemical screening of *M.oleifera root* starch.

Parameter	Result
Carbohydrate	+
Terpenoids	-
Flavonoids	+
Resin	-
Saponin	+
Alkaloids	-
Sterols	-
Glycosides	+
Tanin	-
Cardiac glycoside	-
Tanin	-
Cardiac glycoside	-
Anthrancene	-
Plobatanin	-
Phenol	-
Volatile oil	-
Carbohydrate	+

focus-diverg. Slit-100 mm; step size°2Th -0.0040, scan step time - 8.8900 s. The samples were incubated in a chamber at 100% RH for 24 h and then packed tightly in a circular aluminum cell. The samples were exposed to the X-ray beam from an X-ray generator running continuously at 40 kV and 30 mA and scanning regions of the diffraction angle, 2θ, were 9.9991 to 40.9831°, which covered most of the significant diffraction peaks of the starch crystallites. Duplicate measurements were made at ambient temperature. Radiation was detected with a proportional detector. The XRD pattern was generated from the data acquired using Microsoft Office Excel 2007 application.

RESULTS AND DISCUSSION

Yield and nature of the starch

The starch obtained was found to be a pure white, crystalline, non-hygroscopic powder with a yield of about 53%. The yield is therefore comparable with previous work on some native starch such as *Icacina trichantha* (76.8 %) and *Anchomanes difformis* (21%) (Omojola et

al., 2010).

Antioxidant analysis

The DPPH test provides information on the reactivity of the test compounds with stable free radical and it gives a strong absorption band at 517 nm in visible region. When the odd electron becomes paired off in the presence of a free radical scavenger, the absorption reduces and the DPPH solution was decolorized as the colour changed from deep violet to light yellow. The starch extract is not a good antioxidant because the colour did not change even at lower concentrations. It also showed higher absorbance of the reaction mixture indicated lower free radical scavenging activity and the degree of increment in absorbance measurement is an indication of the radical scavenging power of the extract as shown in Table 1.

Flavonoids and tannins are phenolic compounds and plant phenol is a major group of compounds that act as primary antioxidant or free radical scavengers (Polterait, 1997). The biological functions of flavonoids include protection against allergies, inflammation, free radicals scavenging platelets aggregation, microbes, ulcers, hepatoxins, viruses and tumors (Ayoola et al., 2008). It is worthy to note that these phytochemicals responsible for the mentioned activities must have been lost during the starch processing as revealed in Table 2.

Infrared analysis

FT-IR is a powerful technique for elucidation of structural changes in samples, with the ability of discovering differences not seen by certain other techniques because it has a unique region known as the finger print region where the position and intensity of bands is specific for every polysaccharide. The FT-IR evaluation of starches in four main regions helps in the successive interpretation of the key bands. These regions are as follows: below 800 cm[-1], 800 to 1500 cm[-1] (the finger print region), the region between 2800 and 3000 cm[-1] (C-H stretch region) and finally the region between 3000 and 3600 cm[-1] (O-H stretch region). The FT-IR spectrum of the starch showed the following bands as indicated in the Table 4.

Table 3. The results of elemental analysis of *M. oleifera* root starch.

Metal	Copper (Cu)	Nickel (Ni)	Chromium (Cr)	Zinc (Zn)	Calcium (Ca)	Iron (Fe)	Manganese (Mn)
Conc. (mg/g)	0.002755	BDL	0.02	0.01	BDL	21.51	BDL

BDL: Below detection limit.

Table 4. FTIR analysis result of *M. oleifera* Lam root starch.

S/no.	Peak	Intensity	Corr. intensity	Base (H)	Base (L)	Area	Corr. area
1	621.1	30.272	9.321	678	339.48	139.468	37.891
2	751.3	28.509	5.838	831.35	678.97	76.091	5.414
3	849.67	37.358	0.112	872.82	832.31	17.295	0.029
4	1023.27	23.611	2.872	1057.99	873.78	100.319	4.323
5	1106.21	23.565	2.301	1267.27	1058.96	118.903	3.881
6	1357.93	25.504	12.302	1562.39	1268.24	143.42	27.321
7	1647.26	35.48	17.516	1856.55	1563.36	89.374	14.154
8	2143.95	56.447	3.067	2313.69	1857.51	106.344	4.298
9	2916.47	24.657	9.082	3007.12	2313.69	261.573	12.862
10	3116.11	24.583	0.615	3129.61	3008.09	69.782	1.123
11	3177.83	24.133	0.604	3231.84	3130.57	61.958	0.538
12	3277.17	24.625	0.35	3345.64	3232.8	68.3	0.359
13	3465.23	24.88	0.345	3440.16	3346.61	56.202	0.281
14	3465.23	25.3	0.404	3536.6	3441.12	56.195	0.343
15	3577.11	26.347	2.834	3897.3	3537.57	142.823	2.56
16	4002.43	49.548	0.891	4181.81	3898.27	84.896	1.092
17	4661.14	50.299	0.419	4700.68	4521.29	52.811	0.343

3116.11 to 3577.11 cm^{-1} represent (O-H stretch); 2916.11 cm^{-1} represent (C-H stretch); the absorption peak at 3465.23 to 3577.11 cm^{-1} represent OH stretch of alcohol, 3385.18 cm^{-1} represent OH broad of carboxylic acid and phenol; 3116.11 cm^{-1} represent =CH stretch of alkenes; 1647.26 cm^{-1} represent C=C of stretch of alkenes; 1023.27 cm^{-1} represent C-O stretch. Aromatic absorption is absent in the diagnostic region (1600 and 1500 cm^{-1}) but medium intensity absorption at 1644 cm^{-1} is due to water absorbed in the amorphous region of the starch. 1357.95 cm^{-1} represent CH_2OH.

The absorption peak at 1106.21 cm^{-1} represents coupling mode of C-C and C-O stretching vibrations while the band at 1106.21 cm^{-1} represent C-O-H bending vibration. The absorption at 849.67 cm^{-1} vibration is typical of the system (C-O-C), skeletal mode vibration of α-1,4-glycosidic linkage while 621.1 cm^{-1} represent the skeletal mode of pyranose ring; 1106.21 cm^{-1} represents C-O and C-C stretch. The spectra of starch show complex vibrational modes at low numbers below 800 cm^{-1} due to skeletal vibration of the glucose pyranose ring (Sekkal et al., 1995). The absorption peak at 849.67 cm^{-1} represents C-H out of place of aromatics (Brandon, 2012). The region between 800 and 1500 cm^{-1} (finger print region) is the empirical proof of identity characteristics of the sample identity and the pattern of vibration and band location is unique for starch sample. Although it provides complex and overlapping spectra at this region, making the exact assignment of band difficult. But the IR spectrum of polysaccharides in this region originates from the vibrational state of its monomer glucose (Cerna et al., 2003). Therefore information obtained from glucose spectra is used in the assignments of wave numbers corresponding to the vibrational mode of starch.

Since starches exhibit very similar spectra characteristics with glucose in this region. Therefore in this study, the major bands below 800 cm^{-1} from 625-581 cm^{-1} and minor bands between 560 and 400 cm^{-1} in the FTIR spectra of the starch was attributed to the skeletal modes of the glucose pyranose ring, since starch exhibit very similar spectra characteristics with glucose in this region (Kemas et al., 2012).

Elemental analysis

As shown in Table 3, it was observed that *M. olifera* starch contain the following elements in their various concentrations: Cu (0.002755 mg/g), Cr (0.02 mg/g), Zn (0.01 mg/g) and Fe (21.51 mg/g).The trace metals like copper, iron and zinc are essential cofactors for a number of biological processes, including mitochondrial oxidative

Table 5. Peak list.

Pos.[°2Th]	Height [cm]	FWHM [°2Th]	d-spacing [Å]	Rel.Int.[%]
11.3175	52.61	0.4408	7.81860	7.26
15.1251	272.06	0.6298	5.85781	37.55
17.1776	724.55	0.2204	5.16223	100.00
19.6726	46.92	0.5038	4.51279	6.48
22.2002	197.08	0.6298	4.00437	27.20
24.3275	189.65	0.3149	3.65883	26.18
26.2960	69.56	0.7557	3.38922	9.60
38.2726	28.72	0.6298	2.35173	3.96

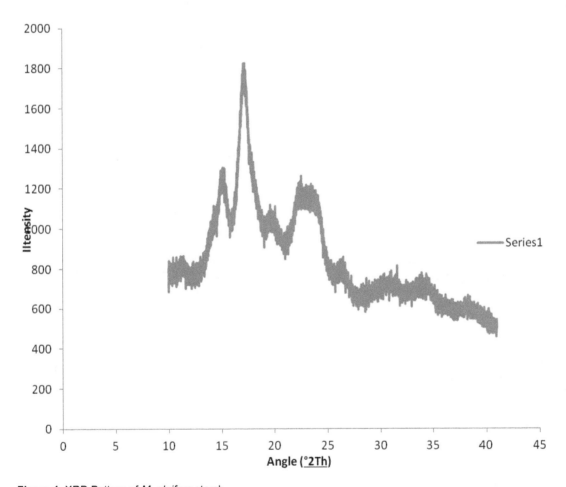

Figure 1. XRD Pattern of *M. oleifera* starch.

phosphorylation, free radical detoxification, neurotransmitter synthesis and maturation and iron metabolism.

X-ray diffractometer analysis

From the XRD pattern shown in the Figure 1 and Table 5, eight peaks were identified; six of these peaks can be seen as major peaks. The reflections at 17.18°, 15.13° and 22.2° correspond to the reflections in yam starch (generated from library) at 17.04°, 14.9° and 22.2°, respectively. Within experimental error, all the major peaks in the yam starch match with the major peaks in the sample. The high background is due to the amorphous nature of the starch. It was also observed that iron complex ($C_{24}H_{16}FeN_{10}$) was recorded as one of the compounds detected. X-ray diffraction has offered academia a potent tool for elucidating molecular structures of crystalline or semi-crystalline materials; however, its use as an analytical tool in the food industry is likely limited somewhat due to the expense associated with the instrumentation. Nevertheless, research has developed methods for measuring the relative percentages of the crystalline and amorphous phases in starches (Nara et al., 1978).

Conclusion

Some instrumental and chemical analyses of *M. oleifera* starch have been examined and the results presented. The percentage yield as indicated previously showed that *M. oleifera* starch is comparable with other native starch isolated. Thus, the starch can be derivatized and characterized with scanning electron microscope (SEM), Rapid visco-Analyzer (RVA) and differential scanning colorimeter (DSC) to really demonstrate its potential as industrial biomaterials.

Conflict of Interests

The author(s) have not declared any conflict of interests.

REFERENCES

Association of Official Analytical Chemists (AOAC) (1990). Official methods of Analysis.15th Ed, Association of official Analytical chemists. Washington D.C. pp. 808:831-835.

Ayoola GA, Sofidiya T, Odukoya O, Coker HAB. (2006). Phytochemical Screening and Free Radical Scavenging Activity of Some Nigerian Medicinal Plants. J. Pharm. Sci. Pharm. Pract. 8:133-136.

Brandon H (2012). Characterization of Starch by Vibrational Spectroscopy. University of Nebraska, Lincoln.

Brand-Williams W, Cuvelier MO, Berset C (1995). Use of Free Radical Method to Evaluate Antioxidant Activity. Lebensmittel Wissenchaft Technol. 28:25-50.

Cerna M, Antonio SB, Alexandra N, Silvia MR, Ivonne D, Jana C, Manuel AC.(2003). Use of FTIR spectroscopy as a tool for the analysis of polysaccharide food additives. Carbohydr. Polym. 51:383-389.

Fagbohun AA, Afolayan M, Ikokoh P, Olajide O, Adebiyi A, Fatokun O, Ayesanmi A, Orishadipe A (2013). Isolation and Characterization Studies of *Moringa oleifera* Root Starch as a Potential Pharmaceutical and Industrial Biomaterial. Int. J. Chem. Appl. 5(2):117-126.

Gebre – Mariam T, Schmidt PC (1996). Isolation and physicochemical properties of Endset starch. Starch 48(6):208-214.

Harbone JB (1973). Phytochemical Methods. Chapman and Hall Ltd., London. pp. 49-188.

Iqbal S, Bhanger MI (2006). Effect of season and production location on antioxidant activity of *Moringa oleifera* leaves grown in Pakistan. J. Food Comp. Anal. 19:544-551.

Iwu MM (1993). Handbook of African Medicinal Plants. CRC Press Inc., Boca Raton.

Kizil R, Irudayaraj J (2008). Applications of Raman Spectroscopy for Food Quality Measurement. In: Irudayaraj, C. Reh (eds.), Nondestructive Testing Food Quality. Blackwell Publishing Ltd, Oxford, UK. 143-163.

Keller S, Löchte T, Dippel B, Schrader B (1993). Quality control of food with near-infrared-excited Raman spectroscopy. Fresenius' J. Anal. Chem. 346:863-867.

Loss PJ, Hood LF, And Graham HD (1981). Isolation and characterization of starch from breadfruit. Cereal Chem. 58(4):282-286.

Nara S, Mori A, Komiya T (1978). Study on relative crystallinity of moist potato starch. Starch 30:111-14.

Omojola M, Akinkunmi YO, Olufunsho KO, Egharevba HO, Martins EO (2010). Isolation and physico-chemical characterization of cola starch; Afr. J. Food Agric. Nutr. Dev. 10(7):2884-290.

Ribotta PD, Cuffini S, León AE, Añón MC (2004). The staling of bread: an X-ray diffraction study. Eur. Food. Res. Technol. 218:219-223.

Sekkal M, Dincq V, Legrand P, Huvenne JP (1995). Investigation of the glycosidic linkages in several oligosaccharides using FT-IR and FT-Raman spectroscopies. J. Mol. Struct. 349:349-352.

Sohn M, Himmelsbach DS, Barton FE (2004). A comparative study of Fourier transform Raman and NIR spectroscopic methods for assessment of protein and apparent amylose in rice. Cereal Chem. 81:429-433.

Scotter CNG (2001). NIR Techniques in Cereals Analysis. In: Dendy DD, Dobraszczyk BJ (eds.), Cereals and cereal products. Aspen Publishers Inc., Gaihersburg, MA. Pp. 90-99.

D. A. V. Dendy BJ, Satin M (2000). Functional Properties of Starches. FAO Agriculture and Consumer Protection Department: Rome. Available at: http://www.fao.org/ag/magazine/pdf/starches.pdf

Sofowora A (1993). Medicinal plants and Traditional Medicine in Africa. Spectrum Books, Ibadan. pp.150.

Trease GE, Evans WC (1989). Pharmacognosy, 13th edn. Bailliere Tindall, London. pp. 176-180.

Viano J, Massoti V, Gaydou EM, Bourrreil PJL, Ghiglione, Giraud M (1995). Compositional characteristics of 10 wild plant legumes from Mediterranean French pastures. J. Agric. Food Chem. 43:680-683.

Xie F, Dowell FE, Sun XS (2003). Comparison of near-infrared reflectance spectroscopy and texture analyzer for measuring wheat bread changes in storage. Cereal Chem. 80:25-29.

32

Evaluation of the gastrointestinal activity of the aqueous root extracts of *Talinum triangulare*

Olufunmilayo Adeyemi[1], Oluwafunmilade Oyeniyi[2], Herbert Mbagwu[2] and Clement Jackson[2*]

[1]Department of pharmacology, College of Medicine, University of Lagos, Lagos, Nigeria.
[2]Department of pharmacology and Toxicology, Faculty of Pharmacy, University of Uyo, Akwa Ibom, Nigeria.

The effect of the aqueous root extract of Talinum triangulare on the gastrointestinal system was evaluated in mice and rats using normal intestinal transit. Castor oil induced diarrhea and castor oil induced enteropooling models. The result obtained showed that, the effects of the aqueous root extract were dose dependent and biphasic in all the models used. The extract (500, 1000 and 2000 mg/kg) produced a significant ($p < 0.05$) dose dependent decrease in propulsion in normal intestinal transit. The extract at 2000 mg/kg produced a significant ($p < 0.05$) decrease in the frequency of defecation, severity of diarrhea and, afforded protection from diarrhea in rats treated with castor oil. Unlike atropine, the aqueous extract (500, 1000 and 2000 mg/kg) significantly ($p < 0.05$) inhibited castor oil induced enteropooling. The extract was found to contain alkaloids, saponins, tannins, combined anthraquinones, cardiac glycosides and phenol when subjected to phytochemical analysis. The extract gave an LD_{50} of 5514 mg/kg when administered orally and 403 mg/kg when given intraperitoneally.

Key words: *Talinum triangulare*, entropooling, biphasic, LD_{50}, phytochemical analysis.

INTRODUCTION

Herbal medicines are naturally occurring therapeutic compounds in biological organisms. The use of natural plant substances (botanicals) to treat and prevent illness has existed since prehistoric times and still flourishes today in many societies and cultures with many plants still in common use (Duke, 1998). Herbal medicine, which is also known as folk medicine, is known from every continent, essentially every tribe and, the world health organization estimates that up to 80% of the world's population relies mainly on herbal medicine for primary health care either in part or entirely (BGCI fact sheet).

It is therefore no surprise that they have become very important all over the world. Those plants used by people medicinally may be used as crude extracts which are relatively unpurified products; or purified extracts which are chemically modified yielding a semi-synthetic substance; or to produce a new totally synthetic drug by using a plant derivative as a model (Duke, 1998).

In industrialized countries, plants have contributed to more than 7,000 compounds produced by the pharmaceutical industry (BGCI fact sheet) and over 25% of common medicines contain at least some compounds obtained from plants. Also, approximately 120 plant-based prescription drugs are in the marked, and these drugs come from only 95 different species of plants (Duke, 1998).

The importance of medicinal plants in pharmacology is very crucial because they contain active constituents (that are used in the management of various disease conditions) such as; quinine for malaria, opioid analgesics for cancer pain, NSAIDS for pyrexia, laxatives for constipation, etc which have side effects both on acute and chronic administration. Hence, their study is important to the development of new and safer drugs.

Talinum triangulare (jacq.) willd. is a herbaceous perennial plant widely grown in tropical regions as a leaf vegetable. It is probably native to tropical America and the crop is grown in West Africa, Southeast Asia and warmer parts of North America and South America. Along with *celosia* species, it is one of the most important leaf vegetable of Nigeria. Common names include; water leaf, leaf ginseng, American ginseng, Surinam purslane, Surinam spinach, Phillipine spinach, Ceylon spinach, Florida spinach, potherb fameflower, Lagos bologi,

*Corresponding author. E-mail: clementjackson1@yahoo.com

sweetheart, poslen, biala, espinafre de ceilao galaghati grasse, krokot belanda, and kumu manus (Pain, 2001). In Nigeria, *T. triangulare* is known as 'gbure' in Yoraba land and 'nte oka', or ofe bekee in Ibo land (Adodo, 2004).

This research work is designed to investigate the pharmacological effects of *T. triangulare* on the gastrointestinal system. The effect of the aqueous root extract of *T. triangulare* was determined on normal intestinal transit, and its antidiarrhoeal effect was also studied. The acute toxicity test and the phytochemical analysis of the plant extract were also carried out.

MATERIALS AND METHODS

Plant materials

The fresh roots of *T. triangulare* were collected from Abule-ado town in Lagos. The plant was identified by Mr. T. K Odewo of the Forestry Research institute of Nigeria (FRIN) Ibadan, where a voucher specimen is preserved (voucher No FHI 107620).

Experimental animals

Swiss mice (15 to 20 g) and Wistar rats (50 to 150 g) of either sex kept at the Laboratory Animal Centre of the College of Medicine, University of Lagos, and the Nigeria Institute of Medical Research (NIMR), Yaba, Lagos, Nigeria, were used. The animals were maintained under standard environmental conditions and had free access to standard diet (Pfizer feeds Plc. Lagos, Nigeria) and water ad libitum

Other materials

These include glass and rubber funnels, cotton wool, beaker, measuring cylinders conical flask (Pyrex, England), syringes and needles, oral cannula, cages, feeding bottle, hot plate (Binatone Ind. Ltd, China) water bath (Techne (Cambridge limited, England), oven (Griffin and George Ltd. London) weighing Balance (Mettler PM 480 Delta range Blotting paper, knife, scissors, razor blade.

Drugs

Castor oil (Bell sons and Co Ltd, South Port, England); liquid paraffin (New health way Co. limited Lagos); atropine (Sigma chemical Co, St Louis MO, USA).

Chemicals

One percent aqueous hydrochloric acid, ferric chloride, benzene, 10% ammonia solution, aqueous sulphuric acid, pyridine, 2% sodium nitroprusside, 20% sodium hydroxide, acetic anhydride concentrated sulphuric acid, chloroform, glacial acetic acid, 5% ferric cyanide.

Reagents

Distilled water, Dragendorff's reagent, Mayer's reagent, Wagner's reagent, Fehling's solution A and B, Benedict's reagent, and ice

(Teaching Laboratories, Department of Pharmacology, Pharmacognosy and Biochemistry, University of Lagos).

Method

Extraction procedure

The fresh roots of *T. triangulare* were washed with distilled water, air dried and then chopped into smaller bits. The chopped roots (200 g) were boiled in 2 L of distilled water for 45 min. It was left for some hours to cool at room temperature. The solution was filtered and the filtrate was evaporated to dryness in an oven set at a temperature of 40°C. The dried extract was weighed and it gave a yield of 8.5% with reference to the chopped roots. It was then dissolved in distilled water to a concentration of 200 mg/ml and stored at 4°C until required.

Acute toxicity test

Five groups of mice consisting of 5 animals per group were each administered orally with doses of 1250 to 10000 mg/kg of *T. triangulare* extract. In the same manner, the extract (125 to 1000 mg/kg) was administered to another group of mice intraperitoneally. The control mice were given distilled water (1 ml/kg) the mice were closely observed for toxic symptoms and behavioural changes for the first 2 h of administration and mortality recorded within 24 h. The animals were observed for a further 7 days for any signs of delayed toxicity. LD_{50} was estimated by log dose-probit analysis (Miller and Tainter, 1944).

Normal intestinal transit

Mice that have been fasted overnight but with free access to water were allotted to different treatment groups. The animals were treated orally with extract of *T. triangulare* (50 to 2000 mg/kg). Distilled water (10 ml/kg) was used as control. 30 min after treatment with the extract, the mice were administered a standard charcoal meal (0.2 ml per mouse of a 10% charcoal suspension in 5% gum acacia) intragastrically.

All the animals in each treatment group were sacrificed 30 min after administration of the charcoal meal, and the small intestine immediately isolated. Peristaltic index for each mouse was then expressed as a percentage of the distance traveled by the charcoal meal relative to the total length of the small intestine (Aye-Than et al., 1989).

Castor oil –induced diarrhea

Rats were divided into different groups and then treated with the extract (50 to 2000 mg/kg), Atropine (2 mg/kg) and liquid paraffin (10 ml/kg), one hour before the administration of castor oil (10 ml/kg). The control group was given distilled water (10 ml/kg). All the dugs were administered orally. Each rat was kept in a glass funnel the floor of which was lined with blotting paper and observed for 4 h. The parameters observed were: the onset diarrhea, number of wet faeces, total number of faecal output and the total weight of wet stools. A numerical score based on stool consistency was assigned as follows; normal stool = 1; semi solid stool = 2 and watery stool = 3. Calculations were made for the respondent percentages and purging index, the latter by comparison with the control group (Awouters et al., 1978).

Table 1. Results of acute toxicity of *Talinum triangulare* root extract (oral) in mice.

Group	No. of animals	Dose (mg/kg)	Log dose	Mortality	% Mortality	Probit
1	5	Control	-	0/5	0	-
2	5	1250	3.10	0/5	0	-
3	5	2500	3.40	1/5	20	4.16
4	5	5000	3.70	2/5	40	4.75
5	5	10000	4.00	4/5	80	5.84

Table 2. Results of acute toxicity of *Talinum triangulare* root extract (intraperitoneal) in mice.

Group	No. of animals	Dose (mg/kg)	Log dose	Mortality	% Mortality	Probit
1	5	Control	-	0/5	0	-
2	5	125	2.10	0/5	0	-
3	5	250	2.40	1/5	20	4.16
4	5	500	2.70	3/5	60	5.25
5	5	1000	3.00	5/5	100	-

Castor oil induced enteropooling

Rats were divided into different treatment groups. One hour after treatment with extract or distilled water (1 ml/kg), rats received castor oil (2 ml per rat) intragastrically. All drugs were administered orally. The animals were sacrificed one hour later. The entire small intestine was removed after ligation at the pyloric end and ileocaecal junction respectively and weighed. The intestinal contents were expelled into a graduated tube and the volume was measured. The intestine was reweighed and the difference between full and empty intestines was calculated (Robert et al., 1976).

Phytochemical examination of the aqueous extract of *T. triangulare*

Phytochemical analysis was carried out on the aqueous extracts (Itarborne, 1973; Trease and Evans, 1989).

Statistical analysis

Results are expressed as mean ± standard error of mean (S.E.M.). Student's t- test and analysis of variance (ANOVA) were used to analyze the significance of the results.

RESULTS

Acute toxicity test in mice

The summary of the acute toxicity study carried out on the aqueous root extract of *T. triangulare* in mice using the method of Tainter and Miller (1944) is shown in Tables 1 and 2. There was no death recorded, following oral administration of the aqueous extract at a dose of 1250 mg/kg. However, oral doses of 2500, 5,000 and 10,000 mg/kg caused 20, 40 and 80% mortality respectively (Table 1). Intraperitoneal administration of the extract at a dose of 125 mg/kg caused no death,

while the doses of 250, 500 and 1000 mg/kg caused 20, 60 and 100% death, respectively (Table 2). Using SPSS Version 17, probit analysis was performed to determine the LD_{50} at probit value of 0.5 (Figures 1 and 2). The value of LD_{50} obtained (for oral route was 5514 mg/kg and for intraperitoneal route was 403 mg/kg.

The behavioural changes observed in the animals after 2 h of extract administration (oral and intraperitoneal routes) were; mouse writhing, mild diarrhea and anorexia. These were observed for all doses used.

Phytochemical analysis

The result obtained after subjecting the aqueous root extract of the *T. triangulare* to phytochemical analysis showed that it contains alkaloids, saponins, tannins, combined anthraquinones cardiac glycosides and phenols. The colour of the extract is dark brown.

Normal intestinal transit

In control animals, the charcoal meal traversed 68.49% of the total length of the small intestine. Low doses of the extract; 50, 100 and 200 mg/kg produced little or no significant ($p < 0.05$) increase in intestinal propulsion relative to control (6.0, 2.69 and 0.07%).

High doses of the extract, 500, 1000 and 2000 mg/kg produced 7.55, 12.26 and 45.07% significant ($p < 0.05$) inhibition of intestinal propulsion relative control.

Castor oil induced diarrhea

Four hours after castor oil administration, the rats in the

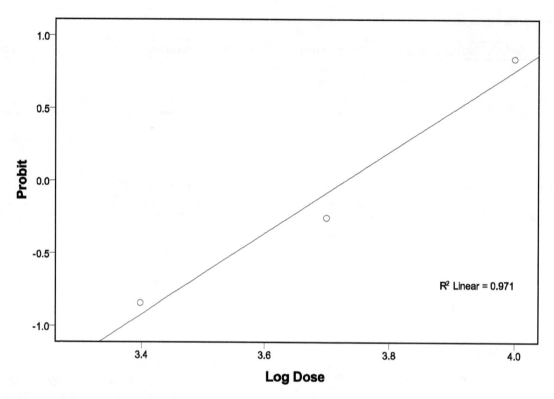

Figure 1. Graph of Probit vs. log dose using SPSS for determination of LD $_{50}$ (oral).

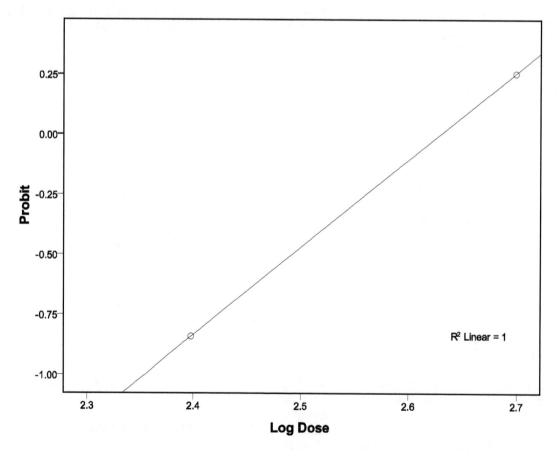

Figure 2. Graph of Probit vs. log dose using SPSS for determination of LD $_{50}$ (intraperitoneal).

Table 3. Effect of low doses of *Talinum triangulare* root extract on normal intestinal transit.

Group	Dose (mg/kg)	Peristaltic index (%)	Propulsion (%)
Control	-	68.49±1.96	-
Extract	50	72.65±4.76	6.07
	100	70.33±1.93	2.69
	200	68.44±3.68	0.07

Values are mean ± SEM of 6 experiments.

Table 4. Effect of high doses of *Talinum triangulare* root extract on normal intestinal transit.

Group	Dose (mg/kg)	Peristaltic index (%)	Propulsion (%)
Control	-	68.49±1.96	-
Extract	500	63.32±18*	7.55
	1000	60.09±2.85*	12.26
	2000	37.62±5.13*	0.07

Values are mean ± SEM of 6 experiments *P < 0.05 vs. control.

control group had copious diarrhea. Pretreatment of rats with low doses of the aqueous extract (50 to 200 mg/kg) score but significantly (p < 0.05) less than the effect produced by liquid paraffin. However, the differences in other diarrhoeal parameters were not dose dependent and not significant. High doses of the aqueous extract (500 to 2000 mg/kg) caused a dose dependent delay in onset of diarrhea, frequency of stooling (reduction in number of stools and total number of wet stools), and total diarrhoeal score. However, only 2000 mg/kg gave a significant (P < 0.05) effect compared to control. .

Low doses of the aqueous root extract produced no significant (p < 0.05) effect on normal intestinal transit (Table 3). High doses of 500, 1000 and 2000 mg/kg of the aqueous root extract produced significant inhibition of intestinal transit (Table 4). Low doses of the aqueous root extract produced no significant (P> 0.05) effect on castor oil induced diarrhoeal (Table 5). Only the 2000 mg/kg dose of the aqueous root extract produced a significant inhibition of castor oil induced diarrhoeal but was significantly (P < 0.05) less than the effect produced by atropine (Table 6).

Castor oil induced enteropooling

There was a dose dependent and non-significant increase in enteropooling, (that is, weight of intestinal content and volume of intestinal content) by low doses of the extract which was less than the effect of liquid paraffin, which produced a significant (P < 0.05 using ANOVA) increase in weight of intestinal content and volume of intestinal content (Table 7). High doses of the extract (500 to 200 mg/kg) produced a dose dependent and significant (P < 0.05 ANOVA) decrease in both weight and volume of intestinal content (Table 8). Their individual anti-enterpooling effects was significantly (P <

caused a dose dependent but not significant (p < 0.05) acceleration in onset of diarrhea and total diarrhoeal 0.05 using ANOVA) higher than that produced by atropine. Low doses of the aqueous root extract produced no significant (p < 0.05) effect on castor oil induced enteropooling (Table 7). High doses of 500, 1000 and 2000mg/kg the aqueous root extract produced no significant (p < 0.05) effect on castor oil induced enteropooling (Table 8).

DISCUSSION

The aim of the work was to investigate the claims made by traditional herbal practitioners on the effectiveness of the roots of *T. triangulare* on the gastrointestinal system. Several tests were employed in evaluating the effect of the aqueous extract of the plant on gastrointestinal motility.

In the normal intestinal transit as in other test models, the activity of the aqueous root extract was dose dependent and biphasic. Low doses produced a slight laxative effect and the greatest effect was shown by 50 mg/kg dose of the extract, which increased the propulsive movement of the standard charcoal meal in the small intestine by 6.07%. However, the result was not significant (P < 0.05) and it cannot be confidently said that, the extract at low doses possess laxative effects.

The result of high doses of the extract on normal intestinal transit showed that, the extract produced a decrease in propulsion movement of the standard charcoal meal in the small intestine, suggesting an antispasmodic activity. This effect was significant (P < 0.05) for all the high doses with the highest effect shown by 2000 mg/kg of the extract; which produced 45.07% inhibition of small intestinal propulsion.

Administration of castor oil causes the release of

Table 5. Effect of low doses Talinum triangulare root extract on castor oil induced diarrhoea.

Group	Dose (mg/kg)	Onset of diarrhoea (min)	No. of Wet stools	Total no. of stools	Weight of wet stools (g)	Total weight of wet stools (g)	Diarrhoeals core	Propulsion (%)
Control	-	92.0±18.65	5.33±0.9	8.17±1.49	2.67±0.48	3.03±0.47	17.17±1.82	-
Extract	50	87.6±10.5	5.80±1.07	8.00±1.14	2.49±0.17	2.76±0.27	17.60±2.77	2.50
	100	88.2±15.96	4.40±0.81	6.40±1.03	1.52±0.39	1.88±0.41	17.40±1.63	1.34
	200	90.2±12.22	4.80.0.37	8.20±1.02	1.80±0.53	2.28±0.55	17.20±1.07	0.17
Liquid paraffin	10 ml/kg	71.2±10.29	7.80±0.49*	9.80±1.39	2.72±0.18	3.19±0.4	23.40±1.6*	36.28

Values are mean ± SEM of 5-6 experiments *P < 0.05 vs. control.

Table 6. Effect of high doses Talinum triangulare root extract on castor oil induced diarrhoea.

Group	Dose (mg/kg)	Onset of diarrhoea (min)	No. of Wet stools	Total no. of stools	Weight of wet stools (g)	Total weight of wet stools (g)	Diarrhoeals core	Propulsion (%)
Control	-	92.0±18.65	5.33±0.49	8.17±1.49	2.67±0.48	3.03±0.47	17.17±1.82	-
Extract	500	110.8±31.44	4.67±1.09	8.83±0.98	1.61±0.46	2.21±0.50	1.65±2.69	3.9
	1000	177.2±32.32	3.80±0.73	7.40±1.5	1.57±0.46	2.10±0.54	13.60±2.6	20.76
	2000	178.0.±28.32*	2.60±0.51*	6.80±1.24	1.42±0.33	1.82±0.46	9.00±1.7*	47.58
Atropine	2	237.6±2.4*	1.00 ±1.0*	1.20±0.97*	0.26±0.26*	0.39±0.26*	2.80±2.56*	83.69

Values are mean ± SEM of 6 experiments *P<0.05 vs control.

Table 7. Effect of low doses of Talinum triangulare root extract on castor oil induced enteropooling.

Group	Dose (mg/kg)	Weight of intestinal content (g)	Volume of intestinal content (ml)
Control	-	2.07±0.1	2.02±0.08
Extract	50	2.07±0.16	2.43±0.17
	100	2.40±0.29	2.35±0.26
	200	2.14±0.09	2.00±0.08
Liquid paraffin	10 ml/kg	2.60±0.38	2.53±0.24

Values are mean ± SEM of 5 experiments.

ricinoleic acid. Ricinoleic acid induces changes in mucosal fluid and electrolyte transport that results in a hypersecretory response and diarrhoeal (Ammon et al., 1974; Gaginella et al., 1975). The aqueous root extract at low doses increase the castor oil in-duced intestinal fluid accumulation (enteropooling) but none of the doses produced a significant (P < 0.05) effect. The standard drug, liquid paraffin, produced a significant (P < 0.05) increase in weight of intestinal content because it retards colonic absorption of water. At high doses, the aqueous extract produced a dose-dependent and significant (P <0.05) inhibition of the castor oil induced intestinal fluid accumulation (entero-pooling).

However, the intestinal content was more viscous in high doses of the extract-treated rats than low doses of the extract-treated

Table 8. Effect of high doses of *Talinum triangulare* root extract on castor oil induced enteropooling.

Group	Dose (mg/kg)	Weight of intestinal content (g)	Volume of intestinal content (ml)
Control	-	2.07±0.1	2.02±0.08
Extract	500	1.72±0.42*	1.6±0.37*
	1000	1.65±0.37*	1.58±0.36*
	2000	1.40±0.45*	1.43±0.47*
Atropine	2	3.42±0.99*	3.13±0.66*

Values are mean ± SEM of 5 experiments *$P < 0.05$ using ANOVA.

and control rats. This increased viscosity could have resulted from the effects of the extract on intestinal transit. Atropine did not inhibit castor oil induced enteropooling and gain in weight of intestinal content suggesting that, mediators other than acetylcholine are involved in castor oil induced enteropooling.

Clinically, diarrhoea may result from disturbed bowel function, in which case there is impaired intestinal absorption, excessive intestinal secretion of water and electrolyte, and a rapid bowel transit (Gurgel et al., 2001). Also, drugs affecting motility, frequency and consistency of diarrhoea also affect secretion (Di Carlo et al., 1994). Low doses of the extract only accelerate the onset of diarrhoea and increase the total diarrhoea score in a dose-dependent manner non-significantly ($P < 0.05$) without any pattern of difference in other diarrhoea.

However, the high doses of the extract produced a dose dependent reduction in the frequency and severity of diarrhoea produced by castor oil.

The total number of stools, number of wet stools, weight of wet stools and total weight of stools, were all decreased in a dose-dependent manner with the highest and significant effects ($P < 0.05$) observed at 2000 mg/kg of the extract. However, the effects of the extract on these diarrhoea parameters were significantly ($P < 0.05$) less than those produced by atropine. The general diarrhoea score of the extract (2000 mg/kg) was 47.58% compared to atropine (2 mg/kg, 83.69%). In this study, atropine produced a significant reduction in the number of stools due to its anti cholinergic effects (Brown and Taylor, 2001). Liquid paraffin produced 36.20% propulsion in general diarrhoea score because; it retards intestinal absorption of faecal water.

Administration of the extract orally, produced toxic effects with an LD_{50} of 5514 mg/kg. Also, the intraperitoneal route produced toxic effects with an LD_{50} of 403 mg/kg. This result shows that, the aqueous extract is better tolerated when administered orally than through the intraperitoneal route. It is relatively safe through the oral route

Conclusion

In conclusion, the investigation carried out proved that, the aqueous root extract of *T. triangulare* does not possess any significant laxative effect but has antidiarrhoeal effect in doses of 500 to 2000 mg/kg. This may account for its use in traditional medicine as an antidiarrhoeal agent. However, further tests need to be carried out to determine the mechanism of action of the extract and *in vitro* effect.

REFERENCES

Adodo A (2004). Herbs for healing. Pax Herbals, Ewu-Ishan, Edo state Nigeria. ISBN 978-8018-48-3, p. 94.

Ammon HV, Thomas PJ, Phillips S (1974). Effect of oleic and recinoleic acid on net jejunal water and electrolyte movement. J. Clin. Invest., 53: 374-379.

Awouters F, Niemegeers CJE, Lenaerts FM, Janssen PAJ (1978). Delay of castor oil diarrhoea in rats: a new way to evaluate inhibitors of prostaglandin biosynthesis. J. Pharm. Pharmacol., 30: 41-45.

Aye-Than JH Kukami W, Tha SJ (1989). Antidiarrhoeal efficacy of some Burmese indigenous drug formulations in experimental diarrhoea test models. J. Crude Res., 27: 195-200.

BGCI Fact Sheet (2000). Plants as medicine. Botanic Gardens Conservation International/British Airways/International Centre for Conservation Education. Www.wwf.org.uk/filelibrary/pdf/useofplants.pdf.

Brown JH, Taylor P (2001). Muscarinic receptor agonists and antagonists. In: Hardman JG, Limbird LE (eds.) Goodman and Gilman's the Pharmacological Basis of Therapeutics, 10th edition. Macgrow Hill New York. Rr, pp.155-173

Di Carlo GD, Mascolo N, Izzo AA, Capasso F, Autore G (1994). Effects of Quercetin on gastrointestinal tract in rat and mice. Phytother. Res., 8: 42-45.

Duke AJ (1998). Strains of medicinal plants. Straney, University of Maryland. www. Life.umd.edu/classroom/bsci124/lec29.html.

Gaginella TS, Stewart JJ, Olsen WA, Bass P (1975). Action of ricinoleic acid and Structurally related fatty acid on the gastrointestinal tract II. Effects on water and electrolyte absorption in *vitro*. J. Pharmacol., Exp. Therap., 195: 355-361.

Gurgel LA, Silva RM, Santos FA, Martins DTO, Mattos PO, Rao VSN (2001). Studies on the antidiarrhoeal effect of dragon's blood from *croton urucarrana* Phytother. Res., 15: 319-322.

Itarborne JB (1973). Phytochemical Methods: A guide to modern techniques of plant analysis. Chapman and Hall, London, p. 279.

Miller LC, Tainter ML (1944). Estimation of the LD_{50} and its error by means of lagarithmic probit graph paper. Sci. Expt. Biol. Med., 23: 839-840

Pain S (2001). The countess and the cure. New scientist, 15 September, 2001. www.wikipedia org.

Robert A, Nezamis JE, Lancaster C, Hanchar AJ, Klepper MS (1976). Enteropooling assay: A test for diarrhoeal produced by prostagulandins. 11: 809-828.

Trease GE, Evans WC (1989). A Textbook of Pharmacognosy, 13th edition. Bailich Tinall Ltd. London.

33

Antibacterial activity of alkaloidal compound isolated from leaves of *Catharanthus roseaus* (L.) against multi-drug resistant strains

Mohammed A. Abd Ali[1], Abdulla H. Lafta[2] and Sami K.H. Jabar[3]

[1]Biology Department, College of Science, Missan University, Iraq.
[2]Biology Department, College of Science, Al basrah University, Iraq
[3]College of Dentistry, Missan University, Iraq.

The following alkaloids were isolated from *Catharanthus roseus L.* leaves from the yellow crystal as white powder at (38°C). The chemical and physical properties were studied by thin layer chromatography (TLC), IR-spectrum (IR), Ultraviolet - visible spectrum (UV) and melting point (mp). Standard strains of bacteria: *Staphylococcus aureus NCTC 6571, Escherichia coli NCTC 5933* and the clinical multidrug resistance (MDR) *S. aureus, E. coli* and *P. aeruginosa* were tested with the alkaloids. The *Catharanthus ruseus (L.)* alkaloids inhibited both type of bacteria strains of gram positive strains *S. aureus NCTC 6571,*S. aureus* and *E. coli* as gram negative strains when concentrations increase (125, 250, 500 mg/ml) with *C. ruseus L.* alkaloids being the most active in (500 mg/ml) concentrations against gram positive *S. aureus* bacteria than gram negative bacteria *E. coli*, while the clinical resistance *P. aeruginosa* showed resistance against *C. ruseus L.* alkaloids in all concentrations (500, 125, 250 mg/ml). The minimum inhibitory concentration (MIC) (μg/ml) of the alkaloidal compound were also determined. Finally, a test was also carried out to examine the cytotoxicity assay methods towards human red blood cells have no cyto-toxicity in all concentration. The good antimicrobial potency of the alkaloidal compound of *C. ruseus L.* indicates the treatment of (MDR) as an alternative to the costly antibiotics.

Key words: *Catharanthus roseus* L. leaves, thin layer chromatography (TLC), alkaloid compound, antibacterial activity.

INTRODUCTION

Infectious diseases account for high proportion of health problems in the developing countries (Sashi et al., 2003). The continuous use of the same antibiotic per disease gave the appearance of resistance bacteria to antibiotic. In particular, emergence of resistance to antibiotics has hampered the pace by which newer antibiotics are being

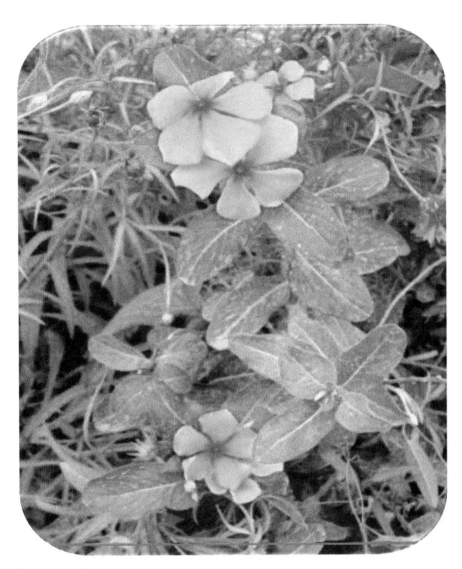

Figure 1. *Catharanthus roseus* (L.) plant.

introduced into the public domain (Russell, 2002). Despite ever increasing advancement in the field of medicine and molecular diagnosis it is estimated that 80% of the world population is still dependent on the plant derived pharmaceuticals. As published, plant natural products or its derivatives accounts for available in the market (Newman et al., 2003). In recent years, many drugs have been isolated from natural source as the modern medicine system treats the symptoms and suppresses the disease but does little to ascertaine the real cause. Medicinal plants are rich source of antibacterial drugs substances (Jaleel et al., 2007). *Catharanthus roseus*, from the family Apocynaceae (Figure 1), is used as plant medicine. Catharanthus roseus alkaloids have anticancer activity (Jaleel et al., 2007). The crude extracts of different parts of *C. roseus*

are used in clinic as a antibacterial agent, it is published that more than 130 of different alkaloids are found in *C. roseus* (Muhammad et al., 2009). The aim of this study was isolation of alkaloids content from the Iraq local medical plant *Catharanthus roseus* (L.) leaves and to study the physiochemical properties and the antibacterial activity of these alkaloids.

MATERIALS AND METHODS

Plant

C. roseus were cultivated and collected at the flowering stage from arboretum garden at Missan in south of Iraq. In this study, the leafs of *C. roseus* were used for testing their antibacterial activity. The plant materials were dried in shade at room temperature (25°C).

Preparation of plant extracts

Material

1. Leaves of *C. roseus* were collected, dried, broken and kept at (4°C).
2. Standard bacteria strains; *S. aureus* (NCTC 5671) and *E. coli* (NCTC 5933).
3. The medical sensitivity for some clinical bacterial isolates, that were isolated from some patients burns in Myssan Public Hospital were tested. These isolates involve *S. aureus*, *E. coli* and *P. aeroginosea*.
4. Ready culture media; culture media (Muller Hinton Agar) was prepared according to information of the manufacturing company.

Isolation of crude alkaloid compound from dry leaves of Catharanthus roseus (L.)

100 mg of finely powdered material and 40 ml of 95% ethanol were refluxed in 100 ml flask for 30 min. The extract was then filtered and then the residue washed twice with 5 ml of ethanol. The washed residues are added to the original filtrate and transfered into a 50 ml standard flask then added ethanol 95% and adjusted to the mark. 5 ml of this solution was pipette into a test tube and ethanol completely removed by evaporation on a water bath, then we treated the residue with 3 ml of 1 N NaOH and then we added acetic acid and the contents transferred to 25 ml standard plates (2 x 9 cm) in a pre-saturated chamber of the mixture of (chloroform: methanol) (0.5: 9.5). The glass plates were dried and the spot which appeared were developed with UV-lamp at (336 to 200 nm), iodine vapor. Melting point electro-thermal is used for the determination of melting point of the isolated compounds (Teresa and Ivan, 2003).

Spectroscopy

1. Inferred spectrum FT-IR spectrum of the isolated compound was recorded with (FT-IR 8400S SHIMADZU- Japan) in the College of Science, Chemistry Department, University of Basrah.
2. Ultraviolet and visible spectra: Ultraviolet and visible spectrum of the isolated compound was carried out in the College of Science, Department of Chemistry, by using ethanol as and the spectrum recorded with the Spectroscan 80D UV-vis spectrophoto-meter UK.

Antibacterial activity

Agar diffusion method (John et al., 1996) was used to determine the antibacterial activity of the isolated compound (30.000 µg/ml) against types of reference strains of gram positive and gram negative bacteria (*S. aureus* NCTC 5671) and (*E. coli* NCTC 5933), *S. aureus, *E. coli* and *P. aeruginosa* as clinical Mullidrug resistance (MDR), clinical strain which are tested using plate of Muller-Hinton agar. The antibacterial activity was defined as the clear zone of growth inhibition (Sashi et al., 2003).

The preparation of alkaloid compound

500 mg/ml (0.5 mg of alkaloid compound soluble into 1 ml DMSO) as stock solution was put in a flask, the volume being to the mark of 10 ml with water. One ml of this solution is equivalent to 1 mg of dry

material, then we finely recrytallized the dry powdered by methanol of 80% and allowed it to dry in room temperature.

Determmination of MIC by agar plate dilution method

According to the methods of National Committee for Clinical Laboratory Standards (NCCLS) (2002), agar plate dilution test was used to determine the minimum inhibitory concentration (MIC) of an antimicrobial agent.

Cytotoxicity assay

According to the methods of Xian-guo and Ursula (1994), human red blood cells were used for toxicity test.

Identification

1. Preliminary qualitative test: The chemical family of the isolated compound was implemented using several test such as:

a) Dragendroff test (Harborne, 1984).
b) Wagner reagent (Harborne, 1984).
c) Mayer's test (Harborne, 1984).

2. Thin layer chromatography (TLC): To determine the purity and relative to front (Rf) of isolated compound, a thin layer chromatography was carried out for 45 min on glass plates (2 × 9 cm) in a pre-saturated chamber of the mixture of (chloroform: methanol) (0.5: 9.5). The glass plates were dried and the spot which appeared were developed with UV-lamp at (336 to 200 nm), iodine vapor (Figure 2).

3. The determination of melting point: Melting point electro-thermal is used for the determination of melting point of the isolated compounds.

4. Spectroscopy:

a) Inferred spectrum FT-IR spectrum of the isolated compound was recorded with (FT-IR 8400S SHIMADZU- Japan) in the College of Science, Chemistry Department, University of Basrah.
b) Ultraviolet and visible spectra: Ultraviolet and visible spectrum of the isolated compound was carried out in the College of Science, Department of Chemistry by using ethanol as the spectrum recorded with the Spectroscan 80D UV-vis spectrophoto-meter UK.

5. The preparation of alkaloid compound: 500 mg/ml (0.5 mg of alkaloid compound soluble into 1 ml DMSO) was used as stock solution.

RESULTS AND DISCUSSION

Qualitative test which describes the appearance of alkaloid is listed in the Table 1 and was isolated from *C. roseus* (L.). The result was similar to that published previously on the leaves of *C. roseus* (L.) alkaloid content (Muhammed et al., 2009). In this study, we did not find saponin, glycoside, amino acid, flavonoid and carbohydrate

Table 1. The qualitative chemical analysis for the isolated compound of Catharanthus roseus (L.).

Reagent	Dragendroff	Wagner	Mayer's
	+	+	+
Alkaloid compound test	Formation	Formation	Formation
	Orange precipitate	Light brown precipitate	White precipitate

Table 2. Thin layer chromatography , Rf value for the isolated compound of *Catharanthus roseus* (L.).

Solvent system	Developers	Number of spot	Rf values	Notes
Methanol : NH4OH 9.5 : 0.5	The eye	1	0.83	Pure compound
	I2 Vapor	1	0.83	Organic nature
	UV- lamp (366 nm)	1	0.83	Conjugated double bond

on *C. roseus*. The thin layer chromatography shows (Table 2) the appearance of one spot using different solvent system and different types of (TLC) plates and diffrenent reagent as spot developer. The Rf value of the peak was 0.83.

Melting point (m.p)

The melting point of the isolated alkaloids shows a sharp melting point peak at 165 to 168°C. These results indicate that the isolated compound is pure. The FT-IR spectra were recorded in KBr on a SHIMADZU 8400S Japan spectrophotometer for the isolated compound as shown in Figure 3 and Table 4. The appearance of a single broad peak at 3411 cm^{-1}, related to the vibration stretching for (-OH) bond which indicated the presence of alcohol group. The band at 2923 to 2856 cm^{-1} related to the vibration stretching for (C – H) bond of aliphatic CH2 and CH3 group (1731 cm^{-1}) is due to the vibration stretching for (C = O) bond of carbonyl group (1441, 1392 cm^{-1}) related to the vibration stretching for (CH3–) bond of aliphatic CH3 group (CH antisymmertic and symmetric). The band at (1060 cm^{-1}) is related to the vibration stretching for (C – O – C) bond of aliphatic ether. The band at 871 cm^{-1} is due to the vibration stretching (-CH) banding of Tri –substitution. 594 cm^{-1} is related to vibration stretching for (C – O – C) bond of ethers bond (Table 4). The result of IR spectrum appeared, the isolated compound is an aliphatic compound containing carbonyl and ether group (Jaleel et al., 2007).

The ultraviolet–visible spectrum (Figure 4), has shown one peak at λ max equal to 300 nm due to the presence of pairs of electrons (non-bonding type π ➡ * n) on the

oxygen atom (Donald et al., 2009; Silverstein et al., 1991). Test for the sensitivity of some clinical bacterial isolates under study life towards some antibiotics was used (John et al., 1996). Isolation bacteria isolated from some patients burns under study were resistant multiple (MDR) as shown in Figure 5 Table 3. Drug susceptibility testing of some bacterial isolates isolated from burns and surgical operations under study for antibiotic showed all of isolation clinical bacteria S. aureus and isolation strain clinical P. aeruginosa resistance to 100% of the direction of six types of antibiotics used as shown in the Figure 5, while it showed isolation clinical strain isolate of E. coli resistance to both antibiotics cephalothine and metronidalzole and rifampin as shown in Figure 5 Table3, thus all of these isolates are multi-resistance to antibiotics multi drug resistance because they showed resistance to more than one antibiotic (Majeed, 1992; Enright, 2003).

The antibacterial activity of isolated compound was determined by using agar well diffusing methods. The results, in Table 5, Chart 1, show that the isolated compound has good antibacterial activity against gram positive and gram negative bacteria which is evaluated for their ability to inhibit the growth against both a standard bacteria S. aureus NCTC6571 and E. coli NCTC 5933, and the multidrug resistant bacterial isolates S. aureus and E.coli studied showed an inhibition activity at 500, 250 and 125 mg/ml in the valuable level (0.01), and the results in Table 6 shows that the MIC value of the isolated compound were 1 µg/ml against gram positive and gram negative bacteria while that of the MIC value of the isolated compound were 1.5 µg/ml against clinical (MDR) S. aureus and E. coli, this may be due to the presence of (OH) group in the structure of the studies which increased the activity of the isolated compound to inhibit the bacteria growth by changing the nature of cell protein (denaturationa), thus increasing the permeability

Table 3. The antibiotic test in this study.

Antibiotic	Symbol	Concentration (µg)
Cephalothen	KF	30
Erythromycin	EA	15
Metronidozle	MET	5
Nalidixic acid	NA	30
Riphampin	RA	5
Streptomycin	S	10
Tetracycline	TE	30

Table 4. The infrared absorption peak and their related functional group for the isolated compound of *Catharanthus roseus* L. leaves.

Frequency rang intensities (cm^{-1})	Group or class	Assignment of remark
3411 (strong)	Alcoholic or phenol	O – H Stretch
2923, 2856 (medium)	Aliphatic CH2 and CH3	C – H Stretch
1731 (strong)	Carbonyl group	Stretch C = O
1441, 1392 (medium)	CH antisymmertic and symmertic	CH3- Stretch
1153 (strong)	Aliphatic ether	Stretch C – O – C
1060 (strong)	Aliphatic ether	Stretch C – O – C
871 (very strong)	Tri - substitution	banding - CH
594 (medium strong)	Ether band	banding C – O – C

Table 5. The bacterial activity for the isolated compound of *Catharanthus roseus* L.

Bacteria strains	Inhibition zone (mm)			
	0.065 µg/ml	125 µg/ml	250 µg/ml	500 µg/ml
Staphylococcus aureus (NCTC5671)	13	19	23	26
Escherichia coli (NCTC5933)	10	19	20	23
*Staphylococcus aureus**	0	13	19	23
*Escherichia coli**	0	10	19	20
*Pseudomonas aerugenosa**	0	0	0	0

*Clinical isolate **three value each number ***diameter of well (8 mm).

Table 6. The minimum inhibition concentration (MIC) for the isolated compound of Catharanthus roseus(L.) leaves.

Bacteria strains	MIC (µg/ml)
Staphylococcus aureus (NCTC5671)	1
Escherichia coli (NCTC5933)	1
*Staphylococcus aureus**	1.5
*Escherichia coli**	1.5

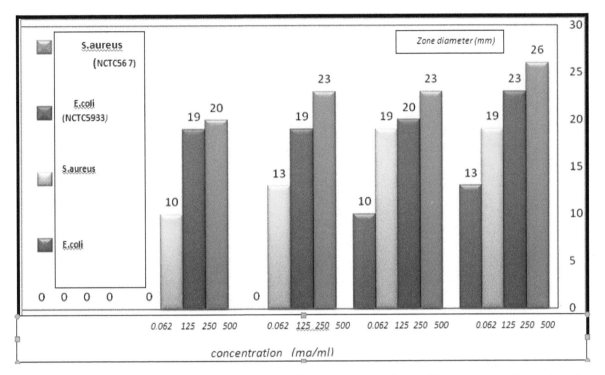

Chart 1. Showing zone of inhibition diameter against different bacteria strains of different concentrations of whole alkaloid compound isolated of Catharanthus roseus(L.) leaves

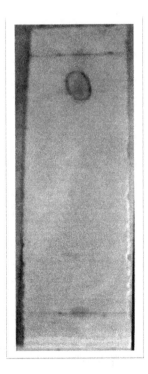

Figure 2. Thin layer chromatography for isolated compound of *Catharanthus roseus L.*

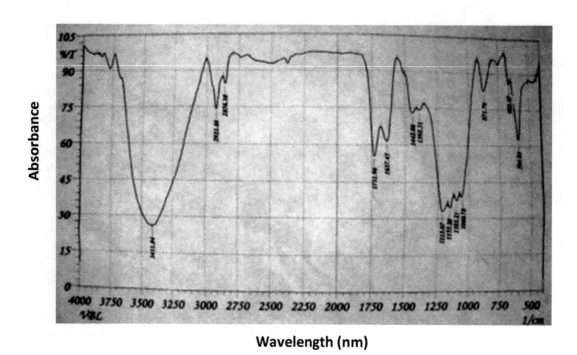

Figure 3. Infared absorption peak and and their related functional group for isolated compound of *Catharanthus roseus (L.)*.

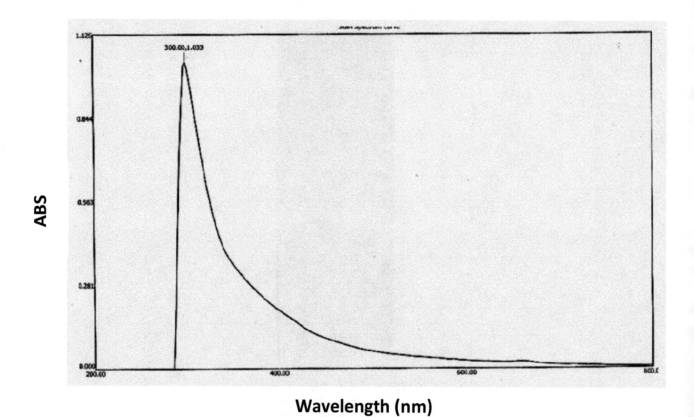

Figure 4. The ultraviolet-visible spectrum for isolated compound of *Catharanthus roseus (L.)*.

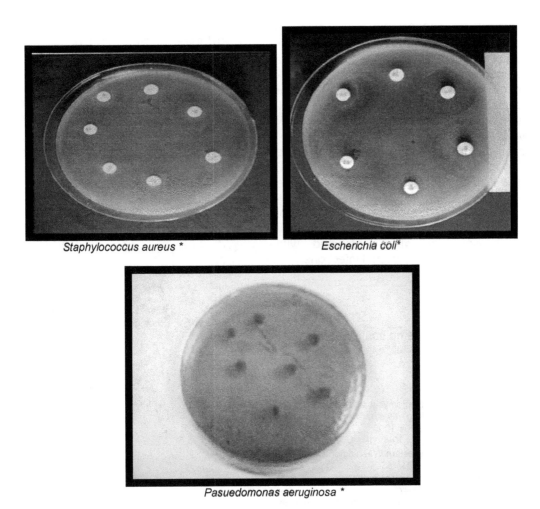

*Staphylococcus aureus ***

*Escherichia coli***

*Pasuedomonas aeruginosa ***

Figure 5. Isolated multi drug resistant (MDR) (*clinical isolate).

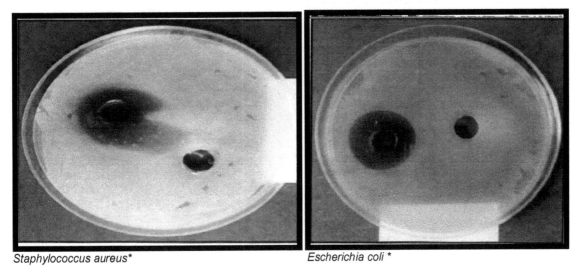

*Staphylococcus aureus**

*Escherichia coli ***

Figure 6. Antibacterial activity of alkaloid compound isolated from Catharanthus roseus leaves against MDR *Staphylococcus aureus and *Eschericha coli.*

of cell membranes (Feeny, 1998), either by increasing the permeability of the membrane cell bacteria. The cell membrane causes loss or leakage of the contents of a cell of bacteria to the outside or through a direct link membrane of cell bacteria, causing the demise of polar membrane of bacteria, which leads to the death of a cell bacteria gradually (Carpenter and Chambers, 2004; Straus and Hancock, 2006).

Finally, a test was also carried out to examine the cytotoxicity assay by using Xian-gou and Ursula (1994) methods towards human red blood cells in which the alkaloid compound of C. roseus (L.) were found that they are not having cytotoxicity on 1 to 500 µg/ml. Results of this study suggested that the alkaloidal compound may be useful either alone or when combined with antimicrobial agents to treat MDR bacterial infections.

Conflict of interest

The authors declare that they have no conflict of interest.

REFERENCES

Carpenter CF, Chambers HF (2004). Daptomycin anther novel agent for treating infections due to drug–resistant gram– positive pathogens. Rev. Anti-infect. Agents 38:994-1000.

Donald L, Pavia GM, Lampman GS, Kris JR Vyvyan (2009). Introduction to Spectroscopy. 4th ed. Western Washington University, U.S.A. 656 pp.

Enright MC (2003). The evolution of a resistant pathogen the case of MRSA. Curr. Opin. Pharmacol. 3(5):474-479.

Feeny P (1998). Inhibitory effect of Oak Leaf tannins on the hydrolysis of proteins by trypsine. J. Phytochem. 8:2116.

Harborne J (1984). Phytochemical methods: A guide to modern techniques of plant analysis. Chapman and Hall, London.

Jaleel C, Manivaqnnan P, Sankar B (2007). Induction of drought stress tolerance by ketoconazole in Catharanthus roseus is mediated by enhanced antioxidant potential and secondary metabolite accumulation. Colloid Surf. B Biointerfaces 60:201-206.

John P, Harley L, Prescott M (1996). Laboratory Exercises in Microbiology. McGraw-Hill, USA. pp. 484, 149 153.

Muhammad IRN, Muhammad AT, Baqir SN (2009). Antimicrobial activity of different extracts of Catharanthus roseue. Clin. Exp. Med. J. 3:81-85.

NCCLS (2002). Performance Standards for Antimicrobial Disk Susceptibility Testing, Twelfth Information Supplement.

Newman D, Cragg G, Snader K (2003). Natural products as sources of new drugs over the period. 1981-2002. J. Natl. Prod. 6:1022-1037.

Russell AD (2002). Antibiotic and biocide resistance in bacteria; Introduction. J. Appl. Microbiol. Symp. Suppl. 92:18-3S.

Sashi K, Ramya M, Janardhan K (2003). Antimicrobial activity of ethnomedicinal plants of Nilgiri Biosphere reserve and Western Ghats. Asian J. Microbiol. Biotechnol. Environ. Sci. 5:183-185.

Silverstein R, Bassler M, Morrill T (1991). Spectrometric identification of organic compounds. 5th ed. John Wiley & Sons Inc, New York, USA.

Straus SK, Hancock RE (2006). Mode of action of the new antibiotic for Gram – positive pathogens daptomycin, Comparison with cationic antimicrobial peptides and lipopeptides. Biochem. Acta. 1758:1215-1223.

Teresa and Ivan (2003). Pharmacology. Translation by Dr. Mansour Bin Sulaiman Bin Saeed and Prof . Mohammed Bin Abdul Aziz al-Yahya and Dr. Nasser.

Xian–Gou H, Ursula M (1994). Antifungal compound from Solanum nigrescens. J. Ethnopharmaacol. 43:173-177.

Permissions

The contributors of this book come from diverse backgrounds, making this book a truly international effort. This book will bring forth new frontiers with its revolutionizing research information and detailed analysis of the nascent developments around the world.

We would like to thank all the contributing authors for lending their expertise to make the book truly unique. They have played a crucial role in the development of this book. Without their invaluable contributions this book wouldn't have been possible. They have made vital efforts to compile up to date information on the varied aspects of this subject to make this book a valuable addition to the collection of many professionals and students.

This book was conceptualized with the vision of imparting up-to-date information and advanced data in this field. To ensure the same, a matchless editorial board was set up. Every individual on the board went through rigorous rounds of assessment to prove their worth. After which they invested a large part of their time researching and compiling the most relevant data for our readers.

The editorial board has been involved in producing this book since its inception. They have spent rigorous hours researching and exploring the diverse topics which have resulted in the successful publishing of this book. They have passed on their knowledge of decades through this book. To expedite this challenging task, the publisher supported the team at every step. A small team of assistant editors was also appointed to further simplify the editing procedure and attain best results for the readers.

Apart from the editorial board, the designing team has also invested a significant amount of their time in understanding the subject and creating the most relevant covers. They scrutinized every image to scout for the most suitable representation of the subject and create an appropriate cover for the book.

The publishing team has been an ardent support to the editorial, designing and production team. Their endless efforts to recruit the best for this project, has resulted in the accomplishment of this book. They are a veteran in the field of academics and their pool of knowledge is as vast as their experience in printing. Their expertise and guidance has proved useful at every step. Their uncompromising quality standards have made this book an exceptional effort. Their encouragement from time to time has been an inspiration for everyone.

The publisher and the editorial board hope that this book will prove to be a valuable piece of knowledge for researchers, students, practitioners and scholars across the globe.

List of Contributors

D. Kubmarawa
Department of Chemistry Federal University of Technology, P. M. B. 2076, Yola, Nigeria

M. E. Khan
Department of Chemistry Adamawa State University, P. M. B. 25, Mubi, Adamawa State, Nigeria

A. Shuaibu
Department of Chemistry Federal University of Technology, P. M. B. 2076, Yola, Nigeria

B. Prasanna Reddy
Department of Quality control, Nosch Labs Pvt Ltd, Hyderabad-500072, A.P, India

K. Amarnadh Reddy
Department of AR and D, Aurigene Discovery Technologies Ltd, Bangalore, India

M. S. Reddy
Department of Plant Pathology and Entomology, Auburn University, USA

Kalpana Joshi
Department of Biotechnology, Sinhgad College of Engg, Pune, India-411041

Shyam Awte
Poona College of Pharmacy, Pune 411029, India-411029

Payal Bhatnagar
Poona College of Pharmacy, Pune 411029, India-411029

Sameer Walunj
Division of Biochemistry, Department of Chemistry, University of Pune, Pune, India 411007

Rajesh Gupta
Division of Biochemistry, Department of Chemistry, University of Pune, Pune, India 411007

Swati Joshi
National Chemical Laboratory (NCL), Pune, India- 411007

Sushma Sabharwal
Division of Biochemistry, Department of Chemistry, University of Pune, Pune, India 411007

Sarang Bani
Indian Institute of Integrative Medicine, Canal Road, Jammu-180 001, India

A. S. Padalkar
Department of Biotechnology, Sinhgad College of Engg, Pune, India-411041

Joshua A. Obaleye
Department of Chemistry, University of Ilorin, Ilorin, Kwara State, Nigeria

Johnson F. Adediji
Department of Chemical Sciences, Ajayi Crowther University Oyo, P. M. B 1066, Oyo, Oyo State, Nigeria

Ebenezer T. Olayinka
Department of Chemical Sciences, Ajayi Crowther University Oyo, P. M. B 1066, Oyo, Oyo State, Nigeria

Matthew A. Adebayo
Department of Chemical Sciences, Ajayi Crowther University Oyo, P. M. B 1066, Oyo, Oyo State, Nigeria

Clement Jackson
Faculty of Pharmacy, University of Uyo, Akwa Ibom State, Nigeria

Emmanuel Ibezim
Faculty of Pharmaceutical Sciences, University of Nigeria, Nsukka, Enugu State, Nigeria

Agboke Akeem
Faculty of Pharmacy, University of Uyo, Akwa Ibom State, Nigeria

Mfon Udofia
God's Glory Computers Institute, Uyo, Akwa Ibom Nigeria

Hilary Odo
Faculty of Pharmaceutical Sciences, University of Nigeria, Nsukka, Enugu State, Nigeria

G. C. Onunkwo
Department of Pharmaceutical Technology and Industrial Pharmacy, Faculty of Pharmaceutical Sciences, University of Nigeria, Nsukka, Nigeria

N. C. Ngwuluka
Department of Pharmaceutics and Pharmaceutical Technology, Faculty of Pharmaceutical Sciences, University of Jos, P. M. B. 2084, Jos, Nigeria

B. A. Idiakhoa
Department of Pharmaceutics and Pharmaceutical Technology, Faculty of Pharmaceutical Sciences, University of Jos, P. M. B. 2084, Jos, Nigeria

E. I. Nep
Department of Pharmaceutics and Pharmaceutical Technology, Faculty of Pharmaceutical Sciences, University of Jos, P. M. B. 2084, Jos, Nigeria

I. Ogaji
Department of Pharmaceutics and Pharmaceutical Technology, Faculty of Pharmaceutical Sciences, University of Jos, P. M. B. 2084, Jos, Nigeria

I. S. Okafor
Department of Pharmaceutics and Pharmaceutical Technology, Faculty of Pharmaceutical Sciences, University of Jos, P. M. B. 2084, Jos, Nigeria

Michael Adikwu
Department of Pharmaceutics, University of Nigeria, Nsukka, Enugu State, Nigeria

Clement Jackson
Department of Pharmaceutics and Pharmaceutical Technology, University of Uyo, Akwa Ibom State, Nigeria

Charles Esimone
Department of Pharmaceutics, University of Nigeria, Nsukka, Enugu State, Nigeria

Oluwatosin K. Yusuf
Department of Biochemistry, Federal University of Technology, Trypanosomosis Research Unit, PMB 65, Minna, Nigeria

Clement O. Bewaji
Department of Biochemistry, University of Ilorin, Ilorin, Nigeria

H. M. Akala
Kenya Medical Research Institute, Walter-Reed Laboratories, P. O. Box 54840 - 00100 G. P.O, Nairobi, Kenya

C. N. Waters
Kenya Medical Research Institute, Walter-Reed Laboratories, P. O. Box 54840 - 00100 G. P.O, Nairobi, Kenya

A. Yenesew
Department of Chemistry, University of Nairobi, P. O. Box 30197 - 00100 G. P. O. Nairobi, Kenya

C. Wanjala
Department of Physical Sciences South Eastern University College (SEUCO) P. O. Box 170-90200, Kitui, Kenya

T. Ayuko Akenga
Office of the Deputy Principal (Academic Affairs), Bondo University College (BUC) P. O. Box 210-40601, Bondo, Kenya

Zhengwu Lu
1006 S De Anza Blvd#K104, San Jose, CA 95129, USA

Peace Ubulom
Faculty of Pharmacy, University of Uyo, Akwa Ibom State, Nigeria

Ekaete Akpabio
Faculty of Pharmacy, University of Uyo, Akwa Ibom State, Nigeria

Chinweizu Ejikeme udobi
College of Science and Technology, Kaduna Polytechnic, Kaduna, Nigeria

Ruth Mbon
Faculty of Pharmacy, University of Uyo, Akwa Ibom State, Nigeria

Musharaf Khan
Department of Botany, University of Peshawar, Pakistan

Shahana Musharaf
Government Girls Degree College S. Malton, Mardan, Pakistan

Zabta Khan Shinwari
Department of Plant Sciences, Quaid-i-Azam University, Islamabad- 45320, Pakistan

Chinedum P. Babalola
Department of Pharmaceutical Chemistry, Faculty of Pharmacy, University of Ibadan, Nigeria

Olayinka A. Kotila
Department of Pharmaceutical Chemistry, Faculty of Pharmacy, University of Ibadan, Nigeria

Patrick A. F. Dixon
Department of Pharmacology, Faculty of Pharmacy, Obafemi Awolowo University, Ile-Ife, Nigeria

Adefemi E. Oyewo
Department of Clinical Pharmacology, Faculty of Pharmacy, Obafemi Awolowo University, Ile-Ife, Nigeria

Clement Jackson
Department of Pharmacology and Toxicology, Faculty of Pharmacy, University of Uyo, Nigeria

Herbert Mbagwu
Department of Pharmacology and Toxicology, Faculty of Pharmacy, University of Uyo, Nigeria

Chidinma Okany
Department of Pharmacology, College of Medicine University of Lagos, Nigeria

Emmanuel Bassey
Department of Pharmacology, College of Medicine University of Lagos, Nigeria

Iniunwana Udonkang
Department of pharmaceutics and Pharmaceutical Technology, Faculty of Pharmacy, University of Uyo, Nigeria

F. C. Nwinyi
Department of Pharmacology and Clinical Pharmacy, Ahmadu Bello University Main Campus, P. M. B. 1045, Zaria 810271, Kaduna State, Nigeria

H. O. Kwanashie
Department of Pharmacology and Clinical Pharmacy, Ahmadu Bello University Main Campus, P. M. B. 1045, Zaria 810271, Kaduna State, Nigeria

P. A. O. Adeniyi
Department of Anatomy, P. M. B 1515, College of Health Sciences, University of Ilorin, Ilorin, Nigeria

A. A. Musa
Department of Anatomy, P. M. B 1515, College of Health Sciences, University of Ilorin, Ilorin, Nigeria

K. M. Ali Gamal
Former Department of Pharmaceutical Services and Planning Manager, Federal Ministry of Health, Khartoum, Sudan

Abdeen M. Omer
Occupational Health Administration, Ministry of Health, Khartoum, Sudan

M. Sheriff
Department of Biochemistry, Faculty of Science, University of Maiduguri, Borno State, Nigeria

M. A. Tukur
Department of Human Physiology, College of Medical Sciences University of Maiduguri, Borno State, Nigeria

M. M. Bilkisu
Department of Medicine, College of Medical Sciences University of Maiduguri, Borno State, Nigeria

S. Sera
Department of Biochemistry, Faculty of Science, University of Maiduguri, Borno State, Nigeria

A. S. Falmata
Department of Biochemistry, Faculty of Science, University of Maiduguri, Borno State, Nigeria

Faisal Hammad Mekky Koua
Department of Biochemistry, Faculty of Science and Technology, Al Neelain University, P. O. Box 12702, Al Baladya St. Khartoum, Sudan

Hind Ahmed Babiker
Department of Biochemistry, Faculty of Science and Technology, Al Neelain University, P. O. Box 12702, Al Baladya St. Khartoum, Sudan

Asim Halfawi
Deparment of Pharmacognosy, Faculty of Pharmacy, University of Medical Sciences and Technology, P. O. Box: 12810, Khartoum, Sudan

Rabie Osman Ibrahim
Department of Biochemistry, Faculty of Science and Technology, Al Neelain University, P. O. Box 12702, Al Baladya St. Khartoum, Sudan

Fatima Misbah Abbas
Commission for Biotechnology and Genetic Engineering, National Center for Research P. O. Box 2404 Khartoum, Sudan

Eisa Ibrahim Elgaali
Commission for Biotechnology and Genetic Engineering, National Center for Research P. O. Box 2404 Khartoum, Sudan

Mutasim Mohamed Khlafallah
Commission for Biotechnology and Genetic Engineering, National Center for Research P. O. Box 2404 Khartoum, Sudan

Clement Jackson
Department of Pharmaceutics and Pharmaceutical Technology, Faculty of Pharmacy, University of Uyo, Akwa Ibom State, Nigeria

Ekaette Akpabio
Department of Pharmaceutics and Pharmaceutical Technology, Faculty of Pharmacy, University of Uyo, Akwa Ibom State, Nigeria

Romanus Umoh
Department of Pharmacognosy and Natural Medicine, Faculty of Pharmacy, University of Uyo, Akwa Ibom State, Nigeria

Musiliu Adedokun
Department of Pharmaceutics and Pharmaceutical Technology, Faculty of Pharmacy, University of Uyo, Akwa Ibom State, Nigeria

Peace Ubulom
Department of Pharmaceutics and Pharmaceutical Technology, Faculty of Pharmacy, University of Uyo, Akwa Ibom State, Nigeria

Godwin Ekpe
Department of Clinical Pharmacy and Biopharmacy, Faculty of Pharmacy, University of Uyo, Akwa Ibom State, Nigeria

A. A. Musa
Department of Anatomy, PMB 1515, College of Health Sciences, University of Ilorin, Ilorin, Nigeria

P. A. O. Adeniyi
Department of Anatomy, PMB 1515, College of Health Sciences, University of Ilorin, Ilorin, Nigeria

Kedar Karki
Central Veterinary Laboratory Tripureswor, Kathmandu Nepal

Sri Agus Sudjarwo
Department of Pharmacology, Faculty of Veterinary Medicine, Airlangga University, Surabaya 60115, Indonesia

Jabbar A. A. Al-Sa'aidi
Physiology and Pharmacology Department, College of Veterinary Medicine, Al-Qadisiya University, Iraq

Mohsen N. A. Alrodhan
Deptartment of Internal and Preventive Medicine, College of Veterinary Medicine, Al-Qadisiya University, Iraq

Ahmed K. Ismael
Physiology and Pharmacology Department, College of Veterinary Medicine, Al-Qadisiya University, Iraq

S. S. Haque
Department of Clinical Biochemistry, Indira Gandhi Institute of Medical Sciences Patna-14, India

A. Sharan
Department of Clinical Biochemistry, Indira Gandhi Institute of Medical Sciences Patna-14, India

U. Kumar
Department of Clinical Biochemistry, Indira Gandhi Institute of Medical Sciences Patna-14, India

A. Bhattacharya
Post graduate Department of Studies in Biotechnology and Microbiology, Karnataka University, Dharwad- 580 003, India

S. Chakrabarty
Post graduate Department of Studies in Biotechnology and Microbiology, Karnataka University, Dharwad- 580 003, India

B. B. Kaliwal
Post graduate Department of Studies in Biotechnology and Microbiology, Karnataka University, Dharwad- 580 003, India

Hashim J. Azeez
Department of Chemistry, College of Education, Salahaddin University, Erbil, Iraq

Kezhal M. Salih
Department of Pharmaceutical Chemistry, College of Pharmacy, Hawler Medical University, Erbil, Iraq

Clement Jackson
Faculty of Pharmacy, University of Uyo, Akwa Ibom, Nigeria

Musiliu Adedokun
Faculty of Pharmacy, University of Uyo, Akwa Ibom, Nigeria

Emmanuel Etim
Faculty of Pharmacy, University of Uyo, Akwa Ibom, Nigeria

Ayo Agboke
Faculty of Pharmacy, University of Uyo, Akwa Ibom, Nigeria

Idongesit Jackson
Faculty of Pharmacy, University of Uyo, Akwa Ibom, Nigeria

Emmanuel Ibezim
Faculty of Pharmaceutical Sciences, University of Nigeria, Nsukka, Enugu State, Nigeria

Musharaf Khan
Department of Botany, University of Peshawar, Pakistan

Shahana Musharaf
Chemistry Government Girls Degree College, Sheikh, Malton Mardan, Pakistan

Mohammad Ibrar
Department of Botany, University of Peshawar, Pakistan

Farrukh Hussain
Department of Botany, University of Peshawar, Pakistan

Fagbohun Adebisi
Chemistry Advanced Laboratory, Sheda Science & Technology Complex, PMB 186 Garki, Abuja, FCT, Nigeria

Adebiyi Adedayo
Chemistry Advanced Laboratory, Sheda Science & Technology Complex, PMB 186 Garki, Abuja, FCT, Nigeria

Adedirin Oluwaseye
Chemistry Advanced Laboratory, Sheda Science & Technology Complex, PMB 186 Garki, Abuja, FCT, Nigeria

Fatokun Adekunle
Chemistry Advanced Laboratory, Sheda Science & Technology Complex, PMB 186 Garki, Abuja, FCT, Nigeria

Afolayan Michael
Chemistry Advanced Laboratory, Sheda Science & Technology Complex, PMB 186 Garki, Abuja, FCT, Nigeria

Olajide Olutayo
Chemistry Advanced Laboratory, Sheda Science & Technology Complex, PMB 186 Garki, Abuja, FCT, Nigeria

Ayegba Clement
Chemistry Advanced Laboratory, Sheda Science & Technology Complex, PMB 186 Garki, Abuja, FCT, Nigeria

Pius Ikokoh
Chemistry Advanced Laboratory, Sheda Science & Technology Complex, PMB 186 Garki, Abuja, FCT, Nigeria

Kolawole Rasheed
Department of Chemistry, Federal University of Technology, Akure, Ondo State, Nigeria

Aiyesanmi Ademola
Department of Chemistry, Federal University of Technology, Akure, Ondo State, Nigeria

Olufunmilayo Adeyemi
Department of pharmacology, College of Medicine, University of Lagos, Lagos, Nigeria

Oluwafunmilade Oyeniyi
Department of pharmacology and Toxicology, Faculty of Pharmacy, University of Uyo, Akwa Ibom, Nigeria

Herbert Mbagwu
Department of pharmacology and Toxicology, Faculty of Pharmacy, University of Uyo, Akwa Ibom, Nigeria

Clement Jackson
Department of pharmacology and Toxicology, Faculty of Pharmacy, University of Uyo, Akwa Ibom, Nigeria

Mohammed A. Abd Ali
Biology Department, College of Science, Missan University, Iraq

Abdulla H. Lafta
Biology Department, College of Science, Al basrah University, Iraq

Sami K.H. Jabar
College of Dentistry, Missan University, Iraq

www.ingramcontent.com/pod-product-compliance
Lightning Source LLC
Jackson TN
JSHW051947131224
75386JS00005B/341